Competency in Home Care

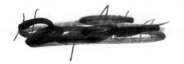

Terasa Astarita, MS, RNC, CCRN

Post Master's Nurse Practitioner Student
Johns Hopkins University School of Nursing
Baltimore, Maryland

Gayle Materna, MPH, BSN, RN

Adjunct Faculty, Community Health
York College of Pennsylvania
York, Pennsylvania

Cynthia Blevins, MEd, BSN, RN

Staff Development Educator
Community Hospital of Lancaster Home Care
Lancaster, Pennsylvania

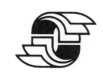

AN ASPEN PUBLICATION®
Aspen Publishers, Inc.
Gaithersburg, Maryland
1998

Library of Congress Cataloging-in-Publication Data

Astarita, Terasa.
Ensuring competency in home care/
Terasa Astarita, Gayle Materna, Cynthia Blevins.
p. cm.
Includes bibliographical references and index.
ISBN 0-8342-1050-9 (pbk.)
1. Home nursing—Quality control.
2. Home care services—Quality control.
3. Clinical competence. I. Materna, Gayle.
II. Blevins, Cynthia. III. Title.
RT120.H65A85 1998
362.1'4—dc21
98-15036
CIP

About Aspen Publishers • For more than 35 years, Aspen has been a leading professional publisher in a variety of disciplines. Aspen's vast information resources are available in both print and electronic formats. We are committed to providing the highest quality information available in the most appropriate format for our customers. Visit Aspen's Internet site for more information resources, directories, articles, and a searchable version of Aspen's full catalog, including the most recent publications: **http://www.aspenpub.com**
Aspen Publishers, Inc. • The hallmark of quality in publishing
Member of the worldwide Wolters Kluwer group.

Editorial Services: Brian MacDonald

Library of Congress Catalog Card Number: 98-15036
ISBN: 0-8342-1050-9

Printed in the United States of America
1 2 3 4 5

We dedicate this book to our husbands:
Salvatore, John, and Jim;
and our children:
Sergio, Liz, Shelby, and Ryan;
all of whom make home the best place to be.

Table of Contents

Contributors

Corrine Parver, JD, PT
Partner
Dickstein Shapiro Morin & Oshinsky LLP
Washington, DC

Joshua H. Soven, JD
Associate
Dickstein Shapiro Morin & Oshinsky LLP
Washington, DC

Foreword

The transformation of health care in the latter part of the 20th century is challenging all health care managers and practitioners. Gearing up for continual change necessitates a review of the process used. This ensures that consumers of all ages receive the highest in care and service quality. Astarita, Materna, and Blevins provide readers with a comprehensive examination of the term "competency" and the process of ensuring the delivery of competent home health care . . . the mission of many organizations.

Traditionally, the presence of a state-granted license indicated the competence of individual practitioners. The mastery of knowledge, skills, and technicalities of the profession were unquestioned as long as a current license could be produced. Now, with Department of Health (Medicare) on-site surveys potentially decreasing to once every three years, measuring the competency within one's own organization has taken on an increasing significance. The government's increasing emphasis on corporate compliance is yet another reason why licensure should no longer be considered a guarantee of competency.

Given the evolution of health care as a result of changing reimbursement mechanisms, organizations find a change in referral patterns from those authorized to pay for the services and those consuming the services. Third party payers demand a high level of competency in the organizations in which they contract. Accreditation is often key to obtaining those contracts, and the accrediting bodies are placing increasing em-

phasis on the competency process. Today's patient profile is much different than that of yesterday's! Specialty services, such as disease state management programs or pediatric rehabilitation services, are becoming the market niche for many organizations. Some find the mean age of their patients has fallen from 76 years of age to 43 years of age. Third party payers prefer "one stop shopping;" therefore, the need may exist for staff to become proficient in the care of the ventilator patient, end stage cardiac patient, and patient with congenital abnormalities. Today, as we think about this diversity, now our norm, it is unrealistic to expect that all practitioners in our employ retain all of the knowledge, skills, and technicalities learned in their professional training and need to support our patient population.

For many of the specialty and care delivery services, basic professional education is insufficient to provide the quality of care desired. Additional course work, certification through national certification programs, skills and assessment training seminars are a few examples of the many avenues available to our professional staff and our organization. These opportunities are designed to increase competency and ensure the delivery of care of the highest caliber.

Aspects to consider in developing a well-planned competency program include external forces, internal support, program development, individual reactions to "testing," organizational needs assessment, principles of adult learning, affordability, and finally the "how to's." The authors of *Ensuring Competency in Home Care* provide a well thought out and very thorough explanation of each of these aspects. As with other operational components, the use of forms and processes directly from a book may not necessarily be in the organization's best interest. Each organization should consider the uniqueness of its internal and external environment, the patient population served, skills demanded by referring physicians, and the expertise of its staff in the development of its individual plan. Orga-

nizations will need to weigh the costs versus benefits and choose those components appropriate to their needs. The value of research, hard work and dedication provided by Astarita, Materna, and Blevins cannot be underestimated. It can serve the organization as a comprehensive resource for the development of an individual competency program to meet the special and unique needs of the patients it serves.

Deborah Anne Ondeck
Barbara Stover Gingerich

Preface

This book is intended primarily for staff development personnel in the home health setting. In addition, it can be utilized as a resource for staff development personnel in other settings, for academic community health faculty, for performance improvement professionals, and for home care managers and administrators. In our experiences as educators in home health, we felt as though we were forging through a forest without a compass when it came to defining our role in home care and developing a competency program. In our search for resources to help us find our way, we were frustrated to learn that there was limited literature available. In addition, when attending professional conferences, we found limited to no discussion of staff development in home care and the issues surrounding competency in the home care setting. We decided to write this book for a number of reasons: to provide an easy resource for how to go about setting up a home care competency program, to show how important the role of staff develop-

ment is in the success of home care organization, to provide suggestions for scholarly inquiry, and to provide a stepping stone for other authors to build upon in the future. It is our hope that this book provide direction for novice educators in home health, and that it provide a foundation from which to build a successful competency program.

We acknowledge and appreciate the work of our contributors Josh Sovan, Esquire, and Corinne Parver, Esquire, both of whom have provided an added dimension to this manuscript. In addition, we are grateful for the encouragement and mentorship of Barb Gingrich and Deb Ondeck, for without their continued support to move forward, completion would have eluded us. Lastly we would like to thank the Visiting Nurse Association of Lancaster for the opportunity to experience and excel in the role of staff development educator and for being the conduit through which lasting personal and professional relationships have developed.

CHAPTER 1

Competency Dynamics

"Wonder is the foundation of all philosophy, inquiry its progress, ignorance its end."
—Baron De Montesquieu

Competent staff are a vital component to the success of any organization providing health care in the home. A home care organization may have an inspired philosophy, visionary administrative staff, and excellent financial management, but will ultimately fail if it doesn't provide high-quality care through competent employees. Competent professional and paraprofessional health care providers are the backbone of any home care organization.

Ensuring the competency of staff has long been an important issue for health care institutions. In recent decades, the exponential growth of medical knowledge and its increasing technological complexity have placed health care providers in a perpetual quest for competency. Also, a complex dynamic of social, political, economic, legal, ethical, and professional forces have created a mandate for staff competency. The aging population, escalating health care costs, increased consumer expectations, increased medical-related litigation, and more stringent professional and regulatory requirements are just a few of the factors creating the need for new strategies for health care delivery and increased accountability for health care providers (Alspach, 1996; Bailey, 1994; Torrens, 1993). A competency-based education program for professional, technical, paraprofessional, and ancillary staff assists a health care organization to reach the goal of providing the highest quality, yet cost-effective patient care. A large body of research-based literature has established

that competency programs improve the skills and knowledge of nurses (McGregor, 1990; Ozcan & Shukla, 1993; Scrima, 1987). In addition to helping patient care staff reach the goals of proficiency, a competency-based education (CBE) program may enhance the operations of many of the health care organization's departments. The competency program itself and the positive outcomes it generates are vital in meeting many of the current regulatory and accrediting requirements (Brent, 1994; Friedman, 1996b; Snow, Hefty, Kenyon, Bell, & Martaus, 1992). Quality assurance and risk management programs are enriched by the information available from competency assessments and training accomplished. The human resources department has easier access to documented employee performance data and to detailed job description data. Staff development can use CBE as a framework for planning, implementing, evaluating, and documenting many of its activities. All of these benefits add to an organization's productivity and commercial viability in a competitive health care services market. Competency programs and activities have been largely concentrated in the acute care setting in the past and only moved to the home health care arena relatively recently. Consequently, the competency literature available was developed largely for the acute care setting. There remains insufficient literature pertaining to comprehensive competency programs developed for the specialty of home care (Astarita, 1996). Most of the existing literature available for home care pertains to the development of competency-based orientation programs transitioning registered nurses (RNs) from the acute care setting to the home care-arena. Ongoing competency education has received little attention for personnel other than nurses in the acute care setting (Snow et al., 1992; Humphrey & Milone-Nuzzo, 1994; Caie-Lawrence, Peploski, & Russell, 1995). However, the existing general and acute care literature may be modified and adapted to the home care setting. This book is an attempt to explain the planning, development, and application of a CBE program for the home health care setting and to demonstrate a comprehensive framework for such a program. Although the focus of this book is nursing competence, other disciplines will also be discussed.

COMPETENCY THROUGH THE YEARS

The term competency first appeared in educational literature in the 1960s in response to the public's demand for increased accountability in the traditional education system. Since that time, CBE programs have been incorporated into many professional and nonprofessional careers as a means to evaluate and improve quality, ensure employee performance, manage liability, and maintain cost-effectiveness (Alspach, 1996; Astarita, Materna, & Savage, in press; Friedman, 1996a). The idea of competence is not new to nursing either. Florence Nightingale wrote of the importance of observing the performance of a nurse's ability to demonstrate a new skill. Traditionally, nurses were primarily trained with a performance-based system in a practical health care setting. Performance of a skill was not measured in the qualitative levels of competency.

As nursing education shifted from the hospital to the college setting, the focus changed from performance attainment to attainment of competency, a subtle but important shift in semantics that indicates effectiveness (Nagelsmith, 1995). Acquisition of beginner- or novice-level competency has become the educator's goal for students. In the late 1970s, Dr. Dorothy del Bueno

introduced a framework of competence tied to a nursing curriculum. She also helped develop competency-based programs for acute care nurses. During the 1980s, models of competency were developed for orientation and the ongoing education of nurses in the acute care setting (del Bueno, Barker, & Christmyer, 1981). The popularity and use of CBE grew dramatically in the acute care and nursing education settings during the 1980s. During this same time period, regulatory and accrediting agencies such as the Joint Commission on Accreditation of Healthcare Organizations (Joint Commission) continued to use standards based on performance rather than competency. The Joint Commission had introduced standards requiring performance appraisals in the 1970s, which were used to evaluate professional and paraprofessional skills. Performance appraisals are similar to competency assessment and may be the same if the performance is tied to a high level of skill. However, the word competence implies a high, proficient level of synthesis of cognitive, affective knowledge and/or psychomotor skills. In 1991, the Joint Commission set a new standard for health care providers by shifting the performance requirements to those of competency (Alspach, 1996; Joint Commission on Accreditation of Healthcare Organizations, 1990).

Competency has become an integral framework for professional and paraprofessional curricula, employee orientation, ongoing education, and evaluation. The Joint Commission standards continue to incorporate the idea of competence into increasingly larger ranges of standards. Similarly, the document stipulating the standards for Medicare certification, the Conditions of Participation (COP), also use the term competency to describe orientation, training, and desired performance level of health care providers. Due to these requirements of competency and those of other accrediting and regulating bodies and the many dynamic forces impacting health care, competency will continue to be a vital issue for health care providers in the foreseeable future (Alspach, 1996; Astarita et al., in press; Friedman, 1996b; Harris, 1996b).

HOME CARE AS A SPECIALTY

Home health care has been one of the fastest growing segments of health care in the United States since the mid-1980s. However, it is also one of the oldest traditions of medicine. Physicians commonly visited their patients in the home before physician shortages and advancements in medical technology made this impractical during the 20th century. Historically, nursing care was usually delivered in the home by informally trained women, charitable organizations, and religious orders before the onset of the Industrial Revolution. In the United States, organized efforts to deliver care in the home by trained nurses began in the 1800s at the Boston Dispensary (Albrecht, 1992; Torrens, 1993). The first visiting nurse association (VNA) began in Philadelphia in 1886 to deliver care to individuals and families in geographical areas known as districts. The goal of these early home care providers was much as it is today: to deliver health care in the home environment and to educate patients and their families in health practices designed to assist them achieve and maintain health.

Despite a great need due to overcrowding, pollution, lack of sanitation, and increased infectious and occupational diseases, the idea of home health care grew slowly with only 21 VNAs in existence by the late 1890s. During the first half of the 20th century, home health nursing was intertwined with models and concepts of public health nursing. Public health nurses generally performed care that was preventative in nature and emphasized patient education. Only a small portion of the work was restorative. Government began to take a larger role in establishing public health agencies and care. However, much early funding for public health and home care was charitable, self-pay, and philanthropic until the growth of health insurance after World War II.

Community hospitals began to develop home health agencies in the 1930s, expanding the presence and role of organized home care (Torrens, 1993). During the economic expansion af-ter World War II, more women entered the work force. As medical knowledge and transportation improved, home care had more opportunity to grow. By 1960, VNAs existed in most large and small cities in America, but most of their care was provided to the poor and needy through nonprofit and public institutions (Milone-Nuzzo, 1995). Home health care nursing was not clearly delineated from public health nursing up to this point. All of this changed dramatically with the passage of Medicare in 1964, which established home health care as a benefit to all citizens older than 65. Home care grew explosively in an effort to fulfill this mandate. Home health care suddenly became a full participant in business economics and the medical care industry (Albrecht, 1992; Milone-Nuzzo, 1995).

Major advances in medical knowledge and technology occurred in tandem with the need for more home health care providers and assisted this sector's growth. This growth also enabled home health care to develop new models of health care delivery, which helped clearly define and delineate itself from public health and community health specialties, which tend to be more general in scope (Milone-Nuzzo, 1995). Home care is currently defined as any health care service or product provided in a person's place of residence. The Department of Health and Human Services defines home health care as part of a continuum of comprehensive health care delivered to patients and their families in their residences designed to promote, maintain, and restore health, and improve their level of functioning (Warhola, 1980). The American Medical Association (AMA), the National League for Nursing (NLN), the National Association for Home Health Agencies, and the National Association for Home Care (NAHC) share similar definitions of home care, seeing it as an integral component of comprehensive care in an often fragmented health care system. Home health care may be delivered by public, government-subsidized agencies and proprietary or private for-profit or nonprofit organizations. These agencies may be hospital affiliated or independent. Increasingly, home care organizations are aligned with large health care networks that include hospitals and ambulatory care facilities. Home care is provided by a wide array of professionals and paraprofessionals such as physical therapists, occupational therapists, speech therapists, medical social workers, home care aides, nutritionists, and homemakers (Albrecht, 1992; Milone-Nuzzo, 1995). Nurses make up the majority of the personnel providing a home health service (American Nurses Association, 1993). Home health nursing is recognized as a specialty component of community health nursing. In 1986, the American Nurses Association (ANA) developed standards for home health care nurses in an effort to ensure a uniform, professional standard of performance and quality of care. In 1993, the ANA Credentialing Center (ANCC) began certifying nurses in home care in recognition of the unique knowledge and skills necessary to provide proficient care (Milone-Nuzzo, 1995). As stated by ANCC president Margretta Madden Styles (Styles, 1996, p. 1), "Credentials assure us of our own special knowledge and competencies." (See Appendix A for ANA standards.)

Caring for patients in their own environments offers the challenges of providing care that is specific and sensitive to their ethnic, cultural, religious, and economic needs. Home care nursing encompasses the skills of a higher level generalist as well as the knowledge and skills of a social worker, financial counselor, dietitian, teacher, case manager, housing inspector, supervisor, and car mechanic (Astarita, 1996; Benefield, 1996a; Harris, 1996b). Knowledge of assessment, intervention, and referral are necessary to handle social issues such as family dynamics, poverty, abuse, neglect, and safety that are now an expected and required component of the plan of care. Excellent communication and teaching skills are necessary to achieve goals of improving health and maximizing independence. Critical thinking skills are required to deliver effective, efficient care in a cost-conscious environment. A nurse must have high-level knowledge and skills in physical and psychosocial assessment, pharmacology, pathophysiology, and high technological care to adequately care for today's more acutely ill clients (Astarita et al., in press; Benefield, 1996a). A solid working knowledge of Medicare, Medicaid, and insurance regulations and documentation are needed by the nurse to manage the plan of care. A thorough background in general legal and ethical standards and those pertaining to home care is also a prerequisite to safe, quality care. And finally, practical skills of time management, driving, map reading, car upkeep, and troubleshooting are needed to get through each day.

COMPETENCY DEFINED

To gain a better understanding of the concepts to be discussed, it may be helpful to define those terms as they will be used throughout this book. Competency, according to Webster's New Twentieth Century Dictionary, is defined as possessing the capacity necessary to fulfill a requirement, or adequate ability and fitness to perform a task. Benner (1982) describes competence as the ability to perform tasks in a variety of real-world circumstances. The ANA *Standards for Nursing Professional Development: Continuing Education and Staff Development* (1994, p. 12) describes competence as the "demonstration of knowledge and skills in meeting professional role expectations." From these definitions, we may deduce that true competence is more than a capability in the cognitive, affective, or psychomotor domain. It is an integration or synthesis of cognitive, affective, and psychomotor skills applied in a situation. Breaking competency down into its component parts may be helpful for designing educational programs and for measuring and assessing outcomes. But true competency is holistic and, thus, is more than the sum of its parts (Alspach, 1996; Astarita et al., in press; Friedman, 1996b). Competency may be further interpreted as the actual concrete performance of a task in relation to an established set of standards. Alspach (1996, pp. 13–14) distinguishes a subtle difference between competence, a "potential" ability, and competency, the "actual" demonstrated capability. Benner (1984) similarly defines competency as the capability to perform in the real, ever-changing world. This distinction may seem minor, but becomes important in accurately assessing an employee. Nurses are deemed competent in the knowledge of congestive heart failure (CHF) if they can accurately demonstrate knowledge of pathophysiology and related pharmacological therapeutics. But they would demonstrate competency when they manage such a patient in the home.

A clearer example might be seen in the following scenario commonly seen in home care. Mr. Smith, a 78-year-old man, is discharged from the hospital with newly diagnosed CHF due to arteriosclerosis. The physician's referral orders request the nurse to assess for all needs. During the admission visit, the nurse finds the patient also manifests moderate deafness, multiple joint osteoarthritis, and benign hypertrophy of the prostate. Mr. Smith is fatigued from mild dyspnea and frequent nocturia, which has increased since the initiation of diuretic therapy. His arthritis and dyspnea make it difficult to walk around the house. The patient lives on a very limited income with his elderly spouse who suffers from insulin-dependent diabetes, hypertension, and diabetic retinopathy. Both have an eighth grade education and a fifth grade reading ability but lively minds and an eagerness to learn. They do not understand Mr. Smith's illness or his new drug, diet, and activity regimen. They have a devoted son who is present during the admission visit and stops by every day.

The nurse writes a plan of care that takes all of these variables into account. She prioritizes all of the patient's needs and those of his family. She organizes the medication schedule so that the Smiths can more easily understand it. She instructs on safety issues and on the emergency signs and symptoms of CHF during the first visit. The nurse listens actively and communicates in language appropriate for Mr. and Mrs. Smith's age, cultural background, social background, and education level. The nurse initiates a multidisciplinary plan of care incorporating a physical therapist, a social worker, and a home care aide for personal care. The nurse begins a program of education for CHF, benign prostatic hypertrophy, and osteoarthritis appropriate to the client's learning abilities. The son's help is enlisted by having him check the medicine tray each evening and call the nurse for any problems. The frequency and duration of visits are based on Mr. Smith's multiplicity of needs. Competency as a home health care RN, a synthesis of a broad range of skills and knowledge, is necessary to adequately accomplish this initial assessment and the subsequent management of Mr. Smith's care.

An example of paraprofessional competencies necessary for home care can be seen in the following scenario commonly encountered by home care aides: Jean, the home care aide, is assigned to assist Mr. Smith in his daily morning care. The RN's plan of care includes daily bathing, shaving, dressing, monitoring intake and output, taking vital signs, and monitoring his use of the medicine box. Within one day of admission to home care, Jean arrives to find Mr. Smith more short of breath and fatigued than usual. She observes that he is too weak to do the regular morning routine and appears less steady on his feet. Jean takes his vital signs and finds little change other than a moderately increased respiratory rate. She notices his ankles are puffy and inquires about his urination since last evening. Mr. Smith assures her it is OK but "forgot to measure it." At this point, Jean checks Mr. Smith's med box and finds most of the pills in Monday's slots, but Tuesday morning's doses are gone. His wife, who appears very anxious, volunteers that Mr. Smith "didn't seem himself, yesterday." Jean realizes there is a problem beyond her capability to solve. She reassures them that things will be worked out. She calls the RN to give her an updated report on the client's condition and receive new orders. From this example, it is apparent that a broad range of cognitive, affective, and psychomotor skills is also needed to provide quality care by paraprofessionals involved in home care. More than just the ability to follow a cookbook style of care is necessary to adequately meet the patient's and his or her family's physical, emotional, and spiritual needs.

Competency Assessment

Competency assessment refers to the process used to verify an individual's ability to meet job performance and regulatory and/or professional standards. It is the mechanism designed to measure and document staff performance in the work environment (Alspach, 1992, 1996). Competency assessment is but one of the components of CBE, which also consists of planning, implementation, and evaluation. Competency assessment focuses on the knowledge, skills, attitudes, and behaviors necessary to fulfill a specific job title or role that is performed in a particular work setting. It distinguishes between various professional roles such as clinical nurse and nurse manager or physical therapist and rehabilitation manager. A distinction is also made between the various settings in which persons with the same job title may work. For example, a clinical nurse may work for the psychiatric team or a maternal–child health team.

An assessment is constructed as a series of competency statements designed to measure a desired performance. The content for these measurable outcome statements is derived from job descriptions, accrediting and regulatory requirements, professional standards, quality improvement criteria, risk management needs, and learner needs assessments. Staff development educators design the assessment program with the input of experts in the field. Evaluation of learner/employee competency is identified by experts in that particular field and by learner self-assessment (del Bueno, Barker, & Christmyer, 1981; McGregor, 1990).

The role of staff development educators is vital in competency assessment. The educators can design the competency assessment by collecting information from sources within the organization, such as job descriptions, learner input, and in-house experts or specialists. Staff development can also network with other facilities to gather expert information and input. By keeping abreast of the latest research literature, health care delivery changes, and the needs of the population, staff development is in an excellent position to identify these specialists and experts. These persons may be persons with advanced degrees and/or vast experience in the field.

Competency-Based Education

CBE is an alternative method of teaching that focuses on the learner's ability to demonstrate job or career requirements. Traditional teaching emphasized the acquisition of cognitive knowledge. CBE emphasizes demonstration of acquired skills and knowledge. It constructs a curriculum framework based on competency measurement and achievement in the three domains of learning: cognitive, affective, and psychomotor. It recognizes that a synthesis of knowledge in all three domains of learning is required to be truly qualified and capable in a variety of real-world work settings (Alspach, 1996; Friedman, 1996b).

CBE uses assessment, planning, implementation, and evaluation as the structural components of its curriculum. All components are geared toward preparing the learner to demonstrate competency of a specific set of outcomes in a specific work setting. The learner is prepared to function optimally in a real-world setting and is often observed in that setting, rather than the ideal setting of a model or lab. Input of experts in the field, staff, and learners is used in all phases of the curriculum planning, implementing, and evaluating (Alspach, 1996; Staab, Granneman, & Page-Reahr, 1996).

CBE also recognizes that a wide variety of learner needs must be addressed to achieve success. From its inception, adult learning theory was incorporated into the competency model (Staab et al., 1996). Adult learning theory was developed by the humanistic educational theorist Malcolm Knowles. Knowles held that adults have special learning needs such as the need to know; the need to be self-directed; the need to know why learning something is necessary; the need to be motivated to learn; the need to be able to apply the new learning to life. This theory also recognizes the unique qualities, experiences, knowledge, and developmental stages adults bring to the learning situation (Abruzzese, 1996). Consequently, CBE incorporates a wide variety of learning strategies into its curriculum. Learners are encouraged to assess their needs, design contracts for learning, and use methods of learning that are effective for their needs. Learners often use self-learning programs and may choose to challenge or test out of topic areas in which they feel competent (Abruzzese, 1996; Alspach, 1996; Staab et al., 1996).

PROFESSIONAL AND PARAPROFESSIONAL ATTRIBUTES IN HOME CARE

Caring for persons in their home environment has become, in recent years, the preferred method of health care delivery for the chronically ill, those clients recovering from an acute illness, their families, and for third-party payers. It is generally recognized that persons tend to live, heal, and thrive better at home than in an institution (Milone-Nuzzo, 1995). The bulk of today's home care population consists of the elderly who tend to have multiple chronic health and social problems. Another large segment is made up of children and young adults experiencing permanent chronic health problems and a wide array of social needs. Health care providers and third-party payers alike recognize that a wide variety of services, products, and caregivers are needed to provide comprehensive, quality health care to this population. These services are carried out through the combined efforts of professionals, such as RNs and physical therapists, and paraprofessionals, such as home care aides and personal care attendants.

Each of the professions involved in the delivery of health care in the home has its own set of standards based on scientific theory and research. After the attainment of a required amount of formal education, the graduate is qualified for testing to obtain licensure or certification. Professionals are then expected to operate autonomously, responsibly, ethically, and within legal bounds to assess, plan, implement, and evaluate patient care within their particular area of expertise. They must also be skilled in coordinating patient care and communicating with other providers on the health care team. Medicare's Conditions of Participation state that their patients must require the skills of a professional to qualify for Medicare-reimbursed services. RNs are the most frequently used professional in the home care setting to manage a client's plan of care. Other professionals qualifying for reimbursement under Medicare as skilled providers are physical therapists, speech therapists, medical social workers, nutritionists, and occupational therapists. These professionals are recognized as an integral component in home health care. These specialties are needed to maintain the continuum of comprehensive health care that is necessary to meet the goals of maximizing health, functional ability, and independence (American Nurses Association, 1993; National Association for Home Care, 1994).

As mentioned above, RNs are the largest group of professionals providing health care services in the home. The RN is often responsible for assessing the patient, designing a plan of care, implementing the plan, recommending other disciplines, coordinating care, supervising paraprofessional staff, and evaluating patient responses. Nurses come to these complex tasks with a wide variety of education, preparation, and skill backgrounds. Nurses entering home health care frequently have worked only in the acute care setting and have no practical work experience in home health (Caie-Lawrence, Peploski, & Russell, 1995). Knowledge and educational background among nurses vary with their level of education. Community health curricula that contain the home health component are often omitted in associate degree and diploma RN programs. The only nursing educational program that requires community health theory and practicum is the bachelor's degree. The ANA (1993) standards recognize that nurses operating in the community health field should hold a minimum of a bachelor's degree for generalized practice. They recommend a further credentialing and/or a master's degree to work in specialty areas (See Appendix A).

Paraprofessional health care providers perform most of the direct patient care in home care (Surpin, Haslanger & Dawson,1994). The ability to meet client and family needs with a paraprofessional is unique to the home care setting. This category of paraprofessionals consists of home care aides/nurse's aides, personal care attendants, and home attendants. The vast majority of these positions are held by women who are often single and a member of a minority. Most do not have education beyond high school. These positions have been low paying and have occupied the lowest rung on the medical hierarchy ladder of patient care providers. These services have been traditionally viewed by the home care industry as low-skilled extensions of women's work (Surpin et al., 1994; Walter, 1996). Consequently, little training or resources have been directed toward this important group of people. These providers of direct care are at the intersection of an organization's philosophy and the product it provides to consumers. Clients usually rate the quality of care based on their experiences with their direct care providers. Hence, the satisfaction clients feel with a home care aide reflects directly on their satisfaction with the home care agency; thus, it benefits home care organizations to place well-trained paraprofessionals in the home (Surpin et al., 1994).

The largest category of paraprofessional patient care providers is the home care aide. These service providers are trained to perform a variety of semiskilled and unskilled duties under the supervision of a professional. These unlicensed personnel are frequently needed to give personal care and perform simple health care tasks as dictated by the nurse's plan of care. Home care

aides, sometimes called the "backbone" of the home health industry, are the fastest growing health care job opportunity (Walter, 1996). Most states have regulations defining a set of core skills and knowledge that must be achieved to become a nurse's aide. These usually include basic personal care such as bathing, positioning, feeding patients, and taking vital signs. Nurses' aides may also perform a wide range of other simple health care tasks for stable, uncomplicated patients. These tasks may include simple dressing changes, routine Foley care, routine colostomy care for a stable stoma, urine and stool specimen collections, etc. These tasks must be able to be performed without the scientific knowledge or critical judgment required of a professional. However, these tasks must be carried out under the supervision of a professional (licensed) nurse (Brent, 1993, 1996; Commonwealth of Pennsylvania, 1993).

Most states use broad guidelines to define the scope of practice for home care aides. This allows each health care organization to specify the tasks within this scope of care that are appropriate for its particular needs and setting. The health care organization is then responsible to train and provide home care aides that are competent to perform those tasks and skills specified. For example, if an agency, following state guidelines, chooses to allow its nurse aides to perform simple dressing changes, then the agency is responsible for safe and appropriate performance of the procedure and to ensure that the RN demonstrates knowledge–appropriate delegation and supervision of the aide. The organization must ensure that ongoing competency assessment is performed for these skills (McHann, 1994). A comprehensive CBE program can help a home care organization and its employees navigate this maze of standards and guidelines. Competency education can help ensure the highest quality patient care by paraprofessionals. This care can enhance an organization's bottom line by increasing efficiency and productivity.

Personal care attendants are allowed to give personal care, such as bathing, dressing, toileting, feeding, and light housework. They are not allowed to do health-related tasks. This group may have a few days of class or only on-the-job training. They do not follow a physician-ordered and nurse-supervised plan of care but perform duties contracted by the client and family. Their work is physically and emotionally demanding. They are often isolated in the field and have little regular contact with the organization or other staff.

Homemakers, volunteers, and respite workers are valuable assets to a home care organization. These nonprofessional staff are able to provide the assistance to patients that enables them to restore their health and maintain independence. Homemakers often contribute to clients' independence by enabling them to remain at home rather than enter long-term care. Volunteers and respite workers are able to give physical, emotional, and spiritual support to clients and their families. For example, hospice volunteers are able to give simple personal care, such as feeding, positioning, and grooming, to the patient. These volunteers are often able to provide unique emotional and spiritual support by active listening and informal counseling for the patient and his or her family. Competency assessment, orientation, and ongoing education can help define the skills needed and assist these valuable personnel to perform at a higher level of proficiency. Paraprofessionals are often seen as having more quality time to spend with clients and families than hospice professionals, such as the RN, who frequently has more tasks and time constraints. Paraprofessionals perform an important service for the patient and to the organization by improving customer satisfaction and easing the burden of the often more time-constrained professionals.

SOCIAL AND ECONOMIC FORCES

Home Health Care Expansion

As discussed previously, until the 1960s most home health agencies consisted of VNAs funded by charities or by public agencies funded through the government. The passage of Medicare in 1965, which contained provisions to fund home care for the elderly, created explosive growth in the numbers of home care agencies. Home health care quickly evolved from a "cottage industry" to big business within a few years. In 1967, there were 1,750 Medicare participating home health care agencies. Most of these were nonprofit and publicly funded. Since then, Medicare has become the largest publicly funded program in the United States (Maurer, 1995b). By 1994, the number of home care organizations totaled 7,500, with the majority being Medicare participating, proprietary agencies (National Association for Home Care, 1994).

During Medicare's first year of operation in 1967, costs totaled $4.7 billion. Total costs by 1992 were $132 billion (Maurer, 1995b). During much of this period, the home health care industry grew faster than any other segment of the U.S. health care system. Growth rates often topped 30% per year. In 1983, in an effort to cut spiraling Medicare costs, the federal government introduced a prospective payment program for hospitalized Medicare patients based on diagnosis related groups (DRGs). This payment plan allots a specified payment amount for a diagnostic category regardless of the length of the hospitalization. This effort to cut medical costs has resulted in shortened hospital stays and the discharge of more acutely ill patients into the community. The number of home health care providers grew dramatically in an effort to meet the needs of this burgeoning population group affected by DRGs. Similar effects are also being felt due to the influence of other prospective payment plans recently introduced by various private insurance groups. The annual costs of the Medicare program continue to grow as does the demand for more home health care. This trend is expected to continue well into the foreseeable future (Bender, 1997; Harris, 1996a; Patel & Rushefsky, 1995).

The Cost of Caring: Health Care Costs in the United States

This explosive growth in Medicare and home health care has paralleled the rise in U.S. health care costs in general. Total U.S. health care expenditures were $42 billion in 1965 and amounted to 4.8% of the Gross National Product (GNP). In the year 2000, the total health care costs are expected to top $1.631 billion, with the costs of Medicare and Medicaid alone requiring approximately 15% of the GNP (Maurer, 1995b; Sonnenfield, Waldo, & Lemieux, 1991). Health care costs have grown faster than the annual inflation rate for decades. These costs have also outpaced the cost increases of most other segments of the economy. Health care is now the third largest industry in the U.S. economy. Consistently, the cost of caring for our health constitutes a larger percentage of the national economy than any other industrialized nation (Koch, 1993; Maurer, 1995a). Unlike many other highly industrialized countries, the United States continued to use a retrospective payment system for the reimbursement of medical costs until recent decades. In a retrospective payment system, reimbursement is made after the care is given and services rendered. Most insurance companies and government programs have traditionally participated in a fee-for-service system of reimbursement. Providers had no incentive to control spending because the costs of operation, plus profit, were covered. This system lacked the competitive forces found in other industries that help control costs and increase efficiency and productivity. By the 1980s, with health care costs spiraling out of control, third-party payers began to look to prospective payment as a method of cost containment (Stanhope, 1992; Koch, 1993).

In contrast to a fee-for-service system of payment, prospective payment occurs before care is rendered. A set payment fee may be designated on the basis of the number of persons covered: a capitated system. Others use a designated payment amount allotted for certain services, or a combination of both. In this system, the third-party payer manages the monetary resources available and the access to health services, as in a health maintenance organization (HMO). Or the payer may contract with a group of providers to give care to its clients for a fixed price, as in a preferred provider organization (PPO). The onus

is on the health care provider to improve productivity and efficiency to make a profit (Maurer, 1995a; Koch, 1993).

Medicare began using a prospective payment system for acute care patients based on DRGs in 1983. Under this system, payment price was fixed based on the type of diagnosis, regardless of the cost incurred by the hospital. Although Medicare costs are continuing to rise, this use of managed care is credited with slowing the rise in overall health care costs. Since the 1980s the use of prospective payment systems has been adopted by most insurance carriers and into most government programs. Managed care has infiltrated most of the acute care settings and is making huge inroads into home care. Retrospective payment concepts are expected to be used increasingly in health care's private, public, acute, and home care sectors (Jones, 1994; Koch, 1993; Linne, 1995). Escalating medical costs and prospective reimbursement are creating a paradigm shift in home health care and the entire health care system. When DRGs were introduced, effectively limiting reimbursement and hospital stays, home care was seen by Medicare and other third-party payers as a less expensive alternative to care in the acute care setting (Harris, 1996a; Maurer, 1995b; Stanhope, 1992). It was also believed that keeping patients in their familiar environments improved recovery time and health outcomes and promoted independence. This was thought to prevent recurrent hospitalizations. Because of advances in medical technology, home care had become a feasible alternative to long hospitalizations. As the numbers of inpatient acute hospital stays decreased, the home care industry grew rapidly in complexity and dramatically in cost. The Health Care Financing Administration (HCFA) estimates that home care will grow 328% by the year 2000 when a projected $60 billion per year will be spent on home health care (Smith, 1997).

Proponents of home care have tried through numerous studies to prove the financial and health benefits. However, many studies have repeatedly shown that health care costs increase with the use of home care. Most studies have also shown that the number of rehospitalizations is not decreased. The other benefits of improved independence and lifestyle have not routinely been found and are short lived when they are (Linne, 1995). Other recent data show that managed care has decreased overall health care expenditures in the United States, due in large part to the savings gained with the use of managed care in the home health arena (Zelman, 1996). Whatever the final outcome of these arguments, there is the general belief that home care is the right thing to do. Most elderly people and their children currently desire the home care benefit, and the demand for home care services is expected to grow. In order to continue this service, providers can no longer rely on the presumption of lowered health care costs. They must learn to provide a cost-effective service to survive the future health care climate of competition and regulation.

There are currently many efforts by third-party payers to reduce the cost of home care. Various prospective methods of reimbursement such as HMOs, PPOs, and capitated systems are moving into the home care sector. The movement of managed care into the home care arena requires providers to become more efficient and productive. They must learn to provide a lower cost, high-quality product (Benefield, 1996b; Bender, 1997; Jones, 1994). This often means doing a better job with fewer staff per patient. Patient care is now frequently accomplished via care maps or critical pathways that reduce the number and length of staff visits in the home, while at the same time expecting highly positive outcomes. CBE has emerged as the preferred technique to prepare and maintain staff quality, productivity, and effectiveness in a cost-conscious manner.

Demographic Influences

The dramatic rise of health care costs may be attributed only in part to the combined effects of the growth of Medicare and Medicaid. Other frequently named forces on the cost of medical care

have been the rapidly expanding over-65 population, the dissemination of medical advances and technology, and the nature of our third-party retrospective payment system (Stanhope, 1992; Torrens, 1993; Van Ort & Woodtli, 1989). These same forces have also influenced the growth of the home care industry's size and operation. These social, political, and economic dynamics have also directly and indirectly propelled the necessity of CBE and assessment in the home care field (Astarita, 1996; Bailey, 1994).

The elderly segment of the population became the fastest growing in the United States after the baby boom of World War II. The population older than 85 is expanding at 232% faster than the rest of the population (U.S. Department of Health and Human Services, 1991). This improved life expectancy is due to advances in public health, nutrition, and medicine. Although people are living longer and healthier, this age group places an increasing burden on the health care system. The elderly suffer from more acute and chronic illnesses than any other segment of our society. Providing quality health care for this large population requires the consumption of a tremendous amount of health care resources. This trend is expected to continue well into the 21st century as life expectancy lengthens and the "baby-boomer generation" ages (Lashley, 1995; Torrens, 1993; Van Ort & Woodtli, 1989). Other late 20th century demographic changes have increased the need for more home care. Women have traditionally cared for the elderly and chronically ill family members. Since the coming of age of the baby-boomer generation, women have entered the work force in ever greater numbers. Today, 65% of all women are employed outside the home. This creates a need for caregivers from outside the home. In addition, the geographic separation of families due to modern technology and employment options has left many elders and chronically ill persons without family caregivers nearby. These trends are expected to continue and increase the demand for home care services (Reif & Martin, 1996).

Consumerism and Health Care

A better informed and educated public has also inadvertently increased the costs of health care. The education policy in the United States holds that everyone is entitled to primary education. Completing 12 years of primary education became the general expectation in the 1900s. And for many, secondary education has become a reality and necessity as well. During this same era, information about medical advances and technological breakthroughs became available to the general population due to the progress of communication systems. This better informed and educated public's expectations of health and medical care changed as they began placing a high value on health care. As consumers, they demanded easy access to high-tech care and the miracles it performed. The public also began to always expect positive outcomes from high-quality care given by highly trained individuals. Increased professional accountability was expected from health care providers and workers, creating a need for further education and credentialing. The efforts to provide all of these services has required a huge input of resources, time, money, and personnel from the home care industry (Bailey, 1994; Stanhope, 1992; Koch, 1993).

In addition, the consumer must be able to choose among the many home health care options available. Among home care agencies, there is enormous variation in the kind of services they offer, the fees they charge, the third-party payers they accept, and the type of clients they serve. Agencies may be public or private, for profit or nonprofit, free standing or hospital based. In addition, agencies may now be part of an integrated delivery network of affiliated health care entities, part of a managed care network, or operating as a free-standing fee-for-service organization. The focus of care may be short-term/episodic care or long-term care, medical-model based or service-model based. Agencies may or may not be licensed as home care providers, certified as Medicare providers, or accredited by the NLN or the Joint Commis-

sion. All of these variables greatly influence the philosophy of care, the organizational mission, and thus its quality of care (Reif & Martin, 1996).

In response to consumer needs and concerns, various regulating and accrediting bodies have evolved that set standards for home care organizations to help ensure quality, patient-focused care. This credentialing and affiliation also enable consumers to make informed decisions about their health care choices.

EFFECTS OF REGULATORY REQUIREMENTS

CBE plays an important role in ensuring that a home care organization meets the requirements demanded by regulating, accrediting, and professional bodies. Meeting these regulations and standards is necessary to function legally and effectively in today's dynamic and competitive health care market. A Medicare-certified home care agency must comply with federal law, such as the Medicare COP. Standards in home care are often driven by Medicare requirements due to the huge role this federal entitlement program plays in general in the home care industry. To increase their standards and competitiveness, an organization may choose to qualify for accreditation by various accrediting bodies such as the Joint Commission and/or the Community Health Accreditation Program (CHAP). These accrediting and regulatory standards require evidence of competence in clinical and administrative areas. In addition, professional specialty organizations, such as the ANA and NAHC, have set standards for home health care delivery only by those deemed competent (Friedman, 1996b; Reid-Webb, 1995; Zink, 1996).

State Law

State law governs the licensure and scope of practice of professionals, such as RNs, physical therapists, and occupational therapists, and para-professionals, such as nurses' aides. State laws usually describe a profession's scope of practice in rather broad terms. A range of skills appropriate to a variety of work settings is allowed to professionals and paraprofessionals. The law allows the health care institution hiring these individuals to delineate the specific tasks they deem appropriate for their situation and client needs. For example: According to the Pennsylvania State Board of Nursing (1985), a professional nurse (RN) is allowed to carry out medical regimens under the auspices of a licensed physician or dentist. An RN is allowed to diagnose and treat health problems through "casefinding, health teaching, counseling and by performing restorative measures" (p. 1). This act excludes medical therapeutics limited to physicians and dentists. This broad definition allows the health care institution to determine the specific tasks their RNs will perform within the legal range of activities.

The health care institution is compelled to ascertain the employees are qualified and trained with the requisite skills and knowledge they will need to perform their duties. Professionals and paraprofessionals are also held accountable to practice within the scope of their practice and within their knowledge and skill base. A CBE program helps ensure the training of a competent employee and documents that training for the employer and the health care providing employee.

Medicare Conditions of Participation

Federal guidelines for Medicare, the Conditions of Participation (COP), have been established through the HCFA. These COPs detail the standards a home care organization must meet to become a Medicare-certified provider. As the largest third-party payer in the home care sector, Medicare has a huge impact on the standards of practice for the entire home health industry. The COPs provide a framework for the structure and functions of home care organizations. The document establishes standards for the qualifications and performance of administrative and clinical personnel. The goals of the COPs are patient-focused. The standards aim to provide high-quality patient care and establish methods for evaluating patient outcomes (Reid-Webb, 1995) (see Appendix A). The COPs designate activities and scope of practice appropriate to professionals, such as RNs, physical therapists, and medical social workers. They also detail knowledge and skills necessary for paraprofessionals, such as home care aides and vocational nurses. The standards establish the qualifications, training, and continuing education necessary to hire and maintain a competent health care worker. Organizations are to document competence at hire and record the ongoing efforts to maintain or improve skill levels.

An excellent example of these requirements can be seen in Condition 484.36, which deals with standards pertaining to the home care aide. The home care agency must ensure and document that all home care aide hires have completed a state licensure, certification, or competency evaluation that meets Medicare requirements. The aide must be competency tested on a specified list of core knowledge and patient care skills, such as giving a bed bath, performing oral hygiene, and taking vital signs at the time of hire. Other tasks within a state's legal scope of practice that range outside of these core tasks must be taught and evaluated as well. Medicare requires that home care aides complete 12 hours of continuing education related to their practice each year. It is also stipulated that home care aides must be competency evaluated in the practical setting with a patient at yearly intervals. The agency is responsible for ensuring this education and testing are completed and accurately documented.

The Joint Commission on Accreditation of Healthcare Organizations

The Joint Commission is a nonprofit organization that endeavors to improve health care services to the public. The Joint Commission and its standards have evolved as a powerful force in U.S. health care. Accreditation is sought by many providers in the acute care and home care sectors as a way of improving organizational performance and public image (Biere & Rooney, 1995; LoGerfo & Brook, 1988). According to the Joint Commission manual of accreditation, the accrediting process assists a health care organization in analyzing and refining the everyday tasks and activities that impact patient care outcomes. Standards governing the administration of the organization and continual improvement are designed to help facilitate overall organizational self-assessment and function. In addition, the standards are divided into sections that deal with various services providing patient care. Chapters include client rights and responsibilities, safety management of the client, infection control, the home health record, equipment services, pharmaceutical services, respiratory services, personal care, and home health care services. Adherence to these standards helps ensure high-quality patient care (Biere & Rooney, 1995).

In 1991, the Joint Commission revised its accreditation requirements to include home health organizations. Standards that had previously required performance-based education and testing for employees were changed to include standards requiring competency for all nursing employees. By 1994, the Joint Commission required evidence of competency for every professional, paraprofessional caregiver, and of all support staff throughout the organization (Alspach, 1996; Astarita et al., in press; Friedman, 1996b). The Joint Commission standards for Human Resources are most pertinent for the discussion of staff competency. Human resources are assigned the duty of providing staff who are competent to meet the peculiar patient care needs of the organization. These standards begin being applied before the hiring process. Written competencies for each job description must be developed throughout the organization. Upon hire, all new potential employees must meet the required educational qualifications and licensure and/or credentialing. All patient care staff must be competency assessed on their professional core skills needed for their new posi-

tion before caring for patients. An orientation to the organization and all new skills must be provided as well. Competency assessment, maintenance, and improvement of all patient care staff must also occur at regular intervals. These continuing education programs must be designed to address the needs indicated from the assessment of staff competency. Staff development educators are usually deemed responsible to carry out these standards. In addition, educators are to keep written descriptions of a competency program, documenting its regular updating, and the assessment mechanisms used. Ongoing records are to be kept documenting each employee's continuing education and competency testing (Alspach, 1996; Joint Commission, 1996).

The Roles of CHAP and NAHC

CHAP has been accrediting home- and community-based care since 1965 and is an independent subsidiary of the NLN. CHAP's organizational philosophy is based on the provision of high-quality health care to the public by improving the performance of health care delivery organizations. CHAP's standards stress management excellence, fiscal reliability, and customer satisfaction. CHAP provides this accrediting information to the public to enable consumers to make informed health care decisions (Bohlen & Mitchell, 1994; Zink, 1996).

CHAP uses comprehensive, outcome-based standards of excellence to evaluate organizations. This requires an organization to measure quality, performance, and outcomes throughout all of its structures and functions. CHAP is seen as a leader in developing benchmarks for excellence in the home care industry due to its deemed status. In 1992, CHAP became the first private accrediting body to achieve this status, which means that earning the CHAP accreditation also confers Medicare and Medicaid certification. CHAP standards meet and often exceed the Medicare COPs.

CHAP has standards of excellence developed for professional and paraprofessional services, and for specialty teams such as infusion and hospice. Standards encourage the use of highly qualified, motivated, and informed employees who produce a top-quality product to consumers. Competent staff at all organizational levels are necessary to meet this commitment to quality (Zink, 1996).

The Influence of the NAHC on Standards for Home Care

The NAHC is the largest organization representing the interests and concerns of the home care industry and the people it serves to federal and state legislative bodies. The NAHC engages in public education, research, and collaboration with other agencies to promote the interests of the home care industry. The voluntary membership has grown to well over 6,000 home care agencies by 1995 (Halamandaris, 1994). The NAHC has established a set of standards that deem it an ethical responsibility for a home care agency to hire qualified, competent health care providers. This directly influences competency assessment programs. In addition, the NAHC standards address the need to provide a high quality of care, a standard that can be met only if staff are competent to perform the duties described in their job descriptions. Thirdly, the NAHC promotes knowledge of and involvement in relevant legislation, which should also be included in competency programs.

THE VALUE OF COMPETENCY IN HOME CARE

CBE can be a powerful tool to enhance an organization's performance and maintain a competitive business edge. CBE can help a home care agency provide competent, efficient, and productive staff necessary in the emerging health care paradigm that demands high-quality care and cost containment. However, as pointed out by del Bueno and Altano (1984), CBE is not a magic solution to an agency's problems. A CBE program is often more time consuming than traditional education programs based on the transfer of knowledge from teacher to student. It requires more input and coordination by the managers and staff development educators to assess needs, develop appropriate competencies, educate staff, and evaluate outcomes. The amount of time required for the orientation of new staff is usually longer but spent more productively in the acquisition of needed job skills (del Bueno & Altano, 1984). In the final analysis, however, CBE is more beneficial than traditional education models due to its far-reaching effects on an organization's ability to meet the ethical, legal, and business demands of today's home health care environment.

CBE can be used as an organizational strategy to improve overall internal and external processes. It can assist internal coordination and communication between departments and interdepartmentally. It may also enhance exterior communication and relationships with customers, such as physicians, clients, and medical equipment and services suppliers. Coordination and clear communication with external clients and partners is vital in today's home care market where health alliances and provider networks are increasingly common (Jones, 1994). CBE enhances the organization's marketability to consumers and third-party payers by providing qualified, productive, and efficient staff educated in these issues (Gingerich & Ondeck, 1997).

CBE can be used as a framework, helping to unite and coordinate organizational departments and activities. Professional and paraprofessional competence can help assure an agency that its employees are functioning at the highest levels, helping to maintain organizational growth and vitality. For example, risk management functions are enhanced when a highly functioning staff commits fewer errors and omissions, resulting in fewer critical incidents. CBE can be used as a framework for staff development and human resources departments. A competency framework can be used as a link and tool of communication and tracking for organizational improvement activities. CBE can improve productivity of staff and cut employee costs by improving staff satisfaction and retention. In short, competency-based assessment and education are one strategy that can help a home health care provider deal with the social, economic, political, legal, and ethical dynamics that influence the medical system today (Alspach, 1996; Astarita, 1996; Bailey, 1994).

Ethical Issues

Moral codes to govern behavior have existed for thousands of years from early Hebrew law and Greek philosophers. Socrates postulated that a person should do no wrong, nor participate in wrongdoing. The philosophy of the art and science of medicine is rooted in these Greek moral codes of caring for humanity compassionately. Both professions of medicine and nursing have long traditions of caring for the ill, promoting health, and relieving suffering. Caring for the needy, regardless of the social, economic, or political circumstances in which the client and caregiver find themselves, has long been a primary tenet of medical care. To uphold high ethical standards and remain competitive economically may seem currently incompatible. However, ethical standards are more important than ever in today's isolating and complex society. Practicing ethical principles can enhance a company's productivity and is actually vital to economic viability and positive patient outcomes (McMaster-Fitzig, 1994).

A comprehensive CBE program helps ensure a qualified, capable staff. This is an ethical necessity in order to give the high-quality, safe patient care. Competency is a professional and paraprofessional standard of care for health care providers. Ethical issues are familiar in all areas of health care but are of particular importance in the specialty of home health care. Caregivers in home health deliver care in an isolated setting, without the influence of peers or the immediate presence of supervisors. In addition, the home care clientele contains disproportionate numbers of the weak, frail, powerless, and disenfran-

chised of our society. This clientele may be easily taken advantage of, becoming victims of mistreatment, abuse, or neglect. Extra attention must be given to staff selection and training to alert staff to these ethical and legal problems and to ensure that staff are ethical and responsible in their treatment of clients (Lashley, 1995).

Because staff often work alone in the field, an agency must be assured that they are qualified to perform not only the cognitive and psychomotor tasks involved within their job description but the affective and critical thinking ones as well. In order to deliver the highest standard of care, there must be a synthesis of this knowledge and skills by caregivers. Only with the use of a highly competent staff can an agency feel confident that its ethical obligation in the delivery of safe, quality care to the public is being met (Lashley, 1995; Reif & Martin, 1996).

Accurate documentation of clients' needs is also important for Medicare compliance and reimbursement. The majority of nurses responding in surveys have reported that they never record false or inaccurate information in the patient chart. However, authorities recognize that some nurses may be tempted to alter documentation to ensure reimbursement and continue care for those clients they deem as needy of more visits. Nurses in the home care setting often find themselves caught between meeting clients' needs and reimbursement issues. During Medicare surveys, compliance with the home care reimbursement criteria of being homebound, having a physician plan of care, or requiring skilled care is often found lacking (McMaster-Fitzig, 1994). Competency training in ethics and case management can assist nurses in making correct legal and ethical choices.

Home health care providers encounter a variety of ethical problems daily. All patients must be assessed in regard to their physical and psychological safety. The home setting often reveals problems of neglect or abuse that are not evident in the acute care setting. All health care staff must be trained to recognize and intervene appropriately in these situations. In addition, the expertise of the RN case manager or social worker is often needed to help clients and their family sort out issues the end of life brings. Decisions about remaining in the home, entering a long-term care facility, discontinuing curative care, and beginning hospice care are issues often encountered by the bulk of home care clients: the elderly. Home care organizations must be sure their staff are well educated in the options available to consumers and have the ability to confront these difficult topics with their clients. A well-trained work force can help ensure the best quality-of-life decisions are made for home care clients.

Performance Improvement

The current home care climate requires a home care agency to have a performance improvement program operating throughout the organization. These programs may be expressed variously as quality improvement (QI), total quality management (TQM), continuous quality improvement (CQI), or quality assurance (QA) in different organizations. These programs all attempt to measure the actual performance of a company against a set of recognized standards and company goals. These activities are vital to a home care organization's success clinically and financially (Harris, 1996a).

There are a number of political, social, and economic forces dictating QA activities. QI endeavors are necessary in part due to federal and state regulations, such as the Medicare COP. Accrediting bodies such as the Joint Commission also have set standards requiring QI activities throughout the organization. Professional standards of many health care disciplines require QI efforts. Consumers also have their own unique definitions of quality. These may include professional high-tech care but also often include convenience, kindness, timeliness, and assistance to the client's primary caregiver.

Competent staff are a necessary ingredient of any QA program. They are the key to carrying out the organizational goals by providing safe, expert care in a cost-efficient manner. Staff

training and education based on the acquisition of competency will enhance any QI program. The very nature of CBE compels staff to improve their performance and, thus, enhance quality. Actual staff performance may be compared to competency statements based on regulatory, professional, and accreditation standards. These performance indicators may be used throughout the organization to improve the quality of internal processes and structure functions. Competency-based expectations enhance the tracking of patient care activities and of quality health care services rendered (Alspach, 1996; Astarita, 1996; Friedman, 1996a).

Findings from the QI program can be used to revise the competency education program. For example, it is found that documentation of diabetic patient education is not performed. QI personnel and the staff-development educators can collaborate to detect the area or areas of difficulty. Expectations may not be clear, and documentation or teaching skills may need to be improved. In addition, an organization can more easily compare its performance to other standards. The interaction of the QI and educational processes gives evidence of systemwide QI initiatives, which is necessary to achieve accreditation (Alspach, 1996).

Risk Management

A CBE program can enhance risk-management efforts of a home health care organization. When a problem is identified in any department, remediation may be done through changes in the competency requirements. Pinpointing targets for alteration is made easier by the clear outcome assessment statements. Workers' tasks or duties may change as a result of risk management information. These changes affect the processes of the organization as well. This interaction of risk management and the education program can decrease risk through all departments. This in turn can decrease the health care organization's legal liability (Alspach, 1996; Brent, 1994; Leidy, 1992).

With the rapid growth of home health care has come increased risk for provider organizations due to changes in client needs and the influx of new employees. The population of clients is more acutely ill, requiring more highly skilled, complex care. A thoroughly educated and skilled staff can give safe technical care and use good judgment and critical thinking skills in complex situations (Jacobs, Ott, Sullivan, Ulrich, & Short, 1997). Large numbers of health care workers have had to leave the acute care setting as the result of downsizing. Home care employers frequently have to hire personnel who are inexperienced in home care (Caie-Lawrence, Peploski, & Russell, 1995). A competency-based orientation helps ensure an adequate introduction to home care (Astarita, 1996; Hefty, Kenyon, Martaus, Bell, & Snow, 1992).

Promoting competence can also assist the collaboration of risk management and quality-improvement departments. Competency provides a framework from which to easily identify, assess, intervene, and evaluate adverse outcomes. This activity assists the work of risk management, QI, and the staff-development departments. The documentation of the interaction of CQI, risk management, and staff competency may assist the defense of an agency in malpractice litigation (Revis, Thompson, Williams, Bezanson, & Cook, 1996).

Staff Development

A staff-development department can use competency as a central framework for its curriculum. This framework can be used to organize all phases of the educational work. The clearly specified outcomes and measurable goals lend themselves to the assessment, planning, implementation, and evaluation of many elements of the staff-development program (Alspach, 1996; Lassiter, Kearney, & Fell, 1985; McGregor, 1990). The competency assessments that are performed upon hire can be used for orientation programs to provide information to formulate the content and instructional methods that prepare employees to meet their position demands. To adequately fulfill the responsibilities of providing competent new staff to the work force, staff development needs to continually monitor the changes and requirements of each employment position. Ongoing revision of competencies must be done to include technological advances, organizational structure, and process changes. The information gleaned during initial competency assessments may be further used to design and update inservice education needs. This allows the inservice program to more adequately address the changing needs of existing employees.

The competency framework can be used effectively to fulfill Joint Commission requirements of regular staff-competency evaluations. Needs assessments from learners, risk management, QI, and professional standard changes may be easily incorporated into competency-based outcome statements. A competency-based curriculum can greatly assist the staff-development department in its efforts to provide proficient workers throughout the organization (Alspach, 1996; Brent, 1994).

Human Resources

The clear delineation of duties and tasks specified in a competency education program can assist the human resources department in the generation of accurate job descriptions. Competency expectations can add to the specificity and detail describing a position's responsibilities. This detailed, updated job description can be used to give prospective employees an accurate picture of the skills, knowledge, and duties required. The competency information is also a valuable source of information for employee recordkeeping activities. Information from competency assessments is helpful in documenting performance evaluations, promotions, or conversely, remedial and disciplinary activities (Alspach, 1996).

Productivity and Cost Benefits from Competency

To some, competency and productivity may be very distantly related; however, ever increasingly, educators are verbalizing possible correlations about their relationship and what meaning if any it has on care delivery in home health care. It is speculated that skills that enhance productivity, such as physical assessment, time management, and communication, are related to the competency level with which they are carried out; however, to date, there have been no measurement devices to prove this assumption. Until recently, home care managers were concerned primarily with the number of patients in a clinician's caseload, which has now been replaced with the archaic concern for productivity, which has been recently defined as the total visits per discipline divided by the paid hours per discipline multiplied by eight (National Association for Home Care, 1997). With the advent of managed care, the push began to develop productivity measurement systems and to perspicaciously analyze monthly productivity reports to identify who was making the most visits and how the organization matched up to the industry standard. Home care clinicians and educators alike are well aware of management's push to increase the average patient visits per day in order to cover the cost per visit. Management, in return of this push, is typically responded to with negativity and "but how can we?" remarks from clinicians. Staff development is then summoned to decrease the number of educational programs or is instructed to cancel the programs altogether so that staff can be in the field. This scenario is a "catch 22" because, in many instances, staff are in significant need of the educational endeavor so that they can add knowledge or skill to their clinical repertoire in order to be more effective in care delivery, which in turn is proposed to increase their productivity. Unequivocally, the visits need to be made, or the business does not survive; however, there can be a collaborative and "win-win" approach in this scenario with

careful planning and development of a competency program that is outcome oriented, based upon the latest research findings and measurement tools, and is supported by management.

Hedtcke, MacQueen, and Carr (1992) set out to identify how home health nurses spend their time. This survey was undertaken because management increased the productivity requirement to match the industry standard and staff responded that it was not feasible to meet such a standard. Upon review of staff logs over a 2-week period, management found that it indeed was not feasible. It was found that nurses spent 47% of their time in direct patient care, 18% of their time documenting care, 12% of their time in other activities, and 22% of their time traveling. Their findings were similar to the findings of Caie-Lawrence (1990). From a management perspective, one would seek inquiry into where inefficiencies may lie so that productivity could be increased. One would assume that it would be in the nondirect patient care activities; however, an aspect that has only minimally been investigated is the time spent in direct patient care. Is it possible that per-visit time could be cut if clinicians were more competent in their care delivery activities and had a solid grasp of the specialty of home care? This question has yet to be answered by scholarly inquiry. Perhaps it is possible to decrease the nondirect care activities by streamlining documentation activities and decreasing travel time by planning assignments by territory; however, the literature shows that there is a lack of inquiry into the impact that competency, the ability to perform the job function, plays in productivity. It must also be acknowledged that sophisticated productivity measurement systems have been difficult to develop because of the large number of intangible variables in home care, and industry standard figures may not be representative of a true picture because of the differences in geography and definitions of the productivity components.

Benefield (1996a) uses effectiveness, the degree to which the RN has accomplished intended agency goals related to managing and providing care to clients in their homes, and efficiency, the production of the home visit and associated activities without time or material waste, as the two primary components encompassing productivity. Her definition of productivity expands upon the traditional calculation of visits divided by time by incorporating the quality component of care delivery utilizing the Benefield Productivity Measurement Classification (1989). This classification was developed as the result of a national descriptive, correlational study using quantitative and qualitative methods of data collection where 360 home health care nurse managers were asked to identify the knowledge and skills of productive nurses. The results identified a profile of 35 areas of knowledge and abilities that are reflective of productive practice (Benefield, 1996a). The 35 areas were then grouped into like categories and developed into the Productivity Measurement Classification (PMC) (Exhibit 1–1). Her study indicates that among agencies considered preeminent, intellectual skills appeared to be of greater importance to productive practice than direct-care skills (Benefield, 1996b). Benefield (1996a) further states that "the PMC can be used by management during the hiring process to identify if candidates portray the identified knowledge and abilities related to the role. If the candidate portrays skill in areas within a category of practice, the RN is considered proficient in that area of practice and is able to function with minimal guidance from management." Benefield (1996a) has produced the first home care productivity measurement tool, one that can be incorporated by home care organizations to screen applicants, utilized as a component of the job description and performance appraisal, and utilized in developing the curriculum for orientation and components of competency-based orientation.

From an acute care perspective, Ozcan and Shukla (1993) investigated the effect on nursing productivity of a competency-based targeted staff development (TSD) system. Competency of medical-surgical nurses was compared with a preestablished standard. The Slater Scale of Nursing Competencies (Wandelt & Steward,

1975) was administered to these nurses. The authors describe TSD as a five-step process that includes nursing assessment, individual feedback, educational offering, behavior modification, and reassessment. The study found that TSD over a 6-month period significantly increased productivity of direct care and decreased insignificant indirect care.

The literature, however limited, shows that there is a correlation between competency and productivity. Productivity may be seen as the difference between the energy and resources expended by a health care provider and the energy and resources gained. However, productivity is more than making reimbursements total more than expenses. True productivity is difficult to measure in health care because of the complexities and intangibles of providing quality care. True productivity suggests both quality and efficiency. Quality infers a value of excellence. Efficiency may be defined as the wise use of time and resources (Humphrey & Milone-Nuzzo, 1994; LoGerfo & Brook, 1988). It is clear from these definitions that an organization needs staff that are proficient in the delivery of care.

CBE has been shown repeatedly to be an effective teaching method for improving the performance of health care workers (McGregor, 1990; Scrima, 1987). An organization can choose to educate staff in areas that enhance productivity, efficiency, and quality. A competent staff can help an agency function at its highest levels of capability, and yet, in a cost-effective manner (Ozcan & Shukla, 1993; Twardon, Gartner & Cherry, 1993). A competency-based orientation program for employees new to the field of home health care can be a cost-effective tool for an organization and can enhance productivity in several distinct ways. An orientation program based on competency uses adult learning theory, which allows learners to challenge out of areas of expertise and to proceed at their own pace. This decreases ineffective use of staff time and allows experienced hires to proceed more rapidly (Bethel, 1992; O'Grady & O'Brien, 1992). The competency approach allows for individual learner styles and adult

Exhibit 1–1 Productivity Measurement Classification Model

Practice management

*Expert in health assessment skills
*Organized in approach to time and tasks
*Able to analyze a situation and develop an appropriate plan
*Able to make independent decisions
*Able to deal with problems in priority order
Able to adjust daily client schedule if unexpected problems occur
Delegates non-nurse tasks to support personnel

Knowledge/skills maintenance

*Hands-on technical skills in area of practice
*Understands how physical processes of illness and associated complications relate to the client
Able to update technical skills and knowledge of unfamiliar diseases and conditions

Written documentation

*Complete paperwork tasks to meet Medicare (and/or other payers) and agency requirement and deadlines

Home health care knowledge

*Understands rules and regulations governing home health care
*Background in principles of teaching/learning for client/family
Knowledge of nutrition teaching

*among most important elements in practice.

Communication

*Good interpersonal communication skills with client/family, staff, colleagues, and physicians
Uses referrals to other agency services and community resources to meet client needs when appropriate
Able to be a "marketing person" for the agency
Keeps supervisor informed of major changes in clients
Understands the structure of the agency

Nursing process

Foundation in formulating nursing diagnoses and measurable goals for client care

Client/family management

*Provides clear direction for clients during visits
Deals in realistic and practical ways with situations confronting clients
Activities are planned and implemented based on treatment goals for the client
Views client as part of a family and community
Encourages client and family independence when necessary
Demonstrates empathy for the client
Recognizes and deals with family concerns related to the client's health problem
During visits, gives time to psychosocial and physical care
Does not force own values on client and family

Source: Copyright © 1989, Lazelle Benefield.

---

needs, which enhances job satisfaction, self confidence, and self-esteem. This can help prevent occurrences of personnel loss within a year of hire, which saves the agency valuable time and money required to hire and train new staff (Lassiter, Kearney, & Fell, 1985).

Competency education for maintaining and improving existing employees' skills, expertise, and professionalism also assists their self-confidence and job satisfaction. A quality continuing-education program can help professionals keep abreast of the rapidly changing medical field.

This also contributes to personnel retention and improved productivity, leading to cost savings (O'Grady & O'Brien, 1992). A competent staff can work more productively and efficiently in the field. Everyday clinical decisions made in the field can impact the efficiency and productivity of the entire organization. For example, nurses who are well informed in Medicare regulations can make more appropriate decisions regarding frequency and duration of care. Medicare denials of payment cost both money and time.

In short, a comprehensive, effective CBE program can allow a home care agency to behave proactively toward the rapidly changing dynamics of the health care system. A competent, productive staff can enhance an agency's market edge and competitiveness. High-quality professional care contributes to increased customer satisfaction, word-of-mouth advertising, and an improved image. This allows a home health care provider to position itself strategically to take advantage of the evolving health care delivery mechanisms. This helps ensure an agency's viability in this age of mergers, health alliances, and affiliations.

REFERENCES

Abruzzese, R.S. (1996). *Nursing staff development: Strategies for success* (2nd ed.). St. Louis: Mosby-Year Book, Inc.

Albrecht, M.N. (1992). The community health nurse in home health and hospice care. In M. Stanhope & J. Lancaster (Eds.), *Community health nursing* (3rd ed.) (pp. 747–760). Philadelphia: Mosby.

Alspach, J.G. (1992). Concern and confusion over competence. *Critical Care Nurse, 12*(4), 9–11.

Alspach, J.G. (1996). *Designing competency assessment programs: A handbook for nurses and health-related professionals.* Pensacola, FL: National Nursing Staff Development Organization.

American Nurses Association. (1993). *Standards of home care nursing practice.* Washington, DC: Author.

American Nurses Association. (1994). *Standards for nursing professional development: Continuing education and staff development.* Washington, DC: Author.

Astarita, T.M. (1996). Competency-based orientation in home care: One agency's approach. *Home Health Care Management and Practice, 8*(4), 38–49.

Astarita, T.M., Materna, G., & Savage, C. (in press). Perceived knowledge level among home health nurses: A descriptive study. *Home Health Care Management and Practice.*

Bailey, C. (1994). Education for home-care providers. *Journal of Gynecological and Neonatal Nursing, 23*(8), 714–718.

Bender, A. (1997). Bringing managed care home: Strategies for success. *Home Healthcare Nurse, 15*(2), 133–139.

Benefield, L.E. (1989). *Productivity measurement for home health care registered nurses.* Unpublished doctoral dissertation. Old Dominion University. Norfolk, VA.

Benefield, L.E. (1996a). Productivity in home healthcare: Assessing nurse effectiveness and efficiency. (Part I). *Home Healthcare Nurse, 14*(9), 698–706.

Benefield, L.E. (1996b). Productivity in home healthcare: Maintaining and improving nurse performance. (Part II). *Home Healthcare Nurse, 14*(10), 803–812.

Benner, P. (1982). Issues in competency-based testing. *Nursing Outlook, 30*(5), 303–309.

Benner, P. (1984). *From novice to expert: Excellence and power in clinical nursing practice.* Menlo Park, CA: Addison-Wesley.

Bethel, P.L. (1992). RN orientation. Cost and achievement analysis. *Nursing Economics, 10*(5), 336–359.

Biere, D., & Rooney, A. (1995). The joint commission's home care accreditation program. In M.D. Harris (Ed.), *Handbook of home health care administration* (pp. 56–64). Gaithersburg, MD: Aspen Publishers, Inc.

Bohlen, S., & Mitchell, M. (1994). Accreditation: Standards of excellence for home care and community organizations. In M.D. Harris (Ed.), *Handbook of home health care administration* (pp. 65–75). Gaithersburg, MD: Aspen Publishers, Inc.

Brent, N.J. (1993). Delegation and supervision of patient care. In M. McHann (Ed.), *What every home health nurse needs to know: A book of readings* (pp. 183–186). Memphis, TN: Consultants in Care.

Brent, N.J. (1994). Orientation to home healthcare nursing is an essential ingredient of risk management and employee satisfaction. *Home Healthcare Nurse, 10*(2), 9–10.

Brent, N.J. (1996). The home healthcare nurse and the state nurse practice act: Gaining familiarity is as easy as 1-2-3. *Home Healthcare Nurse, 14*(10), 788–789.

Caie-Lawrence, J. (1990). *A time study of home care nurses.* Poster presented at the Sixth National Nursing Symposium-Home Health Care, Ann Arbor, MI.

Caie-Lawrence, J., Peploski, J., & Russell, J.C. (1995). Training needs of home health nurses. *Home Healthcare Nurse, 13*(2), 53–61.

Commonwealth of Pennsylvania. (1993). *Title 49. Professional & vocation standards: Chapter state board of nursing. (3676).* Harrisburg, PA: Author.

del Bueno, D., & Altano, R. (1984). Competency-based orientation: No magic feather. *Nursing Management, 15*(4), 48–49.

del Bueno, D., Barker, F., & Christmyer, C. (1981). Implementing a competency-based orientation program. *Journal of Nursing Administration, 11*(2), 24–29.

Friedman, M.M. (1996a). Problematic standards: Improving organizational performance through the plan, design and measure phases. *Home Healthcare Nurse, 14*(4), 277–280.

Friedman, M.M. (1996b). Competence assessment: How to meet the intent of the Joint Commission on Accreditation of Healthcare Organizations' management of human resources standards. *Home Healthcare Nurse, 14*(10), 771–774.

Gingerich, B., & Ondeck, D. (1997). Credentialing and accreditation: What exists for health care provider organizations. *Home Health Care Management and Practice, 9*(4), 67–68.

Halamandaris, V.J. (1994). The national association for home care. In M.D. Harris (Ed.), *Handbook of home health care administration* (pp. 103–108). Gaithersburg, MD: Aspen Publishers, Inc.

Harris, M. (1996a). Medicare as secondary payer. *Home Healthcare Nurse, 14*(1), 51–53.

Harris, M. (1996b). Home healthcare nursing is alive, well, and thriving. *Home Healthcare Nurse, 12*(3), 17–20.

Hedtcke, C.S., MacQueen, L., & Carr, A. (1992). How do home health nurses spend their time? *Journal of Nursing Administration, 22*(1), 18–22.

Hefty, L.V., Kenyon, V., Martaus, T., Bell, M.L., & Snow, L. (1992). A model skills list for orienting nurses to community health agencies. *Public Health Nursing, 9*(4), 228–233.

Humphrey, C.J., & Milone-Nuzzo, P. (1994). Home care nursing orientation model: Justification and structure. *Home Healthcare Nurse, 10*(3), 18–25.

Jacobs, P.M., Ott, B., Sullivan, B., Ulrich, Y., & Short, L. (1997). An approach to defining and operationalizing critical thinking. *Journal of Nursing Education, 36*(1), 19–23.

Joint Commission on Accreditation of Healthcare Organizations (1990). *1991 Comprehensive manual for home care.* Oakbrook Terrace, IL: Author.

Joint Commission on Accreditation of Healthcare Organizations (1996). *1997–1998 Comprehensive manual for home care.* Oakbrook Terrace, IL: Author.

Jones, K.C. (1994). Managed care: The coming revolution in home health care. *Journal of Home Health Care Practice, 6*(2), 1–11.

Koch, A.L. (1993). Financing health services. In P.R. Torrens & S.J. Williams (Eds.), *Introduction to health services* (4th ed.) (pp. 335–366). New York: John Wiley & Sons.

Lashley, M.E. (1995). Health promotion and risk reduction in the community. In C.M. Smith & F.A. Maurer (Eds.), *Community health nursing: Theory and practice* (pp. 403–424). Philadelphia: W.B. Saunders.

Lassiter, C.K., Kearney, M.R., & Fell, R. (1985). Competency-based orientation: An idea that works! *Journal of Nursing Staff Development, 1,* 68–73.

Leidy, K. (1992). The effective screening and orientation of independent contract nurses. *The Journal of Continuing Education in Nursing, 23*(2), 64–68.

Linne, E.B. (1995). *Home care & managed care.* Chicago: American Hospital Publishing Co.

LoGerfo, J.P., & Brook, R.H. (1988). The quality of health care. In S.J. Williams & P.R. Torrens (Eds.), *Introduction to health services* (3rd ed.) (pp. 407–426). New York: John Wiley & Sons.

Maurer, F.A. (1995a). The U.S. health care system. In C.M. Smith & F.A. Maurer (Eds.), *Community health nursing: Theory and practice* (pp. 53–84). Philadelphia: W.B. Saunders.

Maurer, F.A. (1995b). Financing of health care: Context for community health nursing. In C.M. Smith & F.A. Maurer (Eds.), *Community health nursing: Theory and practice* (pp. 110–138). Philadelphia: W.B. Saunders.

McGregor, R.J. (1990). A framework for developing staff competencies. *Journal of Nursing Staff Development, 6*(2), 79–83.

McHann, M. (Ed.). (1994). *What every home health nurse needs to know.* Memphis, TN: Consultants in Care.

McMaster-Fitzig, C. (1994). Ethical issues. In M.D. Harris (Ed.), *Handbook of home health care administration* (pp. 520–531). Gaithersburg, MD: Aspen Publishers, Inc.

Milone-Nuzzo, P. (1995). Home health care. In C.M. Smith & F.A. Maurer (Eds.), *Community health nursing: Theory and practice* (pp. 776–796). Philadelphia: W.B. Saunders.

Nagelsmith, L. (1995). Competence: An evolving concept. *The Journal of Continuing Nursing Education, 26*(6), 245–247.

National Association for Home Care. (1994). *1995 blueprint for action.* Washington, DC: Author.

National Association for Home Care. (1997). NAHC publishes home care and hospice staff productivity report. *Home Care News, 12,* 14–15.

O'Grady, T., & O'Brien, A. (1992). A guide to competency-based orientation: Develop your own program. *Journal of Nursing Staff Development, 8*(3), 128–133.

Ozcan, Y.A., & Shukla, R.K. (1993). The effect of a competency-based targeted staff development program on nursing productivity. *Journal of Nursing Staff Development, 9*(2), 78–84.

Patel, K., & Rushefsky, M.E. (1995). *Health care and policy in America.* Armonk, NY: M.E. Sharpe, Inc.

Pennsylvania State Board of Nursing. (1985). *Professional nurse law and practical nurse law.* Harrisburg, PA: Commonwealth of Pennsylvania.

Reid-Webb, P. (1995). Medicare conditions of participation. In M.D. Harris (Ed.), *Handbook of home health care administration* (pp. 23–55). Gaithersburg, MD: Aspen Publishers, Inc.

Reif, L., & Martin, K.S. (1996). *Nurses and consumers: Parameters in assuring quality care in the home*. Washington, DC: American Nurses Publishing.

Revis, K.S., Thompson, C., Williams, M., Bezanson, J., & Cook, K.L. (1996). Nursing orientation: A continuous quality improvement story. *Clinical Nurse Specialist, 10*(2), 89–93.

Scrima, D. (1987). Assessing staff competency. *Journal of Nursing Administration, 17*(2), 41–45.

Smith, C.J. (1997). Home health care leadership in a changing environment. *Home Health Care Management and Practice, 9*(6), 38–44.

Snow, L., Hefty, L.V., Kenyon, V., Bell, M.L., & Martaus, T. (1992). Making the fit: Orienting new employees to community health nursing agencies. *Public Health Nursing, 9*(1), 58–64.

Sonnenfield, S., Waldo, D., & Lemieux, J. (1991). Projections of national healthcare expenditures through the year 2000. *Health Care Financing Review, 13*(1), 1–27.

Staab, S., Granneman, S., & Page-Reahr, T. (1996, May–June). Examining competency-based orientation implementation. *Journal of Nursing Staff Development*, 139–143.

Stanhope, M. (1992). Economics in health care delivery. In M. Stanhope & J. Lancaster (Eds.), *Community health nursing* (3rd ed.) (pp. 45-68). Philadelphia: Mosby.

Styles, M.M. (1996, Winter). Credentialing: Pretension and realities. American Nurses Credentialing Center, Credentialing News, 1.

Surpin, R., Haslanger, K., & Dawson, S. (1994, April). Quality paraprofessional home care. *Caring Magazine*, 12–22.

Torrens, P.R. (1993). Historical evolution and overview of health services in the United States. In S.J. Williams & P.R. Torrens (Eds.), *Introduction to health services* (4th ed.) (pp. 4–30). New York: Wiley.

Twardon, C., Gartner, M., & Cherry, C. (1993). A competency achievement orientation program: Professional development of the home health nurse. *Journal of Nursing Administration 23*(7/8), 20–25.

U.S. Department of Health and Human Services (1991). *Aging in America: Trends and projections*. Publication No. 7C OA-28001. Washington, DC: U.S. Government Printing Office.

Van Ort, S., & Woodtli, A. (1989). Home health care: Providing a missing link. *Journal of Gerontological Nursing, 15*(9), 1–9.

Walter, B.M. (1996). Home care retention: Building team spirit to avoid employee walkouts. *Home Healthcare Nurse, 14*(8), 609–612.

Wandelt, M., & Steward, D. (1975). *Slater nursing competencies rating scale*. New York: Appleton-Century Crofts.

Warhola, C. (1980). *Planning for home health services: A resource handbook*. Washington, DC: U.S. Department of Health and Human Services.

Zelman, W.A. (1996). *The changing health care marketplace. Private ventures, public interests*. San Francisco: Jossey Bass.

Zink, M.R. (1996). Home care accreditation with the community health accreditation program: Part I: An overview. *Home Healthcare Nurse, 14*(8), 590–594.

CHAPTER 2

Pre-Development Considerations

"Do what you can, with what you have, where you are."
—Theodore Roosevelt

Revising or developing a nonexistent competency program in home care can be a tremendous challenge even for the most seasoned educator. Today, the home health educator faces an era of significant cost-cutting initiatives and the burden of proof for demonstrable outcomes of learning, making program development more of a demanding endeavor. In addition, educators often lead a solitary existence in the home health care environment fulfilling the roles of program manager, educator, consultant, and clinician; and having limited to no professional and paraprofessional staff-development support.

KEY COMPONENTS

There are four key components that are instrumental in planning for the framework of a successful competency program: (1) identifying and assigning responsibility for the competency program, (2) defining and understanding the organizational structure and culture, (3) winning and maintaining organizational support, and (4) recognizing the primary administrative elements (Exhibit 2–1). Each component is equally important and should be explored comprehensively prior to competency program revision or development. A synopsis of each component will be offered in this chapter.

Assignment of Responsibility

Prior to initiating the development of a competency program, assignment of responsibility for the program must be appointed. This may sound elementary; however, if the responsibility is spread among positions that have other primary responsibilities, program development may be fragmented and the outcomes will not be in the best interest of the organization, likewise if the responsibility is given to an individual with no formal or informal education into the specialty of nursing education and staff development. Humphrey and Milone-Nuzzo (1994) state that in many organizations, orientation of new nursing staff is no one's responsibility and everyone's job. The result can be a haphazard and disorganized orientation program.

Home care organizations in this day of expanding regulatory requirements are finding staff development a necessity. As indicated by Gingerich and Ondeck (1997), for home care to remain a competitive force in the managed care setting, attention needs to be focused on the preparation levels and skills of our care providers' staff. These authors further indicate that staff development and education are primary components within the premier home health organization. Formalized staff development programs are somewhat of a new entity in home care and are typically the responsibility of a single individual who functions as the program director as well as the organizationwide educator. The specialty of staff development in the arena of home care is in greater demand due to the rapid growth of the home care industry, a significant increase in patient complexity and

Exhibit 2–1 Key Planning Components of Home Care Competency Framework

- Identifying and assigning responsibility for competency program
- Defining organizational structure and culture
- Winning and maintaining organizational support
- Reorganizing primary administrative elements

acuity, advances in technology, and compliance with regulatory requirements (Astarita, 1996).

Abruzzese (1996) stated that a graduate degree in nursing is currently necessary for educators in nursing staff development; and, as indicated by Hitchings (1996), the minimal formal educational preparation for staff development directors should be a master's degree, and the educational level of other personnel must be considered in determining reporting relationships. The executive to whom staff development reports should also hold a master's degree. Blocker (1992) surveyed 117 staff development departments of hospitals to determine the type of organizational model used. The survey also looked at other components of staff development, including educational preparation. Analysis of educational preparation found dominance of master's level preparation for staff development instructors with the percentage of diploma-only instructors or those with an associate's degree or a doctorate correspondingly low. In comparison, statistics from the National Nursing Staff Development Organization indicate that approximately 116 of its 3,000 members work in either visiting nurse associations or other types of home care setting. Of these 116, approximately 40% have a bachelor of science in nursing degree, and only 25% possess a master of science in nursing degree (R. Rupp, personal communication, April 7, 1997).

Increasingly, the importance of staff development in health care is becoming more apparent. A research study replicated by Stefanik et al.

(1994) examined various components of job satisfaction, including professional development of hospital nurses, and found that the ability of professional development opportunities is associated with nurses' job satisfaction, organizational commitment, and intent to remain. The findings of this study confirmed the findings of Kirsch (1990). Both studies support the premise that staff development is important to an organization's strategic plan, not only because of its influence on the quality of patient care but also because of its relation to work-force satisfaction and stability (Stefanik et al., 1994). It can be proposed that these findings would be similar in the home care setting; however, to date, the research-based literature is lacking in proof of such. Studies such as these need to be performed in the home care setting in order to make visible staff development's contribution to the satisfaction and stability of staff. Of interest is the lack of research-based and professional literature regarding the role of staff development in home care. The majority of the literature referencing staff development is acute care based.

Viewing the organizational table will identify if staff development has formal authority. It is essential that staff development be included on the organizational chart reporting to an executive vice-president (Avillion, 1994). This may be the vice-president of nursing, human resources, or risk management. The reasons for this are multifaceted. First, there is enormous responsibility in being accountable for the learning outcomes of all employees. Second, staff development impacts upon the working relationships, marketing endeavors, job satisfaction, and organizational commitment and retention of staff (Stefanik et al., 1994). Staff development is important to an organizational strategic plan because of its influence on the quality of patient care and its relation to work-force satisfaction and stability (Stefanik et al., 1994). Third, staff development personnel possess a great amount of informal power due to their vast experiential and knowledge base and the fact that they encompass much information about the organization, particularly the culture, beliefs, and values of staff. Fourth, a direct reporting structure to an executive demonstrates a higher value for educational activities than if placed at a lower level in the organization (Hitchings, 1996). Fifth, if the staff development leader is functioning in the role of director by managing a budget, preparing monthly reports, and is accountable for program development and outcomes, then he or she should have a direct reporting relationship to an executive. Lastly, staff development must be given a position of status in the organization in order to achieve educational goals and to carry out their role successfully (Hitchings, 1996).

Today, many home care organizations are placing staff development within the auspices of human resources, primarily because of their responsibility for all occupations, not just nursing (Figure 2–1). Inclusion of staff development within the department of human resources has many potential benefits. First, it may help facilitate consistent screening and hiring practices. Second, a close working relationship may be fostered with human resources personnel, which may help to facilitate a seamless program for orientation and competency evaluation. Third, mutual identification and planning for organizationwide education will be carried out in an orchestrated fashion. Finally, chances are that employee human resource files will be up to date with all competency-related information come survey time; however, human resources staff cannot be accountable for the clinical aspects of staff development.

As the facilitator of organizational learning, staff development should maintain primary accountability for the organization's competency program, whether in a centralized or decentralized structure and regardless of with whom he or she has a direct reporting relationship. Staff development personnel are well versed in educational theories and principles and are experts in assisting learners to translate knowledge, principles, skills, and theories into the practice of health care (Avillion & Abruzzese, 1992).

Organizational Structure

Viewing an organizational table can provide much insight into the status and power of individuals and departments. Organizational structure functionally dictates how interaction occurs among individuals and departments. If rigid in structure, the organization can function as a barrier to responsiveness and collaboration (Gundlach, 1994). In addition, the organization's mission and scope of services may also influence the structure. All organizations have both a formal and informal structure. Formal structures are the planned, official arrangement of occupations, whereas informal structures bear a clandestine character with all personnel having their own assumptions and opinions about the hierarchy. Culture, the usual behavior of a group, is unique in every health care organization. Culture is developed from the beliefs and values of the organization and ultimately impacts upon the perceptions and behavior of staff. Myths, rituals, ceremonies, stories, and metaphors, all part of an organization's culture, both promote understanding of organizational life and help people cope with organizational conflicts (del Bueno & Vincent, 1986).

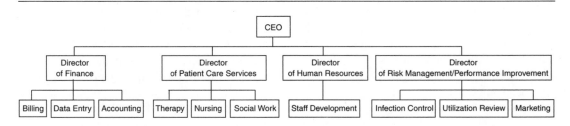

Figure 2–1 Home Care Organizational Chart

The types of organizational structures are varied ranging from line, line and staff, functionalized, and matrix, to arrangements that are customized to meet the specific mission of the organization. As indicated by Gundlach (1994), organizations are fast learning that it is commonly their structural rigidity that has institutionalized their barrier to collaboration, learning, and responsiveness rather than personalities or the infamous enemy, limited resources. In home care, the organizational arrangement is dictated by its size, service provision, mission, and alliances. Home care traditionally embraced a centralized line structure, but today, due to its growth, expanded scope of service delivery, and integration with the private sector and primary care facilities, it has had to move to a more flexible decentralized structure allowing staff to have more authority. This has occurred in part due to the increase in expert job knowledge, skill, and autonomy of the clinical staff. Decentralized structures in home care are proving to be essential, particularly in regard to affecting organizational learning processes and flexibility. Gundlach (1994) summarized this point well by stating that "hierarchical systems that rank instead of link people do not lend themselves to the collaboration essential in our increasingly team-oriented, service-conscious organizations."

It cannot be stressed enough how important it is to thoroughly investigate the formal and informal structures as well as the culture of the organization prior to developing a competency program. The program should be customized based upon the established norms of the organization. In addition, it is crucial to identify if the organization is change focused or if it is more conservative and finite. Avillion (1994) indicates that health care organizations should be viewed as political systems; and, in order to gain insight into the internal workings, one should concentrate on the interdependence of the interests, conflicts, and power among individuals within the organization. Gaining insight into the internal workings of a home care organization is necessary to establish a reality-based competency program.

Organizational Support

The most fundamental component of competency program development is winning support from key administrative personnel. Because of staff development's newness in home care, it can often be a forgotten appendage on the organizational chart. It may often appear to staff development personnel that they need to continually strive to be recognized for their contributions to the organization. In addition, it may become apparent that administrative staff may not understand the role functions of staff development, including what is and is not appropriate utilization of their services. Avillion (1994) indicates that staff development should be visible, viable, and valid and in doing so will demonstrate that they are critical to organizational survival. Staff development also needs to build support within the administration by understanding the management perspective and setting mutual goals (Sheridan, Abruzzese, O'Grady, & Green-Hernandez, 1996).

The successfulness of a home care competency program lies not only with staff development but with all employees of the organization. At various points in time, all staff will have some degree of contact with the competency program, whether directly experiencing having their competency assessed or assisting to assess the competency of others in their role. In doing so, they will develop impressions and assumptions about competency assessment. It is, therefore, important to make a positive impression on all employees surrounding the program. Of critical importance is having the belief and support from the organization's administrative staff. It is essential that key administrative personnel be included from the beginning in all phases of competency program development. One way to immediately foster inclusion is by submitting a proposal demonstrating that the competency program is in line with the organizational goals and objectives. Secondly, the proposal should include the indications for and the tangible outcomes of a successful competency program; and lastly, management personnel should be included in the ongoing decision making and evaluative processes of the program.

Managers can be included directly with competency assessment in their areas of expertise. Some managers may see this as additional work; however, the benefits of participation far outweigh the small amount of time investment. A few possible benefits to participation include being able to identify first hand the competency level of their staff, the admiration and respect staff gain after seeing their manager demonstrate clinical expertise in a certain area, increased staff approval of and respect for the competency program after seeing their manager participate, and managers knowing that their staff have been competency assessed and that they are in compliance with organizational and regulatory requirements.

How does one maintain ongoing support for the competency program? The answers to this will become apparent after program implementation. In most cases, staff will begin to look forward to competency evaluation because it is a time of validation and learning for them. Managers will have identified additional information about their staff, which will assist them in helping to further develop staff or, in some rare instances, sever relationships with staff. In addition, both staff and managers should see improvement in patient care delivery and outcomes, and senior administrative staff will certainly find confidence in the program during survey time when no recommendations are cited regarding the competency of staff. Winning organizational support can be a time consuming and arduous process; however, with good planning and persistence, support will become apparent, and maintaining support will be even simpler.

Administrative Aspects

Organizational strategic plan, curriculum planning, fiscal resources, marketing, and evaluative mechanisms are the administrative aspects requiring pre-development consideration (Exhibit 2–2). The administrative aspects as a whole

Exhibit 2–2 Primary Administrative Elements

• Organizational strategic plan • Curriculum planning • Fiscal resources • Marketing • Evaluative mechanisms

function as an empowering tool for staff development in competency program development.

Strategic Planning

Awareness of the organization's strategic plan is of primary importance. The goals and priorities of the organization are the driving force behind all administrative aspects. Abruzzese (1996) relates that staff development should not be left out of major decisions because it is a major facilitator of change within an organization and that input from the staff development department is critical for any new program or major change. He also indicates that staff development should not be notified after a new program is initiated or a major change has occurred. Strategic planning is important to organizational survival in times of turbulent changes and to day-to-day functioning at a status quo level. Strategic planning is just as essential to a staff development department and should be developed based upon the beliefs, mission, and goals of the organization and the vision of both.

Curriculum Planning

Abruzzese (1996) indicates that curriculum planning helps staff development to focus programs and courses on the organization's mission and goals. Bevis (1982) describes steps to curriculum development. These steps include (1) reviewing the organization's mission and goals; (2) developing a philosophy and conceptual framework; (3) developing curriculum purpose, objectives, and strands; (4) organizing the department's programs, courses, and classes; and (5) developing the program content. Curriculum planning should be based on the learner's needs and on adult learning principles and is the most important pre-development consideration. The importance of curriculum development is summed up best by Abruzzese (1996), "A well-planned and well-organized curriculum focuses on the product, that is, on well-developed nurses. The curriculum should be integrated, comprehensive, continuous and potent so that it can become the blueprint that will encourage innovation, productivity, retention and ultimately patient care at a high-quality level" (p. 221). For more information, refer to Chapter 5 on the educational process.

Fiscal Resources

The second pre-development consideration is being able to develop a budget that is in line with organizational objectives. Collection of data to support the proposed operational and capital budget is needed. The projected costs associated with all elements of the competency program will be required (Exhibit 2–3). The more data one can show to support a cost-benefit position the better. Having an understanding of basic budgetary concepts is necessary and should be explored prior to budget development. Documentation of the cost-effectiveness in order to justify the competency program is imperative. No matter how experienced one is, the development of a budget based upon available fiscal resources and projected expenses is always a challenging undertaking.

Marketing

Identification of how the new or revised competency program will be marketed both internally and externally is the third pre-development consideration. Once again, efforts should be directed toward the organization's mission and goals. Recognition of who will be the customers of the competency program is needed if successful marketing endeavors are to be undertaken. Potential customers include all employees of the organization, employees of other organizations, other staff development departments, accreditation bodies, payers, and, potentially, students. Marketing starts with establishing and maintain-

Exhibit 2–3 Competency Program Cost Components

- Labor—educator, honorarium, secretary
- Supplies—markers, tape, food, copying, tri-fold boards, etc.
- AV equipment
- Documentation software
- Learner salaries
- Rental fees—medical, room, tables
- Maintenance/Housekeeping

ing good relationships with customers. Marketing efforts from this point on are dependent upon the quality of the program and its outcomes. Pre-development phase marketing efforts should be directed toward middle and senior management (the individuals who encompass the majority of the power within the organization) and, secondly, the employees who will have primary contact with the program.

Evaluation

Identification of a program evaluation mechanism is the final pre-development consideration. There are many evaluation methods to choose from. The most commonly utilized in staff development are criterion-referenced methods, whereby everyone must meet the same level of achievement or competency. Developing an evaluative mechanism prior to program implementation is the primary focus (see Exhibit 2–4 for an example). Evaluation should be conducted after each competency endeavor, and data should be collected in order for comparisons and changes to be made through the department's performance improvement/management program (formerly referred to as quality assurance or quality improvement).

Revising or developing a competency program can be made less challenging if there is planned inquiry into the four key components. Thorough identification and exploration of the key components will allow the educator to construct a sound framework for competency program development.

Exhibit 2–4 Competency Program Evaluation Tool

Indicator	Retrieval Source	Indicator Met/Not Met	Comments
Evaluator:_____ Date:_____ Key:+ Met –Not Met			
1. Adult learning principles are utilized			
2. Educators facilitate the process for learners to assume responsibility for self-learning and the maintenance of competence			
3. Learning resources are appropriate to the performance indicator			
4. Performance indicators match the competency statement			
5. Varied learning resources are utilized			
6. Learning is evaluated through a variety of methods			
7. Educators consult with administration on an ongoing basis in regard to the competency program			
8. Learning resources reflect the identified needs of the learners and relate to discipline-specific practice			
9. Orientation plan is based upon the components of employee self-assessment			
10. Plan for ongoing competency assessment is evident			
11. Policies exist to support the functioning of the competency program			
12. Competency program is based upon the philosophy and mission of the organization			
13. Periodic needs assessments are implemented and utilized in competency program revision			
14. Initial competency assessment is completed by the conclusion of the orientation process			
15. A report of the levels of competency is provided to administration at predetermined intervals			
16. Competency records are confidential and are available only to authorized individuals			
17. Competency is documented and records are maintained in compliance with the organizational requirements			
18. Mechanisms are in place that allow for systematic and easy retrieval of data on competency activities and participants			
19. An annual competency plan for the organization exists			

continues

Exhibit 2–4 continued

Indicator	Retrieval Source	Indicator Met/Not Met	Comments
20. Competency evaluations are completed by participants			
21. Results of evaluations, and industry and organization-specific trends, are incorporated into the competency program			
Percent Compliance _____			
Performance Improvement Plan:			

Source: Portions of this exhibit are data from *Standards for Nursing Professional Development: Continuing Education and Staff Development,* © 1994, American Nurses Association.

REFERENCES

Abruzzese, R.S. (1996). Counterpoint: Against certification of staff development educators. *Journal of Nursing Staff Development, 2*(1), 9.

Astarita, T.M. (1996). Competency-based orientation in home health care: One agency's approach. *Home Health Care Management and Practice, 8*(4), 38–49.

Avillion, A. (1994). Political savvy in staff development: Building an indispensable department. *Journal of Continuing Education in Nursing, 25*(4), 152–154.

Avillion, A., & Abruzzese, R.S. (1992). Conceptual foundations of nursing staff development. In R.S. Abruzzese (Ed.), *Nursing staff development: Strategies for success* (2nd ed.) (pp. 30–43). St. Louis, MO: Mosby-Year Book, Inc.

Bevis, E.O. (1982). *Curriculum building in nursing: A process* (3rd ed.). St. Louis, MO: Mosby-Year Book, Inc..

Blocker, V.T. (1992). Organizational models and staff preparation: A survey of staff development departments. *Journal of Continuing Education in Nursing, 23*(6), 259–262.

del Bueno, D.J., & Vincent, P.M. (1986). Organizational culture: How important is it? *Journal of Nursing Administration, 16*(10), 15–20.

Gingerich, B.S., & Ondeck, D.A. (1997). From our vantage point. *Home Health Digest, 3*(4), 4–5.

Gundlach, A.M. (1994). Adapting to change: Reconsidering staff development organization, design and purpose. *Journal of Continuing Education in Nursing, 25*(3), 120–122.

Hitchings, K.S. (1996). Organization of staff development activities. In R.S. Abruzzese (Ed.), *Nursing staff development: Strategies for success* (2nd ed.) (pp. 83–108). St. Louis, MO: Mosby-Year Book, Inc.

Humphrey, C.J., & Milone-Nuzzo, P. (1994). Home care nursing orientation model: Justification and structure. *Home Healthcare Nurse, 10*(3), 18–25.

Kirsch, J.C. (1990). Staff development opportunity and nurse job satisfaction, organizational commitment and intent to remain in the organization: Implications for staff development. *Journal of Nursing Staff Development, 6*(6), 279–282.

Sheridan, D.R., Abruzzese, R.S., O'Grady, T., & Green-Hernandez, C. (1996). In R.S. Abruzzese (Ed.), *Nursing staff development: Strategies for success* (2nd ed.) (pp. 16–29). St. Louis, MO: Mosby-Year Book, Inc.

Stefanik, R.L., Cassandra, K., Edwards-Beckett, J., Gresham-Copeland, S.G., Hoffman, C.M., Hulls, P., Freese, L., Opperman, C., & Timmerman, R. (1994). Perceptions of nursing staff development: A replication study. *Journal of Nursing Staff Development, 10*(3), 115–119.

CHAPTER 3

The Role of Staff Development

"He who learns but does not think is lost. He who thinks and does not learn is in grave danger."
—Confucius

The staff development educator's role in the past has often been one-dimensional and relegated to the periphery of a health care organization's activities. Many home care organizations did not have a position dedicated to education until recently. This condition is illustrated by a recent 1996 survey conducted by the National Nursing Staff Development Organization (NNSDO) on the attributes of staff development educators, such as educational background and area of employment. All of the staff development personnel used in the study were from a type of health care facility specializing in acute care, rehabilitation, long-term care, etc. No educators in the home health care arena were surveyed or mentioned in the study (NNSDO, 1996). Education activities in settings without staff development positions commonly designate to nursing managers and administrators the bulk of the responsibility for orienting and educating their staffs while hiring specialists, vendors, and outside educators to assist with some education duties. However, in today's chaotic health care environment, a specialized staff development position is needed to provide education more effectively and efficiently. The staff development role in home care is evolving as a vital strategy that assists an organization to meet the competency needs of staff and to improve organizational performance through its coordination, consultation, and collaboration activities. This enables a home care organization to more easily meet the demands of consumers and regu-

latory and accrediting bodies. Thus, educators can be an integral part in reaching an organization's mission and goals.

Staff development educators may be seen as partially responsible for nurse recruitment and retention, the professional growth of staff, attainment of excellence in clinical practice and the achievement of positive patient outcomes. These achievements are necessary to assist an organization to deliver a quality product and meet budgetary constraints. An efficient, effective, and widely involved staff development department is an integral component of a home care's success. Experts in the staff development field believe that staff development directors should hold a position that is equal to other nurse administrators on the organizational chart (Sheridan & O'Grady, 1996). This allows staff development to participate fully in organizational decision making and allows a proactive approach in educational planning. A management position allows access to persons and information that is vital to maintain an educational department that helps coordinate with other departments and meets agency goals.

The roles and functions of staff development educators extend beyond those of educator. There are a variety of roles inherent in the nursing staff development educator role, especially for those holding management positions in a staff development department. Staff development educators must be able to perform management, budgetary, research, and consultant functions. The scope of activities involved in performing these roles varies greatly depending on the philosophy, mission, and goals of the employing health care organization. Duties and responsibilities will also vary depending on the size of the organization and the number and types of personnel to be educated. Educators working in a decentralized setting will experience a different set of advantages and disadvantages than those working in a centralized educator department (Hitchings, 1996).

The current efforts in health care to contain costs by downsizing, cross training, and expanding employees' job descriptions have also expanded staff development's roles and functions. Staff development educators must be ready to assume responsibilities for a wide variety of activities involving other departments in the home care organization, such as quality assurance and risk management. Educators once dedicated to the learning activities of nursing personnel may now find themselves involved in a range of education activities for non-nursing staff. These staff may consist of non-nursing professionals, paraprofessionals, and semiskilled employees or volunteers. In addition, the dramatic shift of employees into the home care arena and the rapid advances in technology have also increased the depth and scope of employees' learning needs.

Despite all of these changes, the primary focus of staff development remains on meeting the educational needs of the nursing staff because of their influence and importance in the delivery of care in the home setting. Nursing administration may define the role of staff development as integral and central to the organization's mission of providing quality care, or it may restrict staff development to a few educational functions, such as orientation and inservices. Hence, a staff development educator's functions are also determined by the nursing department's philosophy and goals.

The American Nurses Association (ANA) and the American Society for Healthcare Education and Training (ASHET) have analyzed the activities and functions of staff development personnel. These professional organizations have compiled lists of the predominant job responsibilities appropriate to staff development positions. These organizations group these responsibilities into categories that are similar based on the areas of activities in which educators are frequently involved (Rodriguez & Abruzzese, 1996).

In the ANA's (1994a) guidelines for nursing staff development, the roles and functions of staff development can be grouped into management and administrative; developing and using a budget; assessing learning needs; planning and implementing learning activities; evaluating outcomes; recordkeeping; marketing; research; counseling individual learners; and participating in self-education.

In addition to the above activities, staff development educators may be involved in developing nursing policy and procedure; developing and participating in quality-improvement activities; consulting within and outside of the organization; acting as change agents; investigating new products and procedures; acting as a liaison to nursing schools and other professional schools and their students; community education; and participating on various professional committees and task forces that represent nursing or the health care organization (Rodriguez & Abruzzese, 1996).

The focus of the staff development department and the roles it assumes are also determined by the priorities set by the educator. Professional interests and strengths of the individual influence the roles and activities that the educator assumes. It is impossible to find one person who can fulfill all of the roles discussed previously. The staff development educator must be able to honestly analyze his or her strengths and weaknesses. Activities in areas of weakness can then be delegated to others in the staff development department or to others inside the agency. Expert help may also be obtained from outside sources. Using other experts assists the educator to increase his or her exposure to new knowledge, which adds to his or her own expertise. By utilizing other sources of learning, the educator can then better utilize his or her talents and interests to operate the staff development department efficiently, creatively, and productively.

Staff development departments may also develop their roles and responsibilities by consulting with their consumers, those who utilize the services of staff development (Rodriguez & Abruzzese, 1996). The chief consumers of these services in the home health care setting are nurses and nurse managers. Other customers may be the managers and their employees from other patient care professionals and paraprofessional departments. Home care aides, nutritionists, social workers, and respiratory, physical, and occupational therapists are examples of workers who frequently require the services of staff development educators. Administrators, human resource personnel, and clerical and support staff may also rely on staff development for various services. Collecting input from these persons about what they want and need from staff development can help define and clarify the roles staff development should assume. Gathering this input can contribute to open lines of communication, enhancing collegiality and organizational function.

QUALIFICATIONS AND EDUCATIONAL BACKGROUND

The ideal educational background should be that of the graduate level for staff development educators. This allows the person to be more fully prepared for this highly skilled, multifaceted job. Educators need expertise in clinical nursing issues, education theory, working with groups, and problem solving. The director of a department particularly requires an educational background in these areas that has included leadership theory, management, budgeting, consulting, and research. A bachelor of science in nursing (BSN) degree is preferred by most experts as the entry point for any nurse into the staff educator role. Some baccalaureate nurses may also obtain a minor in education to allow them to pursue a staff education career (Case, 1995; Rodriguez & Abruzzese, 1996).

A staff development educator with a graduate degree in nursing holds many advantages for the employing agency. A qualified, well-prepared educator is necessary to effectively carry out the roles of educator, manager, consultant, and researcher. A competent staff development educator will increase staff productivity and help the organization run more smoothly and efficiently. A master's degree in nursing gives the broad educational background necessary to fulfill this role. In addition, clinical nurse specialists (CNSs) are trained and skilled in clinical areas that are of a particular advantage to many home care education positions. CNSs are also educationally prepared in the practice and theory of teaching-learning, leadership, budgeting, group dynamics, communication, consulting, research, management, quality improvement, and ethics. This background is considered especially helpful to carry out the responsibilities of this position successfully.

Credentialing in staff development education is also a helpful qualification. This ensures an experience and knowledge base in clinical education and adult learning. The American Nurses Credentialing Center (ANCC) has established a program for certification in the field of staff development. Nurses must have a BSN or higher and have practiced a minimum of 4,000 hours in staff development to qualify to sit for the certification exam. In October 1996, 108 staff development educators sat for the certification exam, with 88 persons passing (ANCC, 1996–1997). The NNSDO is a voluntary professional entity designed to assist and promote the role of nursing educator. The NNSDO's *Journal of Nursing Staff Development* is specifically designed to increase the knowledge and professionalism of nursing educators.

Ideally, the staff development educator should possess a set of personal qualities that will enhance job function. These include, but are not limited to, adaptability, good communication skills, problem-solving skills, leadership skills, excellent interpersonal skills, professional enthusiasm, and ability to work autonomously. In addition, the educator should have high professional and personal standards in order to act as a role model for the staff. It is difficult, if not impossible, to find one person with all of these attributes. It is also necessary for educators to be able to self-evaluate clearly and know when to seek outside help and resources to assist them in filling these many roles and attributes.

Educator Competence

The picture of the staff development educator that has evolved in the preceding pages is a complex, multifaceted, and dynamic job description. Many staff development personnel, as noted earlier, are often expert clinical nurses with little or no background in education (NNSDO, 1996). The competence of educators is a genuine concern for home care administrators. Much research and literature have been devoted to the assessment, training, and evaluation of the competency of teachers in academic settings. Very little of this knowledge has been applied to the educators in health care institutions (Lane, 1996). Little formal training occurs for many educators in the home care setting beyond orientation due to the lack of acknowledgment of a learning need by nursing departments and administrators and the solitary structure of staff development departments.

Standards of competency for educators should be developed for the same reasons they are needed for other staff positions. Performance standards can be used to guide the orientation process, assist the planning of educational goals, and help measure the success of the educational outcomes for the orientee to the educator role (Fitzsimmons, Piercy, Noel, & Connolly, 1996). The standards found in the ANA Standards for Nursing Professional Development (ANA, 1994a) may be used as a framework for the development of educator competencies in a home care agency. The agency may group activities unique to its institution under the various roles delineated by the ANA, such as educator, manager, researcher, consultant. Additional categories that may be pertinent to home care may be leadership, resource development, and commu-

nity education; and professional development may be useful (Fitzsimmons et al., 1996). Criteria may be gleaned from Joint Commission standards, Community Health Accreditation Program (CHAP) standards, and the Medicare Conditions of Participation (COP) to develop competencies. The NNSDO has published several guides and lists of standards for professional nurses working in staff development (1996).

Several models may be applied when developing, implementing, and evaluating educator competencies. Benner (1984) identifies five levels of professional nursing practice that range on a continuum from novice to expert. The attributes exhibited at each level, such as decision-making ability, independence, intuitive abilities, and synthesis of knowledge, vary with the amount of experience and learning. Many other models of educator learning and practice exist in the literature and may be applied to the health care educator. For example, the Ohio Department of Education developed an educator model based on a continuum of adult professional development involving ego, cognitive, conceptual, and level of commitment development. Lane (1996) uses a conceptual model based on the work of Killion to devise three levels of instructor development: novice, intermediate, and expert. This model describes the strengths and weaknesses of each level and may be used as a guide to address weaknesses and utilize strengths. The models may also be used to design appropriate competencies and evaluations for staff.

As can easily be seen from these models, it is of benefit for staff development personnel to work with other educators. A staff development department consisting of several persons can give opportunity for preceptoring, mentoring, and supporting the newer members in the field. However, staff development personnel are often a one-person operation in many home care agencies. These educators must facilitate their professional growth with involvement in professional organizations and participation in task forces and committees outside the organization. This exposes the beginner to experts in the field who can act as mentors and advisors. Access to these persons is becoming more feasible as home care agencies affiliate with other institutions and participate in health care networks.

THE EDUCATOR ROLE

Meeting the educational needs of the nursing staff continues to remain the primary role of staff development personnel. This educational focus applies to nurse managers, registered nurse (RN) clinical staff and case managers, licensed practical nurses (LPNs), and home care aides (HCAs). Educators are also increasingly called upon to assist with the educational needs of non-nursing staff, such as other patient care professionals and clerical staff. Educational activities may include, but are not limited to, orientation activities; continuing education for contact hours; product-focused inservices; specialty-specific inservices, such as intravenous or psychiatric teams; teaching cardiopulmonary resuscitation; mandatory requirements such as the Joint Commission fire and safety or Occupational Safety and Health Administration (OSHA) material safety data; preceptor training; leadership training; cultural and gender sensitivity training; patient educator training or material development; and clerical support training (Blocker, 1992). Orientation, continuing education, skills lab training, and inservice education may also be directed toward part-time, per diem, and contract/registry personnel as they continue to become a larger part of the health care team (Shaffer & Kobs, 1997). It is imperative that the educator act as a facilitator in learning and attempt to impart in the learners a sense of responsibility for their own learning. These educational programs are intended to improve the performance of patient caregivers and assist them to attain goals of competency and excellence in practice. Thus, the educator has a direct impact on the quality of patient care and attainment of the organization's mission and goals (Rodriguez & Abruzzese, 1996). The educator's duties are directly impacted by the organizational structure of the staff development department. A central-

ized structure containing a department manager and a staff of educators can allow for a division of duties among members. The opportunity for more collegial interaction occurs, encouraging brainstorming, problem solving, and collaboration. Persons can concentrate on their areas of expertise. The roles of mentoring and leadership are important daily functions of the more experienced members. However, a decentralized structure often allows for a quicker recognition of learning needs and a faster response to those needs. A decentralized structure may be able to be more flexible to learners' schedules and individual needs. In addition, a decentralized structure often allows more interaction between educators and learners, facilitating the evaluation of learning outcomes (Case, 1995).

Staff development personnel in the home care setting frequently find themselves in a combined setting in which the structure of the staff development department contains elements of both structures. A department usually has primary responsibility for meeting the educational needs of the nursing staff, which may include several specialty teams such as maternal-child health (MCH), psychiatric, cardiac, and intravenous. In addition, educators may be responsible for the learning needs of other professionals, such as physical therapists, or they may share responsibilities with that department's manager. As home care organizations continue to cut costs by combining job titles and positions, it will become more common for the staff development educator to acquire increased responsibilities for areas outside of nursing and combine efforts with others in the organization.

The Educational Foundation

To carry out this educator role effectively, the staff development educator needs a solid working knowledge of teaching–learning theory. The process of teaching and learning is represented by various models that often reflect the steps of the nursing process (Buchanan & Glanville, 1988). The components of teaching are assessing and diagnosing learning needs; planning appropriate educational interventions; implementing teaching–learning activities; and evaluating the educational outcomes of the intervention. These steps represent the major decision-making points the educator must perform in this process. These steps may be carried out informally and quickly, as in the case of a brief question-answer session with a nurse requiring immediate feedback about a patient care problem. Or the educational process may be a large, formal series of scheduled activities over many months. The staff development educator must be able to reach these education goals of maintaining and improving staff performance in a timely and cost-effective manner. An education program is more effectively carried out if the educator has a broad background knowledge of assessment strategies, learning theory, teaching strategies, and evaluative mechanisms. This knowledge base helps identify learning needs, plan and carry out teaching interventions, and evaluate learning results. A learning need may be defined as a discrepancy between learner performance or knowledge and a desired level of performance or knowledge (Yoder Wise, 1996; Buchanan & Glanville, 1988). It is imperative that the educator keep abreast of current professional, regulatory, and accreditation standards as a measure of desired performance. Further assessment of learner needs may be accomplished by various methods in the home care setting. Surveys, interviews, the Delphi technique, focus groups, observation of performance, and needs suggested from incident reports are just a few of the effective methods available for data gathering. The most effective and efficient method for a needs assessment varies among home care settings and types of learners. The financial resources, time constraints, and personnel available must all be considered when determining the method(s) of data collection.

A learning diagnosis is formulated from the needs indicated from the assessment data. A learning diagnosis defines objective, measurable goals that the learner should reach after the teaching intervention. A staff development educator needs a good working knowledge of the current professional, legal, ethical, and accrediting body standards to formulate appropriate educational goals. Knowledge of current developments in medicine, nursing, and patient care standards is an important guide in planning educational programs and objectives. The educator must also be knowledgeable about current economic, political, and social trends that affect home care practice. They must also be aware of the home care organization's short- and long-term goals in order to set realistic learning goals and objectives. This helps ensure that the educational objectives are in line with the administration's goals and budget. All of these areas of information may be gleaned from current professional literature and participating in professional and organizational committees and activities

To determine appropriate teaching–learning interventions, the educator should utilize the concepts of classic cognitive, behavioral, and humanist learning theories. To behaviorists such as Skinner and Thorndike, learning is a conditioned response to a stimuli that is easily observed and measured. Cognitive theorists, such as Piaget and Gestalt, see learning as a more complex process that depends on the developmental stages of the learners and their interpretation of events. The humanistic view of learning described by theorists like Carl Rodgers and Abraham Maslow sees learning as an even more comprehensive process involving the biological, cognitive, emotional, and spiritual aspects of the person that cannot be fully measured (Lancaster, 1992). Knowledge of these theories is an essential base in developing learning strategies.

Concepts from these classic learning theories provide a necessary background to understanding the cognitive, affective, and psychomotor domains of learning. An in-depth knowledge of these categories of learning is essential in developing learning objectives and appropriate teaching-learning interventions for health care professionals. For example, a learning deficit may be addressed through self-study or lecture, while a psychomotor deficit requires actual practice in a lab situation.

In addition to these general theories of learning, a staff development educator needs a solid working knowledge of adult learning theories, such as those of Malcolm Knowles, because of the adult target population of the staff development educator. An educator can use these theoretical concepts to plan effective learning strategies for staff and patients that utilize the strengths of the learners and get them actively involved in their own learning process (Knowles, 1980). These teaching–learning processes and theories may be applied to educational programs for new orientees, in-service education, continuing education, annual competency training, and remedial training for professional, paraprofessional, and support staff. This knowledge base acts as a framework upon which to build educational programs that produce positive results for the staff and improve the quality of patient care. This framework also enables the educator to use the resources of employees, time, and materials in a cost-efficient manner.

Roles in Patient Education

The staff development educator also has a vital role in assisting the nurses to become competent patient educators. A vital component of home health care is the education of the client and his or her family to promote wellness and independence. These are the primary and ultimate goals of home health care (Lancaster, 1992). Reaching these goals has become more difficult due to cost-cutting measures that now limit the number and length of nursing visits per patient. Nurses need to teach informally and formally as a part of every home visit. Although teaching is expected of every home care nurse, many are not adequately educated or trained in this role. The inclusion of teaching–learning theory is often limited in basic RN education programs. Few nurses, especially those in acute care settings, have a practical background in patient teaching that is adequate to meet the demands found in home care. Nurses need to be able to assess their clients' learning needs, their level of understanding and literacy, along with

their motivation and ability to learn. A working knowledge of teaching strategies and evaluation of learning outcomes is needed by these visit nurses. Staff development educators can have a positive effect on patient education by educating the visit staff in these processes. Educators may also assist patient education by assisting with the development of patient teaching tools and care pathways, which may be used to guide patient care education.

Role as Change Agent

The educator role ideally integrates the goals of the organization and the needs of the employees into a proactive plan to improve staff performance, the quality of patient care, and organizational performance. Staff development personnel often find themselves responsible for the organization and oversight of educational programs for the entire organization in the home care setting. This requires the educator to revise and develop new policies and procedures that deal directly and indirectly with the education process. This places the staff development educator into the role of change agent. In this role, the educator also initiates change through the development and implementation of new curricula and training programs (Alspach, 1996; Case, 1995).

Change is a constant companion of anyone currently involved in the health care field. Change, according to Lewin (1951), is a three-step process of unfreezing, moving, and refreezing. During the unfreezing stage, the need to change is perceived. The stimulus to change may come from outside the agency, such as Joint Commission regulations or Medicare COP. Or the need to change may become evident from internal events and influences as risk management information indicating areas of poor staff performance. There are restraining forces that impede change, such as conservative attitudes and authoritarian rule. Driving forces, such as a desire to compete for status or for financial gain, can facilitate change (Gillies, 1982). This is a time of increasing tension in the organization as the equilibrium is disturbed. The staff development personnel can facilitate this stage by assisting in a needs assessment and developing a plan of action.

During the moving stage, new methods are tried and tested. The second stage of moving or implementing the change in a home care organization is often assisted to some degree by staff development. Educators can give the staff the information they need to understand the necessary changes and assist in any training needed. Staff development may also assist change by giving emotional support to the staff at this time of increased risk and anxiety. This will help move the staff toward the third and final stage of change. In this stage of refreezing, the change is accepted and becomes part of the status quo. An understanding of change theory will assist the staff development educator to prepare and implement the inevitable changes that will occur.

The staff development educator must work within the bounds of the organization's philosophy and goals to create change. Ideally, educational goals for the staff will be determined with the input and support of the management and administration. This is most easily accomplished if the educator's position in the organizational structure allows his or her regular interaction with department managers and administrative personnel. Access to administrative goals, managerial problems, and solutions will enable the educator to develop and operate an educational program that meets the needs of the staff and the organization. Excellent interpersonal and communication skills are required on the part of the educator to assist in building good working relationships with these personnel who have the power to assist or hinder the educational program.

The educational program should also be built with input from the staff. Information gained from a needs assessment is, of course, necessary to formulate a plan. However, the staff development educator may also use input gained from staff in daily interactions with them. The educator has a unique position in the home care organization, often acting as a bridge or liaison between the worlds of staff and administration. Contact and interaction occur between the educator when he or she attends departmental or team meetings, serves on various committees or task forces, and acts as an advisor or problem solver for individual staff. If the educator has developed trust and respect in her or his professional role, the staff will utilize the educator as a resource for advice and problem solving. The information gained from these encounters can help signal problems or potential problems that need educational attention. Using staff input empowers them, increasing professional and employment satisfaction.

Desirable Attributes in an Educator

Effective communication skills are paramount in all aspects of the educator's role. These skills are vital for productive teaching and lecturing to a wide variety of audiences present in the home health care organization. Audiences vary in size, education, profession, and experience. A properly prepared educator is cognizant of group differences and individual learning needs. A working knowledge of group dynamics and the interpersonal skills to utilize these concepts will enhance the educator's effectiveness. From a practical standpoint, the educator needs solid computer skills to function adequately. Word processing skills are needed to compose course content, reports, and schedules. Computer skills are needed to assist with the staff development department's schedule of offerings and activities. Further computer knowledge and skills are needed to choose and help maintain recordkeeping programs that record staff attendance of educational programs. Various regulatory and accrediting bodies require that home care organizations have current data available on individuals' continuing education status. This is to ensure that employees have completed all necessary continuing educational requirements. Current software programs available document summaries of educational attendance and accomplishments for individuals and track trends in learning and attendance for groups such as nurse aide compliance with Medicare standards.

THE ADMINISTRATIVE AND MANAGERIAL ROLE

The job of a staff development educator includes various inherent managerial roles. This is recognized by the ANA (1994a), which has written an administrative section in its standards for staff development educators. The director of a staff development department has more administrative responsibilities than the rest of the educators. But all educators have certain duties and tasks that require management expertise. The job description of the director of the staff development department should clearly delineate the expected responsibilities, authority level, and administrative duties. This person is usually responsible for many duties, some of which are listed in Exhibit 3–1.

Another category of administrative responsibilities is functions of resource management. These resources include people, money, and materials. Administrators must concentrate their efforts on the department's most valuable resource: the staff educators. Many activities revolve around enhancing departmental communication, collegiality, productivity, and efficiency. The director may need to organize and schedule staffing of the education department and participate in peer reviews and evaluations of staff development personnel. Planning, developing, and organizing orientation and continuing education activities that are compatible with the organization's mission and keep the staff prepared proactively are a necessary function. Planning, organizing, and directing staff meetings on a regular formal and informal basis build departmental strength. In addition, the director must participate at the administrative level in organizational task forces, committees, and projects to facilitate planning of the education programs and enhance organizationwide cooperation and professional collaboration. Scheduling and delegating educational activities may be done to utilize individual strengths and encourage mentoring and professional growth (Rodriguez & Abruzzese, 1996; Case, 1995).

In addition, supervising clerical and secretarial support staff is required of those staff development educators benefitted by such a valuable resource. The educator may need to assist in orienting and training clerical staff who are new to the organization or to staff development functions. The educator may need to instruct support staff about specialized staff development programs, such as recordkeeping systems to track class attendance, the scheduling of educational programs, the oversight of library use, etc. Staff development departments frequently share clerical staff with other managers and departments. These busy individuals who are not solely devoted to staff development may need supervision from the educator to prioritize daily or weekly tasks.

The director of the staff development department is responsible for developing a budget within organization guidelines. He or she is accountable for managing the budget and meeting departmental goals within its fiscal resources. The education department is not a revenue-generating source for the organization. Persons and material resources utilized from the staff development budget should be used judiciously. The "nonproductive" hours visit staff spend in class rather than generating organizational income should be tracked and judged in light of overall agency benefit. The staff development administrator can choose from various cost-accounting models to track costs and revenues. The use of cost-effectiveness or cost-benefit analysis to document positive outcomes to the organization is increasingly required in these days of cost containment. It is often difficult, if not impossible, to compare the cost of an education program to the revenues it generates. Many of the benefits of an education program are intangible and measured in terms of value and quality. However, after the initiation of a new curriculum, such as one based on competency, differences may be measured in terms of staff retention, staff productivity and efficiency, and

Exhibit 3–1 Duties of the Director of Staff Development

- Designing a departmental philosophy and goals that are compatible with the organization's mission and philosophy.
- Formulating the department's strategic educational plan that contains measurable goals. Documenting these goals and their review and annual revision.
- Developing all educational policies and procedures. Documenting an annual review of the policies and procedures and their revision.
- Developing an orientation and continuing education program for the educators. These must be based on current regulatory, accrediting, and professional standards.
- Developing the job description requirements for staff educators. Assisting with the hiring and interview process.
- Developing a system for evaluation and review of staff-educator performance.
- Participating in administrative-level task forces, committees, and activities.
- Developing an annual budget in line with organizational policies. Supervising the allocation of money and resources.
- Developing quality-improvement initiatives for the staff-development department. Assisting in the organization's overall quality-improvement efforts.
- Developing and supervising marketing plans and activities.

Source: Data from *Standards for Nursing Professional Development: Continuing Education and Staff Development,* © 1994, American Nurses Publishing.

improved patient outcomes (del Bueno & Altano, 1984).

Another management responsibility for the educator is the creation of monthly and quarterly reports. These reports are designed to keep the administrator with direct authority over staff development informed of the education activities. Reports commonly contain updates on current activities, planned projects, and potential activities for the future. Accomplishments such as programs developed, research implemented, problem-solving results, and anticipated needs should be included. The director/supervisor of the staff education department should meet regularly with the person accountable for the department activities on an upper administrative level. This allows for open lines of communication, assistance with problems, and opportunities to gain support for educational activities.

The staff development director is usually responsible for developing a system of oversight for all educational materials, audiovisual equipment, reference/library books, lab equipment, etc. The educator often has the responsibility for the library, which lends itself to stocking resources that will promote professional growth

and research among staff. This includes ordering and budgeting for new equipment and keeping it in good repair. The oversight of a system for scheduling equipment and its availability to personnel is usually a manager's duty.

In many home care settings, the duties listed previously will be shared among the members of staff development departments that consist of a few persons of equal rank. All of these activities will be the responsibility of one person where there is only one education position, as is sometimes the case. The home health agency's organizational structure and mission greatly influence the administrative activities and responsibilities of the educator. Many staff development departments are now included as part of the human resources department due to Joint Commission standards. The structure and function of the human resources department impact the position and job expectations of the staff development educator. As discussed previously, it is important that the staff development director have a hierarchical position equal with nursing directors and report to an upper level administrator (Abruzzese, 1996). Holding a management position allows the educator to be involved in administrative activities necessary for the proactive strategic planning approach, which is vital to a staff development department. This level of authority is also necessary for appropriate interaction between the educator and management, visiting staff, and clerical staff. The nature of the educator's job requires that he or she work with administration to formulate educational policy and programs. The educator needs the organizational authority to carry out these programs. To perform adequately at this level, the staff development educator ideally needs a graduate degree giving expertise in management, administration, leadership, communication, and policy making.

The educator working in a management capacity must also learn to work effectively within the informal power structure of an organization. In any situation in which people must work together as a group, a distinct culture and set of norms develop. Various persons within the group take over distinct identities within the group such as leadership (Lassiter, 1992). The staff development educator has a unique position that allows the opportunity to become familiar with the politics of the organization. This insight into the true internal workings of an organization is necessary to gain the support needed to implement a workable, competency-based curriculum.

Centralized Versus Decentralized Education Department Structure

The recent cost-containment efforts in health care that have slashed jobs and broadened job descriptions have similarly affected the management role of the educator. In addition, regulatory and accrediting bodies, like the Joint Commission, now require evidence of organizationwide performance improvement. This has encouraged the development of centralized staff development departments that have the accountability for the education needs of all patient care and nonpatient care staff throughout the organization. For example, the educational needs of the rehabilitation, social work, and clerical departments have traditionally been met chiefly by their department managers. An increasing number of staff development departments are now responsible administratively for these non-nursing departments' educational needs. In this centralized structure, educators may be responsible for general planning, oversight, and recordkeeping as well as assisting to varying degrees with developing orientation and competencies, organizing experts to address specialized learning needs, designing and testing annual competencies, and planning inservices and continuing education. In this centralized framework, staff development educators have primary responsibility for all nursing education-related activities, including specialty areas, such as MCH, intravenous, psychiatric, and hospice. Educators frequently find themselves responsible for the oversight and general administration of paraprofessional patient care providers, volunteers, clerical, data entry, and support staff as well as some general oversight for at least part of the educational needs of the managerial and executive administrative staff as well.

This oversight includes assisting the organization to meet regulatory and accrediting requirements. Educators are responsible for assessing the regulatory material to determine the educational requirements for all job descriptions. They are then responsible for developing the educational curriculum and recordkeeping needed to meet those requirements. Examples of this would be assessing the OSHA regulations, developing safety classes, and administering those classes for every employee. This may also be illustrated when the educator develops competencies based on Joint Commission and licensure guidelines for each job description in the organization.

A centralized pattern of organization allows for better communication among staff-development educators and decreased fragmentation within education activities. It enhances collaboration, collegiality, and mentoring opportunities among educators and other managers and administrators within the organization. It allows more opportunities for role modeling professional leadership and management skills. This system creates less isolation for the educator and gives him or her better access to the formal and informal power structure (Hitchings, 1996).

A centralized staff development department is also usually given more secretarial support staff to assist with the clerical and recordkeeping duties. These staff persons may assist with making appointments, faxing, telephoning, setting up schedules, advertising, and other important tasks imperative to managing a staff development program. This can greatly lighten the educator's burden and allow increased energy and time to focus on the development of staff. In a decentralized structure, the educator may need to carry out these functions of management and maintenance personally.

In a centralized system, care must be taken to address the needs of all departments and individuals. There is a natural tendency to become insulated from the everyday activities of the customers. Regular attendance of various departmental staff meetings helps keep communication lines open and helps gather information needed for educational programs. In addition, frequent communication is needed between the educator and department managers. Staff development personnel also need to set time aside to be available for individual consultations. Accessibility can improve communication and may enhance team building, which facilitates learning and, ultimately, organizational outcomes (Hitchings, 1996).

In a decentralized system of staff development, each educator is assigned the responsibility for specific departments, such as hospice, MCH, or adult health. This model is similar to those often found in large acute care settings in which each unit or specialty, such as cardiac intensive care, has an educator. Decentralization to this extent is only found in very large, metropolitan organizations in the home care setting. In this framework, a director of staff development is used to manage the department and supervise other education staff. The director often takes responsibility for administrative duties, such as attending management meetings, and for oversight of the overall agency educational plan.

The staff development educator working in a decentralized department is able to work closely with the managers and staffs of the assigned departments or teams. More opportunity exists in this system to develop good communication and solid working relationships than in a centralized department. This development of relationships allows for more depth in the assessment of learner needs and performance deficiencies. The closer relationship to staff enhances the educator's ability to assess team and individual stressors and impediments to learning. The educator is often better able to respond more quickly or proactively to the needs of the assigned department. Another advantage of this model is that the educator can become more expert clinically in his or her assigned area (Hitchings, 1996).

There are several easily apparent disadvantages in the decentralized staff development office. It is easy to duplicate services and increase the use of resources. Educators in different areas may be spending valuable time developing similar projects without each other's knowledge, for example. Also, this type of department is rarely given adequate, if any, secretarial or support staff. This requires the educators to perform most of the everyday maintenance tasks. The educators may also feel isolated from their peers (Hitchings, 1996). Many of the problems of decentralization may be addressed by a central manager who assists with overall coordination, communication, scheduling, and recordkeeping. It is vital in this format to maintain regular staff development meetings and communications.

THE ROLE OF CONSULTANT

The role of consultant is also an integral component of the staff development educator. The ANA (1994a) describes consultation as a necessary endeavor to facilitate learning and professional development of various persons involved with health care. Consulting is defined as a process of communication between professionals, in which the consultee requests the assistance or advice of a consultant, a person with expertise in a particular area. It is assumed in this process that the consultant, because of his or her experience, knowledge, or skills, can help find a solution to the problem that has been identified by the consultee/client. The consultee is free to choose whether to follow the advice or solution suggested (Barron, 1989; Nelson, 1996).

Consulting may be simply seen as a way of sharing information between the client/consultee and the consultant/educator. Many times, clarification of a problem or diagnosis of the true problem is all that is needed. The consultant may not even need to suggest solutions or actions (Nelson, 1996). This process frequently occurs informally in the home care situation when nursing personnel have questions regarding daily patient care issues.

Typically staff development personnel are used as consultants for problems relating to staff performance and competence, as individuals and as a group. For example, staff development educators are often requested to help the organization trim costs and improve performance of existing staff as individuals and as a group. They are also frequently used as experts in patient care issues. For example, educators may be asked to help develop efficient patient teaching tools or care pathways and assist with their implementation. As can be seen from these examples, the consultant's job often goes beyond sharing knowledge. The consultant may also need to diagnose problems, recommend several solutions, implement the solutions, and evaluate their effectiveness (Barron, 1989; Case, 1995).

The more complex activities of consulting are performed via a formal process that includes assessment and diagnosis of the problem; planning and implementing an intervention; and evaluating outcomes and follow-up of organizational satisfaction with the process (Alspach, 1996; Barron, 1989). Following this familiar process may be beneficial to staff development consultants when working with complex problems inside the home health agency and for those situations outside the agency. As health care delivery networks become more prevalent, staff development educators are called upon to consult with

other divisions and entities within the network, such as hospital discharge planners or educators.

Assessing the problem thoroughly is necessary for clarification in any consultation. Collecting and gathering pertinent information and data are necessary to fully define or redefine a problem. This data gathering may be done independently or with the assistance of the client/consultee as a collaborator. Collaboration between client and consultant allows both to share their knowledge and input to accurately diagnose the true problem.

The consultant's recommended interventions should be constructed as specific, measurable objectives to be reached within a certain time frame. The consultant should also provide several solutions to the problem. This allows the client to choose the approach that is best for him or her. This decision-making process may be done with other administrators or experts. In the home care situation, it may be especially helpful to obtain input from staff that will be affected by the decision and changes. It is easy for field staff to feel isolated and disconnected from managers and upper administration. Encouraging collaboration will assist implementation of solutions and their acceptance by staff.

For most consultation relationships, the responsibility for carrying out the interventions falls on the client. For example: If a case manager comes to the educator and requests help educating a patient who is blind and has insulin-dependent diabetes, the educator may give the nurse literature on patients with diabetes who are visually impaired, information on products to assist such patients, and patient teaching guides and tools. It is up to the case manager to choose the materials and methods most appropriate for this patient. However, educators acting as consultants may frequently be asked to assist with the implementation of the solutions they devised to improve staff knowledge, skills, and performance. For example, staff development educators are often asked by home care administrators to decrease incidents and errors of visit staff. This would require finding causes for the problem and suggesting and implementing solutions to increase staff competence. Educators/consultants can enhance the implementation process by providing the professional leadership necessary to build a consensus among all levels of personnel involved. The consultant must establish trust and create a positive atmosphere for clear communication to effectively create the change inherent in all interventions (Alspach, 1996; Case, 1995).

The consultant/educator must work collaboratively with the consultee during the evaluation phase of the process as well. Goals and methods to measure the effectiveness of the intervention must be designed that are practical and feasible for the client. Short- and long-term goals allow the consultant to make formative assessments and alter interventions if necessary. If the consultation is external, the client may carry out these evaluations independently. The educator often assists with this phase, as well, when working for internal clients.

An educator/consultant must possess not only a body of knowledge and expertise, but also assertiveness, excellent communication and interpersonal skills, and the ability to build professional relationships with individuals and groups. The consultant must possess characteristics that will engender respect, trust, and credibility.

THE ROLE OF RESEARCHER

Participation in various research activities is also recognized as an integral activity of the staff development educator. The ANA *Standards of Home Health Nursing Practice* (1993) mandates research involvement for all nurses. The standards recognize there will be various levels of involvement in research depending on the nurse's educational background and practice setting. The ANA standards (1994a) further define the role of researcher for the staff development educator as one "that enhances learners' competence to provide quality health and enhances their contribution to the profession" (p. 11). The educator is expected to include research literature in the educational program and facilitate the use of research findings into the staff's

practice. The educator is also expected to participate directly in the research process for problem solving and the generation of new knowledge (ANA, 1994a).

Nursing research is critical to the improvement, advancement, and survival of the profession. Scholarly inquiry into clinical nursing practice is necessary to maintain and extend the research base that is the foundation of all the health care professions. By improving the quality of nursing care, research may also improve patient outcomes (Mottola, 1996). In addition, a work environment that integrates research into daily activities is enhanced by the increased critical thinking and collaboration of professionals. The staff development educator has a unique opportunity to facilitate the use of research throughout the organization. The very nature of staff development's responsibility to evaluate educational intervention outcomes lends itself to problem solving and systematic inquiry. A current knowledge of research-based literature is a necessary framework for education programs, quality assurance efforts, and risk management activities (Nelson, 1996).

Any nurse who has ever questioned if his or her care makes a difference in a patient's long-term health or wondered about any aspect related to nursing care has begun the research process. Research is not an elitist pursuit performed only by highly schooled academicians. Research begins as simple problem solving, evaluation, and questioning of everyday educator and nursing practice (Polit & Hungler, 1995). The ANA (1994b) and Hodgeman (1983), among others, recognize various levels of research involvement for the educator. These levels range from reading, evaluating, and applying the research literature, to actual generation of research projects. The most basic level of research involvement the educator must be involved in consists of reading and evaluating current nursing research literature. The educator should be able to critically analyze the quality of the study by judging its reliability and validity. An effective study generates findings that are applicable to other settings. The educator must be able to interpret the findings and relate their significance to the staff (McGuire & Harwood, 1989). Valid nursing findings should be included in educational programs for staff and patients. The educator has a large role in creating an atmosphere for staff that is enriched by integration of research-based literature into all aspects of the orientation, education, and inservice programs. The educator should choose journals for the library that publish high-quality research for each of the various health care disciplines involved at the organization. The educator should use the teaching-learning process in a manner that facilitates staff attainment of the new knowledge and incorporates it into their health care practice.

The second level of research activity takes the involvement a step further into the realm of utilization of research findings. This level includes the testing of others' research and the application of recent findings to the clinical area (McGuire & Harwood, 1989). This utilization may be a simple, informal test of a small amount of knowledge such as including new information in a patient-teaching packet. Or the utilization may be a more formal testing of a study's findings in your clinical area. An example of this might be developing a new in-home dobutamine infusion protocol based on study findings and comparing patient outcomes to those of the original study. This advanced level of activity obviously requires more planning, knowledge, time, experience, and collaboration within the organization. The educator is again pivotal in the role of facilitating the utilization of research into the clinical practice. The educator may assist department managers or organization administrators with the development and implementation of research-based findings. It is critical to center research endeavors in the staff development department of a health care organization due to the educator's integral involvement with organizational quality assurance, management, and evaluation and risk assessment activities (Nelson, 1996).

The third and most advanced level of research activity includes active participation in the generation of knowledge through a range of activities. These include precepting student researchers, replicating research projects, collaborating with others in research projects, or independently conducting original studies (McGuire & Harwood, 1989; Hodgeman, 1983). The educator who acts as liaison between the home care organization and educational facilities is in a prime position to facilitate and foster scholarly inquiry by acting as a preceptor or advisor to students conducting research projects. Replication of the research first carried out by others may be done to explore the ability to generalize the findings to other settings. The educator may find this a more appropriate alternative to developing original projects. Using a previous study may save time and labor by cutting development time and preventing some of the errors or problems encountered in the first study. The educator may become involved in original research by collaborating with others within the organization or other medical professionals outside the agency. External collaboration is growing increasingly feasible with professionals from entities within health care alliances affiliated with home care organizations. The educator may also conduct studies independently depending on employment circumstances and personal attributes.

A word about ethics at this point is appropriate. Any person contemplating involvement in any level of research must do so with a solid knowledge of the ethical considerations involved. Educators/researchers must use principles of beneficence, which hold that no harm or exploitation should be done to any of the clients or staff in a study. Any potential harm that may arise from a study should be weighed with the considerations of the benefits to all as a result of the research. All investigations must ensure clients' privacy and fair treatment. All test subjects must give informed consent to participation in a study, meaning they are capable of understanding the implications of their consent. All research investigations must be reviewed by the home care organization's research/ethics committee, and approval must be given.

Any level of research involvement is dependent in part on the educational background and personal attributes of the staff development educator. Although all basic educational programs for nurses now contain a research component, actual exposure and experience with research are often limited (Bower, 1994). Educators without an advanced degree may find themselves inadequately prepared to function beyond the basic level of reading and interpreting of studies. Educators with graduate-level education are better prepared to participate in more complex research activities. Some nursing authors contend that only doctorally prepared nurses are adequately trained to carry out scientific investigations. The ANA's Guidelines for the Investigative Functions of Nurses (1981) recommended that master's prepared nurses identify research problems, provide clinical consultation to other researchers, collaborate in research activities, and evaluate quality assurance activities but do not conduct independent investigations. However, in the ensuing time period, many nursing authors have supported independent inquiry for master's prepared nurses and CNSs (Fawcett, 1985; Oberst, 1985; McGuire & Harwood, 1989). Staff development educators with a master's degree in nursing or education may identify a study topic, formulate the research question, design the research method, and collect and analyze the data as independent researchers.

In addition to appropriate educational background and training, the educator involved in research needs a variety of knowledge and skills to function effectively. Clinical expertise is needed as a solid grounding to launch nursing research. A broad knowledge of research methods, measuring techniques, and statistical methods that extends beyond the introductory research courses in most basic nursing programs is needed for the advanced levels of research activity. Ability to analyze and think abstractly and critically are also necessary skills. Writing skills are needed to document the study. The educator also needs a knowledge of the ethical issues involved with research and his or her organization's guidelines for research before beginning a project (Case, 1995; McGuire & Harwood, 1989).

In addition to technical skills, the researcher requires a set of personal attributes, values, and beliefs, not only to facilitate the research process, but to create the possibility of systematic inquiry. The educator must first have a belief in the usefulness and value of research-based knowledge to improve clinical practice and patient outcomes and as a necessary base for the profession of nursing (McGuire & Harwood, 1989). A belief that research is an expected and vital role for staff development educators is a necessary component to initiate any research activity. The educator/researcher must also have intellectual curiosity and energy to work through the barriers inherent in conducting research activities within the home health care organization. Strong interpersonal skills and creative problem-solving ability are necessary to facilitate this process (Case, 1995; McGuire & Harwood, 1989). Educators who view research as an exciting dynamic process that enriches their professional life will create an organizational atmosphere that stimulates professional research utilization in all aspects of administrative and clinical care.

Barriers to the Utilization of Research

The demand for nursing practice that is research based has grown steadily over the past decade, and nurses have answered with a steady increase in the quantity of published and unpublished studies. However, the transfer of these research findings into daily nursing practice has not occurred (Polit & Hungler, 1995). Several nursing authors have addressed this problem and its possible causes (Hunt, 1987; Bower, 1994; Mottola, 1996). Three barriers that have been commonly reported in the literature as a cause for a lack of utilization and diffusion of nursing findings are lack of availability of research findings, the attitudes of nurses, and the lack of environmental support in the workplace (Mottola, 1996).

Although authors in the early 1980s complained that there was a lack of availability of research articles or journals in their area of expertise, a current analysis of nursing and scientific medical literature shows an avalanche of knowledge now available through numerous specialty journals and professional databases (Mottola, 1996). The ease of access for most individuals and institutions to the wealth of information on the Internet has created the problem of information overload. However, it is recognized that some health care professionals may not have this access due to lack of organizational computer support or due to computer illiteracy. Some authors have suggested that lack of utilization is not unavailability of information but the inability to understand much of the research-based literature (Hunt, 1987) due to a lack of depth in research instruction in basic nursing programs (Bower, 1994). Others have asserted that lack of utilization is due to the use of high-tech language and lack of meaningful analysis that is easily transferable to clinical practice (Funk, Champagne, Wiese, & Tornquist, 1991). The educator holds a pivotal role in solving all of these problems. The staff development educator often has Internet access via the organization's computer system that the staff may not share. The educator with an advanced degree or with the help of additional research classes beyond basic schooling will be able to assist the clinical staff navigate this maze of research findings, assist them with the interpretation of findings, and help facilitate their use in clinical practice.

The attitudes of nurses toward research has also been seen as a barrier to utilization of research. Again, the lack of emphasis on research activities throughout the basic nursing curriculum limits nurses' view of research to a responsibility of doctorally prepared nurse academicians (Burns & Grove, 1995). Those nurses with advanced degrees may have found the dissertation process so difficult that they are discouraged from pursuing it after graduation (Bower, 1994). Others have found that nurses often view the nursing research of the past, which emphasized education, nursing models, and history, as irrelevant to their daily clinical practice (Lekander, Tracy, & Lindquist, 1994). The educator can also play a vital role in changing the

attitudes of clinical staff toward research. The research base of all classes and inservices must be emphasized. Distributing pertinent research findings or posting articles helps integrate research into everyday activities. Inservices surveying literature in light of patient and clinical problems can be conducted with staff input for ideas of clinical application from the group (Mottola, 1996). The educator can help make research a part of the organizational culture by including research in all activities, by having a positive attitude, and by making research relevant in clinical practice for each discipline.

The third most frequently cited barrier for a lack of utilization of literature is lack of environmental support (Mottola, 1996). Support of research activity by the organization's administrators is needed for all levels of involvement (McGuire & Harwood, 1989). Research is often viewed as a time- and money-consuming venture with little revenue-generating potential by business-minded administrators. The barriers to engage in research endeavors named most frequently by nurses surveyed by Funk and colleagues (1991) included lack of time on the job, lack of support from other nurses, lack of cooperation from physicians and administrators, and lack of time to read the literature. Educators will find themselves with heavy workloads that aren't compatible with the thoughtful atmosphere required for the creative thinking necessary for research. Budgeting the resources necessary to conduct original research or facilitate utilization may be difficult. Finding expert help and mentoring may also prove problematic.

Organizational policy toward research is a major factor influencing the research environment. Administrative staff must believe in the value of research efforts in order to designate organizational resources to it. The educator can enhance environmental support by using the formal and informal channels of power present in any organization. The educator's job description should contain responsibilities for research activities at all levels of involvement. This helps legitimize those activities in the organization. If the staff development educator shares a position on an equal hierarchical level with upper management, the educator will have more opportunities to work with administrators developing policies that influence research activities. Being involved in task forces and committees at various organizational levels will give the educator opportunities to work within the formal channels of power to design research-friendly plans and activities. Educators may also build their own informal power by gaining the respect of those in power. Influence can be gained by excelling personally and professionally and holding high ideals and standards. This requires strong interpersonal and communication skills. The educator may still need to work for support to gain time and financial resources to conduct complex levels of research. The educator/researcher must be able to document the costs and the benefits of projects to the organization. Some of the cost benefits of research may be improved patient outcomes, increased referrals, and improved staff longevity. Research benefits may often be intangibles, such as improved staff morale, increased collaboration within health alliances, and enhanced public opinion. The educator/researcher may offset some of the costs of research by applying for public and private grants.

The educator can overcome barriers from nursing and other caregiving staff by providing a positive role model. The educator who views research as a fun, creative, stimulating endeavor will have a positive influence on the staff. By including research articles, topics, and information in all educational activities and making the information accessible and meaningful to clinical staff, the educator can create a research-friendly environment.

Various projects and models have been developed to enhance the utilization of research. These models attempt to systematically overcome the barriers and resistance to research and diffuse the knowledge among clinical staff. Models such as Stetler/Maran and the CURN project identify various factors that affect research and recommend a set of steps designed to enhance research activities (Mottola, 1996). It is not within the scope of this work to explore these

models fully. Readers are encouraged to explore these models to choose the one(s) that are beneficial to their situation in an appropriate nursing research text.

The roles of the staff-development educator are varied and multidimensional. The person who assumes this responsibility must prepare himself or herself educationally, experientially, and personally. Regardless of how talented and prepared, educators will fail unless they learn to collaborate effectively with other members at all levels of the organization to meet the demands of today's challenging home health care field.

SHARED RESPONSIBILITIES FOR COMPETENCY

A successful competency-based education (CBE) program requires more than the efforts of the staff development educators. To develop, implement, evaluate, and constantly update a competency program requires the collaboration and support of many individuals and disciplines within the home care organization. It is imperative that the educator obtain the support of administrators, managers, and staff to design a program that is in keeping with their collective values and needs. Only then can the educator provide an education program that will be accepted and effective in creating the desired changes and goals (Martaus, Bell, Kenyon, Snow, & Hefty, 1993).

The role of administrative personnel should not be viewed solely as one of program approval. Administrators should be consulted for direction in guiding the educational strategic plan during pre-development planning and evaluation phases. Upper-level management may also be a resource for expert advice and input in various phases of the program.

The educator must also collect pertinent data from each manager of affected departments, such as physical therapy and nursing. This is imperative in the common situation of a staff development educator designing a CBE program or orientation for another specialty. These managers should be involved in developing the content for all phases of the CBE activities in which they will be participating.

Input must also be obtained from clinical staff to develop education programs that are meaningful and valuable to them. This helps increase their self-esteem and motivation to learn and participate in the programs. Staff input and feedback allow for a reality-based competency program. Regular feedback from the managers is necessary to allow the educator to make accurate formative and summative evaluations. Feedback from all of these parties is necessary to allow the educator to make formative and summative evaluations of the competency-based programs.

Home Care Expectations

A CBE program is expected to provide the home care organization with clinical staff who "possess the skills, knowledge and capacity" (Costello, 1991, p. 277) to perform their jobs in a competent manner. There are various definitions of competency in nursing literature. McGregor (1990) defined staff competency as the ability to deliver safe, professional care to clients. Katz and Green (as cited in Nagelsmith, 1995) believe competence to be a proficient level of skill. Proficiency implies the ability to think critically and apply theory into everyday practice (Swendsen-Boss, 1985). However, Benner (1984) had placed competence third on a hierarchy of five levels of clinical nursing performance. According to Benner's framework, the levels are denoted as novice, advanced beginner, competent, proficient, and expert. At the competent level, nurses are expected to perform capably with an increasing ability to integrate knowledge and situations into a holistic framework. As can be seen by these definitions and the discussions earlier in the book, competency may be viewed differently. Each organization must define competency for its particular situation in keeping with legal, regulatory, and professional standards (Nagelsmith, 1995).

What CBE content is of most benefit to the home care organization and the clinical staff? Content must be based on current professional or paraprofessional standards, federal and state legal requirements, and on the standards of accrediting bodies such as the Joint Commission. Each agency must select its core competency skills for each clinical discipline, based on its focus of care. This can be done by assessing the staff, quality assurance, and risk management issues. Valuable information may also be gleaned from the professional literature to help develop a realistic content for a CBE program (Astarita, 1996).

What skills and knowledge are needed for the clinical home care staff to perform their jobs competently? The skills and knowledge required for home care nursing are unique to that setting (Caie-Lawrence, Peploski, & Russell, 1995; Milone-Nuzzo & Humphrey, 1992). A home health nurse must combine the knowledge and skills specific to home health with those of basic nursing and community health nursing and practice at an advanced level (Astarita, 1996; Colucciello, 1993). Specialized documentation, communication, organizational, and interpersonal skills are needed by all clinical staff. Researching the literature of each discipline is helpful in determining what skills are necessary to include to meet your organization's particular needs. Although this section focuses on nursing, the largest professional group delivering home health care, the assumptions may be applied to other professions and paraprofessionals.

Decisions must also be made as to who will be expected to be competent. Will the expectations for part-time, per diem, and contract staff be the same as for full-time staff? These part-time and contract personnel are becoming an ever-increasing portion of the home health care force (Leidy, 1992). As competition and cost-containment efforts grow, this trend is expected to continue. Concerns about the quality of care and the management of risk and liability are very real. These part-time clinical staff are not normally oriented or trained in the organization's policies or procedures, nor possibly for the population served. Competency-based orientation (CBO) and training may be difficult due to costs and scheduling conflicts. A collaborative decision between administration, middle management, and staff development must be made about solutions, such as mini orientations and performance evaluations.

When will the learning needs of staff be addressed? Many concerns are most conveniently addressed during the orientation process when time, money, and personnel are devoted to enhancing the competency of a new employee. Evaluations of competency at regular intervals are then mandated by regulatory and accrediting bodies such as federal law and the Joint Commission. For example, nurse aides must be performance evaluated annually according to the Medicare regulations. An annual competency skills lab allows clinical staff to update core competencies and be performance evaluated while fulfilling regulatory demands. In addition, evidence of regular inservices and continuing education participation must be documented for clinical disciplines to fulfill regulatory mandates.

The home care organization also has expectations about the cost of a CBE curriculum. The organization desires a competent staff at the lowest possible cost. Some authors have pointed out that CBE is more costly than traditional methods of education (del Bueno & Altano, 1984). Other authors have pointed out that CBE can focus on real learning needs, decrease redundancy, and use education hours more effectively (Lassiter, Kearney, & Fell, 1985). Most authors believe that the long-term benefits to the individual and organization produce cost savings and increase revenue (del Bueno & Altano, 1984; Astarita, 1996).

Orientation

A high-quality orientation program is a critical component in any health care organization. Orientation is defined by the ANA (1994a) as the "means by which new nursing staff are introduced to the philosophy, goals, policies, procedures, role expectations . . . needed to function in a specific work setting" (p. 13). A formal introduction and training process for a new job position is considered so important that orientation is mandated by state and federal law (Brent, 1994). Accrediting and regulating organizations such as the Joint Commission (1996) mandate orientation for all patient care staff before they assume patient care responsibilities. Orientation is a core requirement for the CHAP (National League for Health Care, 1993). The home care agency may also view orientation as a method to reduce liability and risk (Brent, 1994). CBO has been shown to be an effective method to ensure safe provision of nursing care (Snyder-Halpern & Buczkowski, 1990). Properly prepared staff are less likely to make errors in the provision of care. Proper training also enhances long-term employee effectiveness and productivity.

Orientation serves multiple purposes for the employees, as well. New employees feel better prepared for their new responsibilities. This enables the professional or paraprofessional to maintain standards of accountability. Orientation allows the new employee to become familiar with organizational norms and enhances the socialization process (ANA, 1994a). This can lead to greater personal and professional satisfaction (Abruzzese & Quinn-O'Neal, 1992; Caie-Lawrence, Peploski & Russell 1995; O'Shea, 1994).

The content of a CBO program to a home care organization must include those elements that are unique to home health. Nursing orientation must address clinical skills, documentation skills, supervision of aides, quality assurance, productivity, ethics, legal aspects of home care, reimbursement guidelines, and various high-tech skills (Caie-Lawrence, Peploski, & Russell, 1995; Colucciello, 1993; Milone-Nuzzo & Humphrey, 1992). Most other disciplines would benefit from a similar list of topics. It is easy for the new orientee to feel overwhelmed with this avalanche of new information. CBO has the advantages of limiting the content based on each individual's needs and clearly stating what is expected of the orientee. The competency format also allows the orientee to receive immediate feedback, which can lessen anxiety. Problems that may arise if the orientee has difficulty with accurate self-assessment include using self-learning modules or being motivated to learn (del Bueno, 1978). These problems must be addressed chiefly by the educator with assistance from the other members of the orientation team. The new employee, his or her department manager, the staff development educator, and another staff member/preceptor all participate in the implementation of CBO. In response to adult learning needs, the plan emphasizes self-learning in the orientee's preferred style. The manager helps direct, support, assist, and evaluate the orientee throughout the process. The staff personnel are usually "buddied" with the orientee to give real-life training on home visits and management of patients. Ideally, this clinical piece will be done by a trained preceptor, which is discussed below. Staff development coordinates all of these persons, providing resources for learning, feedback, and support. The outcome-focused goals and CBO framework allow for easier implementation for all parties involved.

The evaluation phase of the CBO is also a collaborative effort of the manager, preceptor, educator, and orientee. CBO eases the task of evaluating the acquisition of knowledge and skills by requiring a performance-based outcome (Abruzzese, 1996). Formal and informal feedback mechanisms should begin in the prehiring phase and continue throughout orientation to allow for formative evaluation of the orientee and the CBO (Grant, 1993). Evaluation of outcomes should be done for each orientee at regular, prearranged intervals. Short- and long-term goals allow for flexibility and real-world contingencies. Evaluation of the orientee, the CBO, and self-evaluation by each participant should be performed at summation. In addition, the educator should evaluate the success of each CBO and track the effects of the CBO on groups of hires. Evaluation of long-term organizational effects such as staff retention, productivity, quality assurance, and risk management should be completed yearly by the staff development educator.

Preceptorship in Competency-Based Orientation

The use of preceptors has been widely applied and formalized in nursing and recognized as an enhancement tool for the orientation of new graduates and new employees (Abruzzese & Quinn-O'Neal, 1992; Stevenson, Doorley, Moddeman, & Benson-Landau, 1995). A preceptor is more than a "buddy" or someone the orientee just "shadows" or follows through the day. A preceptor is an experienced staff nurse who is designated and trained to introduce a new employee to the work setting (Abruzzese & Quinn-O'Neal, 1992; Alspach, 1996). Working with an experienced person in the clinical area allows a first-hand introduction to the formal rules, policies, and procedures. Preceptors also facilitate the socialization of the new hire to the informal expectations, politics, and cultural norms found in any work environment. Another vital component of the preceptor's function is to act as a role model for the orientee. Preceptorship naturally lends itself to the CBO framework, allowing the broad, yet specialized format necessary for home care.

Staff-development educators and managers choosing clinical staff as candidates for preceptor training must look for the various professional qualities and personal attributes recommended to fulfill the role, such as competent clinical performance, professionalism, desire and ability to teach, effective interpersonal and communication skills, and flexibility (Meng & Conti, 1995; Young, Theriault, & Collins, 1989). The skills of an expert clinician may seem most desirable but, as Meng & Conti (1995) point out, the expert practices on such an intuitive level that it may be difficult for him or her to break down the decision-making processes. A competent nurse who still deliberately plans activities and care is recommended as being a more appropriate teacher.

Training for preceptors usually lasts a few days and may have a continuing education component for updates and advancement. Learning content should contain much of the following: adult learning needs, assessing learning needs, evaluation of performance, teaching techniques, communication techniques, conflict management, organizational skills and priority setting, and socialization theory (Alspach, 1996; Meng & Conti, 1995; Modic, 1989; Nederveld, 1990; O'Shea, 1994). The preceptor must be introduced to the orientation program itself, including participants, scheduling, and expectations for the orientee and the preceptor. Preceptor training and competencies should be conducted by those in the education department with expertise in this area.

The orientation process should be a collaborative effort among the nursing (or other discipline) manager, the preceptor, the orientee, and the staff development educator. A regular schedule for meetings and feedback should be made between all the participants. The educator should support the preceptor by making himself or herself readily available to answer questions and address any problems as they evolve. The orientee spends anywhere from a few days to 6 or more weeks with a preceptor, depending on agency policy and clinical discipline involved. At the end of this period, an evaluation of the process by all involved parties is necessary to revise and improve the program. The preceptor should evaluate the preceptee's outcomes and make recommendations for remediation if necessary.

CBO and preceptorship can enhance the effectiveness of the orientation process by setting clear goals and reducing anxiety of learners through one-on-one teaching and demonstration in the home setting. Preceptors may be rewarded for their efforts with internal factors, such as increased interest in their discipline, increased self-esteem, increased personal and professional growth, or external factors, such as extra time off, shift preferences, etc. (Stevenson et al., 1995). In addition, preceptor programs may have a positive influence on organizational professionalism and growth. The organization may also gain through improved nurse recruitment and lower staff turnover (McLean, 1987).

Continuing Education

Continuing education may also be built upon a competency framework. Continuing education is defined by the ANA (1994b) as "those learning experiences intended to build upon the educational and experiential bases of the professional nurse for the enhancement of practice, education, administration, research or theory development to improve the health of the public" (p. 5). The ANA views continuing education as a lifelong endeavor that is essential to maintain and increase competence. Increasing the nurse's knowledge and performance base is seen as a responsibility of the professional nurse. Nursing educators are charged with the responsibility to provide opportunities and facilitate continuous learning (ANA, 1992).

The Medicare COP require evidence of ongoing education for all professional disciplines and paraprofessional home care staff (Department of Health and Human Services, 1991). Similarly, the Joint Commission (1996) and the CHAP (National League for Health Care & CHAP, 1993) standards require evidence of continuing education for all home care staff. The concept of improving professional performance has a long tradition in nursing and is a core belief in other health care disciplines.

The need for continuing education has grown as the influx of acute care nurses into the home care setting has increased. Many of these nurses are unprepared experientially for the new range of skills required for community-based nursing (Caie-Lawrence, Peploski, & Russell, 1995; O'Shea, 1994). In addition, the ANA and many experts feel that only an RN with a baccalaureate degree has the educational background to prepare for this role (ANA, 1993; Culley, Courtney, Diamond, & Bates, 1996). Few educational programs exist to help nurses develop the skills necessary to practice safely and competently in the home care setting. Continuing education offers a viable solution to this problem (Culley et al., 1996) by allowing more in-depth study and specialty training needed beyond orientation.

Opinions differ as to the benefit of continuing education in the nursing literature. Some studies have indicated learning may be internal and not transferred into improved performance (Ferrel, 1988; Oliver, 1984). But the survey of continuing education literature done by Rath, Boblin-Cummings, Bauman, Parrott, and Parsons (1996) showed that a majority of study findings concurred in the effectiveness of continuing education; that is, knowledge was gained, and nursing practice was improved. The survey found no particular framework for continuing education was uniformly recommended by the studies as being more effective.

Staff development educators are usually given the responsibility to supervise, monitor, and document the external continuing education activities attended by staff. Educators control the budget allotted for staff and help fairly determine eligibility for attendance. Educators also are expected to post upcoming classes and sometimes negotiate price. By offering a large attendance or assistance with the program, a discount may be given. Most importantly, it is the educator's responsibility to critically evaluate the quality of programs and their pertinence or usefulness for visit staff. Staff development may also have the option to develop their own continuing education classes offering education units to internal and to external customers if they have the time, staff, and administrative support to allow such an endeavor. Creating a consortium of several area home care agencies to collaboratively develop continuing education programs may be an advantageous source of ideas, assistance, and marketing. This approach allows the lone staff development educator or small department larger resources and professional networking.

The ANA (1992) recommends that the principles of adult learning be used in developing, implementing, and evaluating continuing education. CBE lends itself readily to this recommendation and may be adapted as a framework to develop continuing education classes. Staff development can begin this approach by conducting a survey to assess learner needs and interests. This adds a necessary real-life dimension to a competency program. Individual needs may also be addressed by self-assessment tools for the identification of learning deficits (Rath et al., 1996). Including these adult learners in the process adds to their sense of control and may serve to increase their participation and influence learning (Billie, 1979). Involvement of learners in the development stages can also serve to boost marketing by stimulating learner interest and awareness (Meyer & Elliot, 1996). Learning needs may also be obtained by conferring with staff mangers and experts from various clinical and health-related fields. Information gathered from the professional literature and analysis of the organization's most frequent billing diagnoses are rich sources of information. Indicators obtained from the organization's quality assurance programs and risk management reports are vital to the integration of education into overall organizational improvement.

Implementation is enhanced by the competency framework, which provides clear, measurable goals. These objectives provide guidance to the educator, facilitator, and student in the process of teaching and learning. Implementation of continuing education may be performed in a variety of ways to address differing learning styles and maintain interest. The staff development educator must consider the overall costs in terms of people, time, and money to conduct any continuing education offering. Given the current economic environment in health care, it may be wise to use some of the inexpensive, less formal methods of learning. Traditional lectures, classes, and large training sessions may not always be feasible. Competency-based learning can be accomplished in a variety of simpler methods that not only reduce costs but may add methods that better suit individual learning styles. Videos, computer-assisted instruction, posters, and self-learning modules may be utilized by the learner with a paper and pencil test afterward. Self-evaluation may also be done for changes in knowledge, skills, and attitude.

The evaluation of staff achievement is also facilitated by a competency framework. Acquisition of the measurable learning objectives can be accomplished more easily. Care must be taken to have competent assessors evaluate staff outcomes. True evaluation of competency requires more than using a checklist of skills. To judge the quality of a performance, a person needs a tacit knowledge that allows him or her to use the staff's verbal answers and behavioral cues (Percival, Anderson, & Lawson, 1994). Managers and clinical experts must be educated and evaluated as well in their ability to assess learner outcomes. Formative evaluations should occur throughout the continuing education process as a means of finding and correcting problems. Short- and long-term goals should be chosen during the initial stages of planning most projects. Evaluation of programs for effectiveness, learner satisfaction, and learner application is critical for the development of future offerings (Rath et al., 1996). Documentation of all continuing education program topics, methods of implementation, and attendance is necessary for the accrediting, regulatory, legal, and professional bodies mentioned earlier. Topics, content, attendees, and evaluation results are a vital component of quality assurance and risk management activities.

If the true goals of continuing education are the enhancement of professional growth, improved nursing care, and the improvement of patient care, then an evaluation of the program's effects must be done. In a review of the literature, Koyama et al. (1996) found that studies on the evaluations of continuing education focused chiefly on learner outcome with little emphasis on learner behavior changes or patient impact. When studies were conducted, they were usually nonexperimental designs (74%). There currently exists a great need for research-based inquiry into the effects of continuing education. Staff development educators need to use scholarly methods of evaluation to solidly ground their programs, improve their endeavors, and truly impact client health and professional growth.

Inservice Education

Inservice education is defined by the ANA (1994b) as those "activities intended to help nurses acquire, maintain or increase the level of competence in fulfilling their assigned responsibilities" needed to perform a particular job description. Inservice education is mandated by the ANA, the Joint Commission, CHAP, and in the Medicare COP (Yuan, 1995). Inservice education is viewed by these regulatory, accrediting, and professional bodies as necessary to provide professional and paraprofessional staff with the current knowledge and skills necessary to provide safe, quality patient care.

Inservice education is a collaborative effort with the educator utilizing input and assistance from the organization's management, administration, staff, and experts in all phases of developing, implementing, and evaluating programs. The initial development stage for inservice education may often be more informal than other CBE endeavors. Ideas may be generated by reading the literature and conversations with other educators or professionals internal or external to the organization. The educator must be cautious and use inservice time wisely. Yuan (1995) suggests that the educator consult with an interdisciplinary committee to develop a strategic long-term plan for organizational inservices. There is currently an explosion of new products, techniques, and services being offered in the home care arena. Before jumping into an inservice training, the educator must assess the product's or service's viability and usefulness to staff, patients, and the organization. This decision making must be made in conjunction with administrators and experts in the pertinent field.

Elements of CBE are applicable to inservice education. The same steps of assessment of need, implementation, and evaluation are followed. Adult learning principles should be applied, but may be limited in some instances. Frequently, an outside expert or a product representative conducts a lecture or hands-on learning lab for new products or services. The educator should provide materials and literature to complement these inservice situations and to allow self-study time for learners who prefer those methods. The educator must ascertain that the implementation is done by experts in the field or those trained by the expert.

Evaluation of learner competence, satisfaction, and ability to apply the new skill or knowledge is a necessary step for remediation and follow-up. The educator may also be involved in developing policies and procedures for the new product lines or patient services. Some new skills and knowledge should be added to the employee's job description and included in the yearly competency testing and the orientation program. The educator is responsible for the documentation record of staff attendance and competence for regulatory, quality assurance, and risk management activities.

REFERENCES

Abruzzese, R.S. (1996). Evaluation in nursing staff development. In R.S. Abruzzese (Ed.), *Nursing staff development: Strategies for success* (2nd ed.) (pp. 242–258). St. Louis, MO: Mosby-Year Book, Inc.

Abruzzese, R.S., & Quinn-O'Neal, B. (1992). Orientation for general and specialty areas. In R.S. Abruzzese (Ed.), *Nursing staff development: Strategies for success* (2nd ed.) (pp. 259–280). St. Louis, MO: Mosby-Year Book, Inc.

Alspach, J.G. (1996). *Designing competency assessment programs: A handbook for nurses and health-related professionals.* Pensacola, FL: National Nursing Staff Development Organization.

American Nurses Association. (1986). *Standards of home care nursing practice.* Kansas City, MO: Author.

American Nurses Association. (1992). *Roles and responsibilities for nursing continuing education and staff development across all settings.* Washington, DC: American Nurses Publishing.

American Nurses Association. (1993). *Standards of home health nursing practice.* Kansas City, MO: Author.

American Nurses Association. (1994a). *Standards for nursing professional development: Continuing education and staff development.* Washington, DC: American Nurses Publishing.

American Nurses Association (ANA). (1994b). *Standards for continuing education in nursing.* Kansas City, MO: Author.

American Nurses Credentialing Center. (1996–97). ANCC Certification examinations, October 1996. *Credentialing News,* Winter, 3.

Astarita, T.M. (1996). Competency-based orientation in home care: One agency's approach. *Home Health Care Management and Practice, 8*(4), 38–49.

Barron, A.M. (1989). The CNS as consultant. In A.B. Hamric & J.A. Spross (Eds.), *The clinical nurse specialist in theory and practice* (2nd ed.) (pp. 125–146). Philadelphia: W.B. Saunders.

Benner, P. (1984). *From novice to expert: Excellence and power in clinical nursing practice.* Menlo Park, CA: Addison-Wesley.

Billie, D.A. (1979). Successful educational programming: Increased motivation through involvement. *Journal of Nursing Administration, 9,* 36–42.

Blocker, V.T. (1992). Organizational models and staff preparation: A survey of staff development departments. *Journal of Continuing Education in Nursing, 23*(6), 259–262.

Bower, F. (1994). Research utilization: Attitude and value. *Reflections, 29*(2), 4–5.

Brent, N.J. (1994). Orientation to home healthcare nursing is an essential ingredient of risk management and employee satisfaction. *Home Healthcare Nurse, 10*(2), 9–10.

Buchanan, B.F., & Glanville, C.I. (1988). The clinical nurse specialist as educator: Process and method. *Clinical Nurse Specialist, 2*(2), 82–89.

Burns, N., & Grove, S. (1995). *Understanding nursing research: Conduct, critique, and utilization.* Philadelphia: W.B. Saunders.

Caie-Lawrence, J., Peploski, J., & Russell, J.C. (1995). Training needs of home healthcare nurses. *Home Healthcare Nurse, 13*(2), 53–61.

Case, B. (1995). Roles. In *Certification for staff development.* Symposium for the Medical College of Pennsylvania and Hahneman University, Philadelphia.

Colucciello, M.L. (1993). Learning styles and instructional processes for home healthcare providers. *Home Healthcare Nurse, 11*(2), 43–50.

Costello, R. (Ed.). (1991). *Webster's college dictionary.* New York: Random House.

Culley, J.M., Courtney, J.A., Diamond, L.M., & Bates, E. (1996). A continuing education program to retrain registered nurses for careers in client-focused community healthcare. *Journal of Continuing Education in Nursing, 27*(6), 267–273.

del Bueno, D. (1978). Competency based education. *Nurse Educator, 5*(3), 10–14.

del Bueno, D., & Altano, R. (1984). Competency-based orientation: No magic feather. *Nursing Management, 15*(4), 48–49.

Department of Health and Human Services. (July 18, 1991). Medicare program: Home health agencies: Conditions of participation: Final rule. *Federal Register, 56,* 32967–32975.

Fawcett, J. (1985). Typology of nursing research activities according to educational preparation. *Journal of Professional Nursing, 1*(2), 75–78.

Ferrel, M.J. (1988). The relationship of continuing education offerings to self-reported change in behavior. *Journal of Continuing Education in Nursing, 19*(1), 21–24.

Fitzsimmons, B., Piercy, J., Noel, L., & Connolly, C. (1996). Nurse educator performance standards. *Journal of Nursing Staff Development, 12*(4), 247–251.

Funk, S., Champagne, M., Wiese, R., & Tornquist, E. (1991). Barriers to using research findings in practice: The clinician's perspective. *Applied Nursing Research, 4*(2), 90–95.

Gillies, D.A. (1982). *Nursing management: A systems approach.* Philadelphia: W.B. Saunders.

Grant, P. (1993). Formative evaluation of a nursing orientation program: Self-paced vs. lecture-discussion. *Journal of Continuing Education in Nursing, 24*(6), 245–248.

Hitchings, K.S. (1996). Organization of staff development activities. In R.S. Abruzzese (Ed.), *Nursing staff development: Strategies for success* (2nd ed.) (pp. 80–105). St. Louis, MO: Mosby-Year Book, Inc.

Hodgeman, E.C. (1983). The CNS as researcher. In A.B. Hamric & J. Spross (Eds.), *The clinical nurse specialist in theory and practice* (pp. 73–82). New York: Grune & Stratton.

Hunt, M. (1987). The process of translating research findings into nursing practice. *Journal of Advanced Nursing, 12,* 101–110.

Joint Commission on Accreditation of Healthcare Organizations. (1996). *1997–1998 Comprehensive Manual for Home Care.* Oakbrook Terrace, IL: Author.

Knowles, M. (1980). *The modern practice of adult education: Andragogy versus pedagogy* (2nd ed.). Chicago: Follett Publishing.

Koyama, M., Holzemer, W.L., Kaharu, C., Watanabe, M., Yoshii, Y., & Otawa, K. (1996). Assessment of a continuing education evaluation framework. *Journal of Continuing Education in Nursing, 27*(3), 115–119.

Lancaster, J. (1992). Education models and principles applied to community health nursing. In M. Stanhope and J. Lancaster (Eds.), *Community health nursing: Process and practice for promoting health* (3rd ed.) (pp. 180–199). Philadelphia: Mosby.

Lane, A. (1996). Developing healthcare educator: The application of a conceptual model. *Journal of Nursing Staff Development, 12*(6), 252–259.

Lassiter, C.K., Kearny, M.R., & Fell, R. (1985). Competency-based orientation: An idea that works! *Journal of Nursing Staff Development, 1,* 68–73.

Lassiter, P.G. (1992). Working with groups in the community. In M. Stanhope & J. Lancaster (Eds.), *Community health nursing: Process and practice for promoting health* (3rd ed.) (pp. 180–199). Philadelphia: Mosby-Year Book.

Leidy, K. (1992). The effective screening and orientation of independent contract nurses. *Journal of Continuing Education in Nursing, 23*(2), 64–68.

Lekander, B., Tracy, M., & Linquist, R. (1994). Overcoming obstacles to research-based clinical practice. *Maternal-Child Nursing, 3*(2), 115–123.

Lewin, K. (1951). *Field theory in social science.* New York: Harper & Row.

Martaus, T.M., Bell, M.L., Kenyon, V., Snow, L., & Hefty, L.V. (1993). Realities of developing community health orientation programs. *Public Health Nursing, 10*(3), 173–176.

McGregor, R.J. (1990). A framework for developing staff competencies. *Journal of Nursing Staff Development, 6*(2), 79–83.

McGuire, D.B., & Harwood, K.V. (1989). The CNS as researcher. In A.B. Hamric & J.A. Spross (Eds.), *The clinical nurse specialist in theory and practice* (2nd ed.) (pp. 169–204). Philadelphia: W.B. Saunders.

McLean, P.H. (1987, Winter). Reducing staff turnover: The preceptor connection. *Journal of Nursing Staff Development, 3*(1), 20–23.

Meng, A., & Conti, A. (1995). Preceptor development: An opportunity to stimulate critical thinking. *Journal of Nursing Staff Development, 11*(2), 71–76.

Meyer, R., & Elliot, R.L. (1996). Pathway to excellence: A peer based program in continuing education. *Journal of Continuing Education in Nursing, 27*(3), 104–107.

Milone-Nuzzo, P., & Humphrey, C.J. (1992). Home care nursing orientation model: Content and strategies. *Home Healthcare Nurse, 10*(6), 18–25.

Modic, M.B. (1989, May–June). Developing a preceptor program: What are the ingredients? *Journal of Nursing Staff Development, 5*(3), 78–82.

Mottola, C.A. (1996). Research utilization and the continuing/staff development educator. *The Journal of Continuing Education in Nursing, 27*(4), 168–175.

Nagelsmith, L. (1995). Competence: An evolving concept. *The Journal of Continuing Nursing Education, 26*(6), 245–247.

National League for Health Care, Inc. & Community Health Accreditation Program, Inc. (1993). *Standards for excel-*

lence in home care organizations. New York: National League for Health Care.

National Nursing Staff Development Organization. (1996). Staff development survey results. *Trend Lines, 7*(2), 4–6.

Nelson, M.J. (1996). The nurse executive's expectations of staff development. In R.S. Abruzzese (Ed.), *Nursing staff development: Strategies for success* (pp. 65–78). St. Louis, MO: Mosby-Year Book, Inc.

Oberst, M.T. (1985). Integrating research and clinical practice roles. *Topics in Clinical Nursing, 7*(2), 14–17.

Oliver, S.K. (1984). The effects of continuing education on the clinical behavior of nurses. *The Journal of Continuing Education in Nursing, 15,* 130–134.

O'Shea, A.M. (1994). Transitioning professional nurses into home care: A 6-month mentorship program. *Journal of Home Health Care Practice, 6*(4), 67–72.

Percival, E., Anderson, M., & Lawson, D. (1994). Assessing beginning level competencies: The first step in continuing education. *The Journal of Continuing Education in Nursing, 25*(3), 139–142.

Polit, D.F., & Hungler, B.P. (1995). *Essentials of nursing research: Methods and applications.* Philadelphia: J.B. Lippincott.

Rath, D., Boblin-Cummings, S., Bauman, A., Parrott, E., & Parsons, M. (1996). Individualized enhancement programs for nurses that promote competency. *The Journal of Continuing Education in Nursing, 27*(1), 12–16.

Rodriguez, L., & Abruzzese, R.S. (1996). Enhancing human resources for staff development. In R.S. Abruzzese (Ed.),

Nursing staff development: Strategies for success (pp. 106–117). St. Louis, MO: Mosby-Year Book, Inc.

Shaffer, F., & Kobs, A. (1997). Measuring competencies of temporary staff. *Nursing Management, 28*(5), 41–45.

Sheridan, D.R., & O'Grady, T. (1996). Nursing staff development. In R.S. Abruzzese (Ed.), *Nursing staff development: Strategies for success* (pp. 15–27). St. Louis, MO: Mosby-Year Book, Inc.

Snyder-Halpern, R., & Buczkowski, E. (1990). Performance-based staff development: A baseline for clinical competence. *Journal of Nursing Staff Development, 6*(1), 7–11.

Stevenson, B., Doorley, J., Moddeman, G., & Benson-Landau, M. (1995 May–June). The preceptor experience: A qualitative study of perceptions of nurse preceptors regarding the preceptor role. *Journal of Nursing Staff Development, 1*(3), 160–165.

Swendsen-Boss, L.A. (1985). Teaching clinical competence. *Nurse Educator, 10*(4), 8–12.

Yoder Wise, P.S. (1996). Learning needs assessment. In R.S. Abruzzese (Ed.), *Nursing staff development: Strategies for success* (pp. 183–202). St. Louis, MO: Mosby-Year Book, Inc.

Young, S., Theriault, J., & Collins, D. (1989 May–June). The nurse preceptor: Preparation and needs. *Journal of Nursing Staff Development, 5*(3), 127–131.

Yuan, J.R. (1995). Staff development in a home health agency. In M. Harris (Ed.). *Handbook of home health care administration* (pp. 401–410). Gaithersburg, MD: Aspen Publishers.

CHAPTER 4

Constructing Competency Programs in Home Care

"Failing to plan is a plan to fail."
—Effie Jones

LAYING THE FOUNDATION

The first question to answer before constructing a competency program is "Why do it?" An organization is most likely motivated because of regulatory or accrediting standards. Other answers would include (1) risk management issues, (2) the desire to provide safe, quality care in a setting that is largely unsupervised, (3) continuous performance improvement, (4) organizational or departmental philosophy, (5) to expedite the orientation process in a cost-effective manner, (6) to provide a mechanism that will allow staff to receive the same education and training, (7) to prepare new staff to function as productive individuals within a predetermined time frame, and (8) perhaps to expand the scope of practice for a particular role (Exhibit 4–1). Competency program development can be troublesome. It requires careful consideration of the pre-development issues presented earlier as well as strategic planning and continuous quality monitoring. This chapter will attempt to map out the fundamental steps required to be successful at developing and maintaining a high-caliber competency program in home care.

There are many competency models from which to choose. Abruzzese (1996) describes six models, many of which overlap one another (Exhibit 4–2). The competency-based model has been chosen as the most functional model for home care and is best utilized as the foundation or core aspect in competency program development. In this era of managed care with the primary focus on outcomes, competency-based methods best fit the regulatory requirements at this time. Aspects of the other six models are incorporated into the competency-based framework. Because of adult learners' varied preferences for learning styles, it is best to utilize a combined approach to competency program development.

DETERMINANTS OF COMPETENCE

Various determinants and/or disciplines are responsible for setting standards for competent practice. They either direct how to measure competence or specifically dictate what to measure. The determinants and disciplines include regulatory and accrediting bodies, such as Medicare, Community Health Accreditation Program (CHAP), the Joint Commission, professional standards, and standards of care for specific patient populations, practitioners, and home care organizations. Each will be explored in order to provide a comprehensive overview and understanding of the collective determinants of competency.

Regulatory and Accrediting Bodies

The three entities that are well known to the home care industry include Medicare Conditions of Participation (COP) for Home Health Agencies, the Joint Commission, and the CHAP.

Exhibit 4–1 Reasons To Develop a Competency Program in Home Care

- Regulatory or accrediting standards
- Risk management issues
- Desire to provide safe, quality care
- Continuous quality improvement
- Organizational or departmental philosophy
- Expedition of orientation process in a cost-effective manner
- Provision of consistent education and training
- Preparation of productive individuals
- Expansion of the scope of practice

Exhibit 4–2 Orientation Models

- Traditional lectures and buddy system
- Contracts and self-directed study
- Internships and rotations
- Preceptors and mentors
- Competency-based orientation
- Performance-based development system

Source: Reprinted with permission from R.S. Abruzzese, & B. Quinn O'Neill. Orientation for General and Specialty Areas, in *Nursing Staff Development: Strategies for Success*, R.S. Abruzzese, ed., p. 263, © 1996, St. Louis, MO, Mosby-Year Book, Inc.

Each is unique, yet similar in requirements for monitoring the quality of care delivery in the home care industry. CHAP and the Joint Commission are the two independent organizations accrediting home care, while Medicare functions to provide a framework on which services and policies may be based and serves as the minimum standards for the home care industry (Warner & Albert, 1997). The competency requirements of each entity will be explored.

The Medicare COP speak to the competency of all clinical disciplines to various degrees. For all disciplines, the COP define the required personnel qualifications, such as the years of clinical experience, education, eligibility for National Registration Examinations, duties, and membership in professional organizations. These, in essence, can be considered parts of competency, whereby the competency process truly begins during the pre-employment period when the aforementioned information is collected and reviewed.

The training, ongoing competency requirements, and inservice training for home care aides are specifically defined in the Medicare COP. It also speaks of the qualifications of the instructors who are responsible for training the home care aides and to the competency determinations and documentation requirements. The Medicare COP have truly been a forerunner in establishing comprehensive competency re-

quirements of a paraprofessional role. It is assumed that this has occurred in part because of the nature of home care being largely unsupervised and because the role of a home care aide is not licensed or governed by a professional body. The Medicare defined home care aide competency components can be viewed as core elements or skills and only as the foundation for an aide competency program (see Appendix C). Additional competencies should be identified based upon the patient population being cared for and scope of practice defined by the organization.

CHAP is a consumer-driven accrediting body in business for more than 30 years and is an independent subsidiary of the National League for Nursing. CHAP functions to serve the public by providing disclosure of both profit and not-for-profit home care organizations' measurement of standards (Zink, 1996). The CHAP 1993 *Standards of Excellence for Home Care Organizations* contains minimal reference to clinical competency for professionals. The two areas identified fall under CIII, which states that

the organization has adequate human, financial, and physical resources which are effectively organized to accomplish its stated purpose. CIII.1h. indicates that an annual formal performance evaluation is completed on all employees by the appropriate supervisor and is signed by each employee including a statement that indicated the supervisor's assessment of employee fulfillment of job requirements including home care aide skills or competency evaluation. The second area CIII.1i. relates that the organization provides for staff development through orientation, inservice education and continuing education programs (CHAP, 1993).

CIII.1h. merely mentions the word competency but does not expand upon how or what to assess. CIII.1i. indicates that a formal orientation program exists for all disciplines, that current information be provided specific to the discipline, and that staff integrate new knowledge in the performance of their responsibilities when applicable. CHAP does speak to the competencies of paraprofessionals under AIII. The paraprofessional services program has adequate human, financial, and physical resources effectively organized to accomplish its purpose (CHAP, 1993). The standard contains the requirements for hiring, training, and competency assessment and almost mirrors the Medicare COP for home care aide services. In addition, CHAP speaks to the training requirements for personal care, environmental support, and chore service personnel. Overall, the CHAP standards are quite exiguous in regard to directing a home care organization in developing and monitoring competency of its professional staff.

The Joint Commission's 1997–1998 *Comprehensive Accreditation Manual for Home Care* (1996) demonstrates the importance of individual competency on the ability of home care organizations to deliver high-quality patient care within the "Management of Human Resources" chapter. The preface of this chapter states that the goal of the management of human resources' function is to identify and provide the right number of competent staff to meet the needs of patients served by the organization. It also implies that the experience, education, and abilities of

staff are confirmed, that a process is designed to assess competence on a periodic and ongoing basis, and that staff competence is maintained and improved through educational endeavors that are provided by the organization. Hence, a competency program in home health care is essential for successful accreditation and is just plain old good practice in our litigious society and in this era of managed care. And of all premises, the most important is to help ensure that quality patient care is being delivered.

Six of the most significant Management of Human Resources standards are worthy of comment as they impact greatly upon competency program development. They include HR.4, HR.4.1, HR.4.2, HR.5.1, HR.6, and HR.6.1.

HR.4: All staff members are oriented to the organization, and their responsibilities provide the minimum criteria that must be incorporated in an employee's orientation. Using these criteria as the foundation for an orientation program is an excellent place to begin. The criteria can be made into competency statements effortlessly. Additional content can then be built onto this framework (Exhibit 4–3).

HR.4.1: Personal care and support staff complete appropriate training before providing patient care. This signifies the components of training and the importance of proficiency of aide staff. The Joint Commission requirements mirror those of the Medicare regulations for home care aides.

HR.4.2: When changes in patient assignments occur, the organization orients newly assigned staff members or volunteers to their responsibilities and to patient needs, providing a safety net for staff who have no education or experience with a specific patient population, procedure, or skill. This standard has broader implications in that it assists to protect the patient from harm and the employee and organization from risk management quagmires.

HR.5.1: The organization provides ongoing education, including inservice training and other activities, to maintain and improve staff competence. This standard signifies the importance of developing mechanisms that provide assessment

Exhibit 4–3 Core Clinical Competencies for All Disciplines

Competency

1. Demonstrate strategies to minimize safety risks in the community.
2. Demonstrate correct bag technique.
3. Demonstrate standard precautions against blood and body fluid pathogens. (Use of PPE)
4. Demonstrate handwashing.
5. Demonstrate timely and accurate communication with colleagues.
6. Demonstrate an effective working plan for time management and organization.
7. Demonstrate at least minimal documentation proficiency.
8. Demonstrate, organize, and effectively complete at least one home visit.
9. Incorporate cultural, age-appropriate, family, and environmental data into care, teaching, and assessment.
10. Successfully complete and/or report data appropriately.
11. Successfully demonstrate effective map reading and navigational skills.
12. Monitor and/or report patient response to therapeutic interventions.
13. Complete mandatory inservice requirements as outlined by organization.

of learning needs and provision of inservice and continuing education to meet the identified needs and improve competence. The organization determines the number of educational programs that staff must attend each year. Many mechanisms exist to provide learning such as lectures, computer-assisted instruction, journal articles and clubs, audiovisual resources, and self-instruction.

HR.6: The organization assesses, maintains, and improves the competence of all care and service staff members. HR.6 is the essence of a competency program. It indicates that there should be a qualified individual to assess competency in a systematic, measurable, and objective way and a way to identify what competencies to assess. The competencies must be documented, and in addition to the orientation requirements, the frequency of competency assessment needs to be defined.

HR.6.1: The organization collects, aggregates, and analyzes data on staff competence to identify and respond to staff learning needs. This standard provides insight into the type of information that is needed to develop and maintain a quality competency program. Data can be obtained from a number of sources such as supervisory visits, results of needs assessments and performance improvement studies, patient care needs related to new or changed processes, or needs related to operation or maintenance of medical equipment.

The Management of Human Resources standards discussed are applicable to all employees, contracted staff, and volunteers whose job duties and responsibilities include patient care or whose job duties and responsibilities impact patient care. This includes nursing directors, supervisors, and coordinators who make home visits to provide patient care services or conduct patient assessment and educational activities over the telephone (Friedman, 1996). As an accrediting body, the Joint Commission does not specifically dictate which competencies need to be assessed. Instead, it provides a broad structure of what should be included in the competency program. It is the home care organization's responsibility to define how it operationalizes its competency program and its competencies and performance improvement processes, including the frequency with which measurement will occur. In short, make sure that what you plan to do matches what your policies state you should be doing.

Professional Standards

Professional standards should also be used as determinants of competency. The licensing body for professional disciplines is the most logical entity from which to obtain professional standards. In addition, the majority of professional organizations maintain written standards that describe competent practice. The standards are used to guide professional practice. For example, the specialty practice of home care nursing abides by the American Nurses Association's (ANA) *Standards of Home Health Nursing Practice* (Appendix A). The ANA states that "the purpose of *Standards of Home Health Nursing Practice* is to fulfill the profession's obligation to provide a means of improving the quality of care provided to consumers. Standards reflect the current state of knowledge in the field and are therefore provisional, dynamic, and subject to testing and subsequent change" (ANA, 1986). It is highly recommended to review professional licensing standards such as individual state nurses' practice acts and professional organizational standards prior to designing competencies. Doing so will provide insight into criteria for practice, components of practice, practice behaviors, and entry into practice competencies of both the generalist and specialist. For unlicensed positions, resources can include governmental agencies, accreditation bodies, professional organizations to whom the unlicensed position reports, and industry standards (e.g., National Association for Home Care).

Standards of Care

The standards of care for specific patient populations and disease processes are excellent references to employ in developing competencies. For example, exploring and adapting the American Association of Critical Care Nurses' standards of care to the competencies of a high-tech home care team would be a very credible and inquisitive approach. Likewise would be to apply the Nurses' Association of the American College of Obstetricians and Gynecologists standards of care to the competencies of a maternal-child team. Professional organizations' standards of care are by and large seen as industry standards of care and are, therefore, always a first-rate resource for competency development.

Practitioners

Practitioners are utilized as determiners of competency. Various practitioners, in addition to staff development personnel, should be utilized as resources when developing competencies. They include proficient to expert staff in the role being assessed, managers and administrators, clinical nurse specialists, nurse practitioners, physical and occupational therapists, medical social workers, speech therapists, quality assurance and improvement personnel, and possibly even physicians. The practitioners should be utilized in their area(s) of expertise. Practitioners from various disciplines can bring a wealth of knowledge and real-life meaning to the competencies being identified and assessed. Often a multidisciplinary approach can lead to better outcomes for the competency program.

Home Care Organizations

Home care organizations set the preliminary determinants of competence during the hiring process. It is during this time that issues of credentialing are explored, such as licensure and certification. In addition, educational background and clinical experience particular to the identified job function are explored. Information is gathered during the interview process to further identify whether the candidate meets the qualifications of the job description or has the potential ability to do so. The candidate may be requested to complete a self-assessment of his or her skill ability or complete an examination to measure his or her knowledge of particular aspects of home care or care delivery. For example, an examination that would determine the applicant's comprehension and synthesis of the concepts of pharmacotherapy and administration would be utilized. It is essential that the disciplines involved in the hiring process work within a seamless framework. These disciplines include management, human resources, and staff development. It is to the organization's advantage if criteria are set in advance, identifying the personal characteristics that would best match the position. Management, human resources, and staff development must present a united effort, working like a hand in glove in order to find the best candidate and fit for the organization.

A second responsibility of home care organizations is to collect and utilize preexisting data to identify competencies that are organization specific. Data from infection control monitors, incident reports, patient surveys, and other performance improvement initiatives should be identified as critical competencies and form the foundation for annual competency development and evaluation.

The determinants of competency are not to be used in isolation of one another; instead, they are to be integrated into a comprehensive resource to be referenced by staff development. The integration of the determinants will lead to a better quality product and respect from administrative and clinical personnel, regulatory bodies, and payers.

EVALUATORS OF COMPETENCE

The ideal primary evaluator of competence should be staff development. Staff development's inherent role is that of competency program planner, developer, implementor, and evaluator. In the home health care setting where there may only be one individual provided with this responsibility, it is a common practice for staff development to seek out the assistance of advanced practice clinicians or clinical managers to assist with the development and implementation of the competency assessment process. In addition, clinical staff who demonstrate expertise in a specific area based upon certification, advanced education, or years of clinical experience would qualify as evaluators of competency as well.

Job titles should not always be a guarantee of competency. For instance, it should not be assumed that just because an individual carries the title of clinical manager that clinical competency is automatically bestowed upon the manager for

the identified skills. After identifying the skills to be assessed, staff development should seek out evaluators based upon their education, certification, and experience with the identified skills. In doing so, the competency evaluation program will be better developed and will demonstrate quality learning and assessment techniques. It should also be noted that evaluators should be observed and deemed competent by a like discipline prior to evaluating others (Ondeck, 1997). Evaluators of competence do not have to be employees of the organization. As long as the aforementioned criteria are met, individuals from other organizations, including organizations outside of the home care arena, can be utilized. The driving force will be the identified skills that have been chosen to be assessed. To help clarify this point, consider that one of the competencies identified is wound debridement. Wound debridement was identified on the annual needs assessment because of an increase in the volume of patients being seen with venous stasis ulcers. If there were no individuals within the organization who were considered proficient or expert at this task, then an individual outside of the organization would need to be solicited to assist with the competency program. An enterostomal (ET) nurse or wound care specialist from an acute care setting or outpatient setting would be a fine choice. Staff development could develop the competency requirements based upon the industry standards in collaboration with the ET nurse or wound care specialist, and then the ET nurse or wound care specialist could educate, demonstrate, and assess competency of wound debridement. Today, with the increase in the number of mergers and alliances being formed, staff development may have access to clinical experts in many disciplines and settings who can assist with competency evaluation at no added cost to the organization.

COMPETENCY MEASUREMENTS

The synonyms of competence—capability, capacity, ability, efficiency, and proficiency—all have similarities and dissimilarities in their definitions. Examining the word competence from an educator's perspective would lead one to question its intent. If a home health care provider demonstrates ability (physical, cognitive, interpersonal) to perform a specific skill or task in isolation, does it necessarily mean that he or she is proficient at that skill or task in the home care setting? The premise here is that the word *competence* can be viewed from many different perspectives and paradigms; therefore, prior to designing a competency program, the words *competence* and *competency* should be bestowed a definition that matches the mission and goals of staff development and the organization as a whole. Alspach (1992) relates that "having the capacity to perform effectively is not the same thing as actually performing effectively, describing that the validation of knowledge and skill components of competence only tell whether an individual has the potential to function effectively at the bedside, not whether [he or she functions] effectively" (p. 10). She further states that "because competence and competency are not synonymous we need to shift semantically and operationally from the notion of competence to the notion of competency." Competency definitions by del Bueno, Barker, and Christmyer (1981); ANA (1984); Benner (1984); or Alspach (1996) can be individualized to meet the organization's needs prior to program development and competency measurement determination.

Competency measurements can be considered mechanisms that allow for demonstration of a level of skill and knowledge, critical thinking ability, and interpersonal persona that meets the job requirements set forth by the organization. Competency is the synthesis of the aforementioned and demonstration of the ability to perform or fulfill the job requirements in clinical practice as defined. The criteria set forth by the evaluators are based upon the organization's specific determinants of competency. From a staff development perspective, competency measurement should be based upon two important premises: managerial aspects and dimensions of competent performance. Managerial as-

pects include such considerations as the time allotment for competency measurement, number of individuals being assessed, fiscal resources, teaching and learning resources and style, and motivation. The managerial aspects can be viewed as the backdrop for competency measurement. They set the stage for the testing environment, coloring the perceptions, actions, and abilities of the individuals being assessed. Each is highly important in assisting the educator/ evaluator to facilitate an environment that is conducive to learning and in enabling the individual who is being tested to excel to his or her fullest potential.

The dimensions of competent performance include three components: technical skills, interpersonal relation skills, and critical thinking skills (del Bueno, Weeks, & Brown-Stewart, 1987). Technical skills are those identified for assessment based upon such things as frequency of performance and organizational and patient care needs. Critical thinking skills are divided into a subset that includes clinical decision making, priority setting and revising, problem solving and troubleshooting, and care planning (del Bueno et al., 1987). Critical thinking skills are often overlooked as an essential aspect of competency evaluation and must be evaluated in respect to the skill being performed. Case (1995) describes critical thinking as "a process and cognitive skill that functions in identifying and defining problems and opportunities for improvement; generating, examining and evaluating options; reaching conclusions and decisions, and creating and using criteria to evaluate decisions" (p.101). Interpersonal skills include those personality behaviors that are demonstrated during patient interaction. Interpersonal skills, just as critical thinking ability, are essential components of competency achievement.

In order to be effective, competence-measurement techniques should take into consideration the aforementioned premises. Competence measurements include computer and paper and pencil tests, exemplars, role playing and scenarios, gaming, and observation of simulated practice, whereas competency measurement includes direct observation of clinical practice. Competence measurement occurs during or after the following learning activities: lecture, computer-assisted instruction, self-learning modules, audiovisual programs, case-study presentations, direct patient care, or simulation of care. Learning activities are discussed in more detail in Chapter 5. The reader is also referred to Gianella (1996) for a detailed description of each. Recognizing and understanding the variations of competence and competency measurements will enable the educator to select the most appropriate measurement mechanisms based upon the learning need, available resources, and organizational goals.

COMPETENCY ASSESSMENT IN THE HOME

Competency assessment of professional staff is new to home health care. With the advent of accreditation bodies' regulations, home care organizations began scrambling to develop competency programs or at least put individuals in place to develop such programs. Traditionally, home health care competence assessment occurred in a simulated lab, as in the case of home care aide competency assessment. It never seemed feasible to competency assess home care aides in the home setting due to the associated costs that could be attributed to the decrease in productivity, the complexity of scheduling, and the possible infringement on patients' time. However, today, after rethinking this concept, competency assessment is a feasible alternative and carries with it many benefits. It is a viable alternative, particularly for the home care aide staff, for the professional staff during orientation while they are buddied with a preceptor, and on a limited ongoing basis for all disciplines during supervisory visits. The research-based literature is virtually nonexistent surrounding the premise of competency assessment in the home for home health care providers and is in need of scholarly inquiry.

The benefits of in-home competency assessment include (1) direct observation of competency in clinical practice, (2) opportunity for

teaching and learning through direct observation, (3) opportunity for direct identification of incompetence and immediate remediation, (4) intangible marketing benefits (e.g., patient and family admiration and confidence in the home care organization's commitment to assessing its clinical providers' level of competency), and (5) decrease in cost of competency assessment (e.g., the costs associated with not having to remove staff from the field to participate in simulated lab evaluation) (Exhibit 4–4). Evaluation occurs during the patient visit, affecting productivity minimally or not at all. An example of a home care aide in-home competency assessment will be provided to clarify how such a program can be implemented.

In-Home Competency Assessment of the Home Care Aide

Core competency skills such as those identified by the Medicare COP are placed onto a competency template (see Appendix B). The aide staff are provided with a copy of the template and are instructed that it is their responsibility to have the core skills evaluated in the home by a registered nurse (RN). The time frame for completion is 1 year. Upon completion of the template, it is then forwarded to staff development and the aide's manager for review and filing in the human resources file. The premise of this in-home competency evaluation program is that the home care aide is given the accountability to complete his or her annual core competency assessment within the identified time frame. This accountability itself offers many benefits, including increased job satisfaction, learning, and self-esteem for the aide, and less responsibility and work for staff development. The aides are instructed to plan ahead and to identify skills that will be completed during an upcoming home visit. He or she contacts the RN for a joint supervisory visit. During the visit, the RN observes the identified core skills and documents satisfactory or unsatisfactory completion of the skill. Staff development obtains a "buy-in" from management and staff,

Exhibit 4–4 Benefits of In-Home Competency Assessment

> - Most reliable measurement of competency in clinical practice
> - Opportunity for teaching and learning through direct observation
> - Opportunity for direct identification of incompetence and immediate remediation
> - Intangible marketing benefits
> - Decrease in cost of competency assessment

educating both on program components and dynamics prior to the start of the program. It is essential that the RN staff be educated on the program components. They must promptly evaluate and notify management and staff development of findings for remediation purposes. In-home aide competence assessment is particularly valuable in the home care setting, where care delivery is largely unsupervised on a day-to-day basis.

The potential for in-home competency assessment is immense. The success of such a program depends primarily upon support from management and staff. Bearing a creative sense and the ability to take risks are essential elements in the quest to develop programs that are more cost-effective and less burdensome to the organization. Such programs are certainly worth exploring in this era of cost-cutting initiatives, quality care endeavors, and achievement of admiration and respect from the community, physicians, and payers.

A successful competency program in home care is dependent upon strategic planning, identification of the determinants and evaluators of competence, selection of competency measurements, and development of a plan for how competency assessment will be carried out within the home care organization. Providing adequate time for thorough thoughtfulness and planning will result in a structured foundation upon which an honorable competency assessment program can be developed.

REFERENCES

Abruzzese, R.S. (1996). Evaluation in nursing staff development. In R.S. Abruzzese (Ed.), *Nursing staff development: Strategies for success* (2nd ed.) (pp. 242–258). St. Louis, MO: Mosby-Year Book, Inc.

Alspach, G. (1992). Concern and confusion over competence. *Critical Care Nurse, 12*(4), 9–11.

Alspach, G. (1996). *Designing competency assessment programs: A handbook for nurses and health-related professionals.* Pensacola, FL: National Nursing Staff Development Organization.

American Nurses Association. (1984). *Standards for continuing education in nursing.* Kansas City, MO: Author.

American Nurses Association. (1986). *Standards of home health nursing practice.* Kansas City, MO: Author.

Benner, P. (1984). *From novice to expert: Excellence and power in clinical nursing practice.* Menlo Park, CA: Addison-Wesley.

Case, B. (1995). Roles. In *Certification for staff development.* Symposium for the Medical College of Pennsylvania and Hahneman University, Philadelphia.

Community Health Accreditation Program. (1993). National League for Health Care Inc. and Community Health Accreditation Program, Inc. *Standards of excellence for home care organizations.* New York: Author.

del Bueno, D., Barker, F., & Christmyer, C. (1981). Implementing a competency-based orientation program. *Journal of Nursing Administration, 11*(2), 24–29.

del Bueno, D.J., Weeks, L., & Brown-Stewart, P. (1987). Clinical assessment centers: A cost-effective alternative for competency development. *Nursing Economics, 5*(1), 21–26.

Friedman, M.M. (1996). Competence assessment: How to meet the intent of the Joint Commission on Accreditation of Healthcare Organizations' management of human resources standards. *Home Healthcare Nurse, 14*(10), 771–774.

Gianella, A. (1996). Effective teaching and learning strategies. In R.S. Abruzzese (Ed.), *Nursing staff development: Strategies for success* (2nd ed.) (pp. 223–241). St. Louis, MO: Mosby-Year Book, Inc.

Joint Commission on Accreditation of Healthcare Organizations (1996). *Accreditation manual for home care, Vol I: Standards.* Oakbrook Terrace, IL: Author.

Ondeck, D.A. (1997). Competency assessment for maternal-child nursing. *Home Healthcare Management and Practice, 9*(3), 78–80.

Warner, I., & Albert, R. (1997). Avoiding legal land mines in home health care nursing. *Home Health Care Management and Practice, 9*(6), 8–16.

Zink, M.R. (1996). Home care accreditation with the community health accreditation program: Part I: Overview. *Home Healthcare Nurse, 14*(8), 590–594.

CHAPTER 5

The Educational Process Applied to the Home Care Setting

"Not only is there an art in knowing a thing, but also a certain art in teaching it."
—Cicero

This chapter reviews the basic components of the educational process. Those who are asked to assume the role of educator in home care organizations may have little or no formalized training, education, or experience in education to prepare for this role. The challenge is to plan activities for learning that promote critical thinking, commitment to excellence, problem solving, and accountability (Green, 1994). Clinical specialists' roles have evolved to include more educational functions, and a study revealed that most clinical specialist preparatory programs do not address principles of adult learning, teaching and learning strategies, curriculum planning and development, or even how to perform measurement and evaluation (Radke & McArt, 1993). Although it is important that the nurse who is acting as educator has some experience in the home care setting and is proficient in basic home care skills, these qualities are not sufficient alone. Without a working knowledge of the educational process, there is greater potential for ineffective educational programs, unmet learning needs, staff frustration, and educator burnout. Knowledge of educational process alone is also not sufficient, for home care is truly a specialty that must be well understood. This chapter will explore the basics of good teaching and its application to the home care setting.

PHILOSOPHICAL FOUNDATION AND RESOURCES

Educators should have a purpose, philosophy, and departmental objectives. A well-run staff development department can motivate, challenge, encourage, and mentor. A poorly run department can be the downfall for the home care organization. At some agencies, the educator has responsibilities in addition to staff development, but where possible, at least in larger agencies, this should be avoided. Several excellent resources are available to the staff development educator. The National Nursing Staff Development Organization (NNSDO) offers a newsletter and reduced subscription price for the *Journal of Staff Development* to its members. There are texts available that are written especially for staff development educators. As of today, only two of those publications are for educators in home care. As mentioned previously, there are articles that discuss competency and inservice issues, mostly in the acute care setting. And lastly, educators can utilize materials targeting non-health educators as a resource. Some of the leading nursing educational theorists have adapted frameworks to nursing that were created by non-nursing educators (Benner, 1984).

Although at this time there is no association for home care educators, it is probable that some type of organized network or special interest focus group will be developed in the future. At the National Association for Home Care and Home Health Nurses Association conventions, there is frequently a gathering and networking of educators, sharing ideas and support. Another potential source of support might be the educators at other home care organizations in the area, although the organizations are usually in competition with one another.

NEEDS ASSESSMENTS

The educational process begins with a needs assessment. Needs assessments save time and resources by ensuring that time will not be wasted teaching what is already known. Adult learning principles dictate that the learner benefit from providing input about his or her education (Knowles, 1984). Adults will weigh the benefits of an educational program before deciding whether or not to participate (Abruzzese, 1996). To define a learning need, the learner must have a clear idea of what his or her job requires. According to the American Nurses Association's 1994 staff development standards, needs assessments help identify the discrepancy between what is desired and what exists. Although staff usually know which areas need the most education, it is helpful when managers let staff know when they are making errors, rather than waiting for an annual performance evaluation. This enables the staff member to have a perception of his or her own needs and strengths. Eight full-time acute care registered nurses over the age of 50 were interviewed to determine how they felt they were perceived by others and how they perceived their own competence (Wheeler, 1994). Based on the results of the study, as nurses mature, it is possible that they have a better sense of their competence.

Needs assessments provide a valid way to form educational plans. There are different needs assessment models. A needs assessment should be a priority for any staff development educator, for it is the basis for measurement of his or her efficacy and can be used to market educational programs to staff and management (Green, 1994). Education must first be done for all staff regarding the purpose and importance of needs assessments. Educators must teach staff that they are responsible for their own learning and allow them to be self-directed (Abruzzese, 1996). A literature review demonstrates that there are many opposing views about the value

and methods to conduct a needs assessment (Krisjanson & Scanlan, 1989). Based on a review of 132 books and articles about needs assessments, there are four broad themes in the literature about needs assessments (Krisjanson & Scanlan, 1989). This section will discuss two of these themes: the need to define the construct "need" and the methodology for conducting needs assessments. Then, this section will discuss interpretation of needs assessments.

Definition: What Is a Need?

There are many indicators of learning needs, from requests for specific information to an increase in incident reports related to a certain piece of equipment. Needs assessments are the next step, when a judgment is made to prioritize learning needs and take into account the learner's perception of needs. If any of the employees in a home care organization were asked to identify educational needs, responses would probably vary depending on their most recent experiences. For this reason, it is best to present a scripted list to focus their responses, so that another pressing need that has not been evident recently will not be overlooked.

There are many different types of learning needs. Home care nursing has many demands, requiring knowledge and skills that are expansive. Although staff may have an interest in a particular topic, that alone does not justify the expense and labor of planning an inservice. The goal of the educator is to help the learner identify what learning priorities are. The needs assessment must be presented to clarify what an actual need is. Overanalysis of responses given on a needs assessment is time consuming and unnecessary, but there are some considerations. According to Puetz (1987), individuals may have trouble distinguishing needs from wants. The staff should be taught the difference between a *genuine educational need* and just a *perceived need* (Atwood & Ellis, 1971). Learners should be assisted to distinguish a need from a want using the following criteria. First of all, if this need was met, would they be better able to perform their job? Secondly, is this the most important need? Lastly, does this perceived deficit affect quality of care frequently? Hopefully, learners also want to learn the skills that they know they need to learn more about, or the educational experience will not be mutually enjoyable. Certainly, one would expect professionals employed in home care to be able to distinguish which aspects of their job need the most attention, but it is possible that learners can be blind to some areas of weakness in their own practice (Krisjanson & Scanlan, 1989). Organizational needs for education can also be used to develop learning objectives. Needs of an organization are revealed through accreditation surveys, customer input, performance review (quality assurance and quality improvement), or manager and administrator input. An educational need is more than just a deficit between staff performance and supervisor expectation, because it is possible that supervisors may not have expectations that are realistic, and their opinion that there is a deficit may not be based on empirical data (Krisjanson & Scanlan, 1989).

Methods for Conducting a Needs Assessment

The Joint Commission (1996) requires the educator to provide education based on needs that have been demonstrated. There are many ways to collect data to determine educational needs. Formal data collection, semiformal, and informal approaches can be considered (Dyche, 1988). The most typical needs assessments are formal approaches that include using documents, audits, department minutes, questionnaires, and other systematic forms of data collection. Formal needs assessments require the most resources of time and money. The methods that are the most applicable to home care include subjective/objective data collection through questionnaires and Delphi techniques. If a questionnaire is used, it is a challenge to develop a creative way to motivate all staff members to complete and return their needs assessment tools. Considering how infrequently some contract staff are available, perhaps mailing the tool

with a memo explaining it could be useful. Management must support the needs assessment tool and complete one as well. Delphi techniques are used when an expert panel is consulted through the use of a questionnaire, the results are tabulated and distributed to the panel, a follow-up questionnaire is sent, and the cycle repeats until satisfactory data are obtained. Semiformal techniques for collecting data are random checks of staff performance, document sampling, or staff request (Dyche, 1988). Other semiformal sources of data to determine educational needs include committee minutes, performance improvement data, utilization review, and incident/accident reports (NNSDO, 1994). Semiformal techniques save time, but may not provide a complete representation of what educational needs are. Informal assessment is unstructured, coming from overheard statements, inferences, and indirect sources, such as physicians, patient surveys, peer groups, literature, management recommendation, organizational policy and procedural changes, and so on. A focus group can be utilized effectively and is usually quicker to implement than a full organizationwide survey (Puetz, 1987). Changes in professional standards, patient populations, technology, or delivery patterns must all be considered when assessment for needs is conducted (NNSDO, 1994). Lastly, the skills self-assessment completed by all new orientees within the past 3 to 6 months should be summarized to check for clusters of weak areas.

Creating a Needs Assessment Questionnaire

Educational goals evolve not only from the philosophy of the educational department, but from the organizational goals as well. Priorities between organizations may differ. Organizations may adapt the sample needs assessment provided as they wish. Generally, the needs assessment is created with the following goals in mind: (1) Staff will increase their continuing education; (2) Specific educational needs will be identified related to topics such as disease process, disease state management, new procedures, new equipment, and new types of clients; (3) Individual needs and resultant education records will be maintained in human resources files; (4) Staff competence will be self-evaluated using a specified framework; and (5) An educational intervention will be developed based on needs assessment findings and other analyses (McAnnally & Barnett, 1997). Other organization-specific goals might include that the use of needs assessment findings will "assist in development of a buddy system to mentor less experienced nurses" or "assist in selection of specialty teams."

With the appropriate goals in mind, the needs assessment can be developed. Job analysis, expert consensus, professional standards, and scope of practice can all be used to develop needs assessment tools. Job analysis may alone identify all the components necessary for job performance (Garland, 1996). Ironically, one flaw of the needs assessment is that it isolates aspects of job performance; staff tend to evaluate their competence based on caring for a patient with one isolated diagnosis. Patients seldom have such a simple disease process. Also, obtaining consensus "from the experts" alone can lead to designing an incomplete list or one that is too broad (Garland, 1996). A current textbook of the discipline to be assessed and relevant policies and procedures can also be consulted. Lastly, the performance improvement data from the organization, informal observations, and supervisor interviews all can have an impact on assessment tool development.

There are some needs assessments already designed, such as Benner's Nursing Expertise Self Report Scale (Garland, 1996). Although this model has much merit, it is not specifically created for home care nurses. When developing a needs assessment, a framework is helpful. Benner's (1984) competencies identify some excellent measures that might otherwise not be considered such as "crisis management" (Garland, 1996). There are numerous frameworks that can be utilized, such as the Albrecht model (1990). This model was adapted to home care and was administered to a group of 95 registered nurses (Astarita, Materna, & Savage, in press). The data that were collected were easily formatted into a competency program.

Another way of constructing a needs assessment tool is to identify the basic body systems and corresponding disease processes, with relevant skills listed below. For example, the basic systems are cardiovascular, gastrointestinal, genitourinary, integumentary, musculoskeletal, neurological, and respiratory. This list could be adjusted based upon the most frequent diagnoses served by the organization (Astarita et al., in press). Under the basic heading "cardiology" could be written the most common diagnoses for which the organization cares, for example, angina, atrial fibrillation, cardiac tamponade, congestive heart failure, hypertension, myocardial infarction, pericarditis, and so on. Beneath the diagnoses, the most commonly needed job-related skills are listed, such as cardiac assessment, risk factor assessment and teaching, and other skills. The skills that are done on a daily basis and are low risk should not be included, for they can be implied with licensure or certification in most cases (Kobs, 1996).

A close-ended questionnaire contains a list of topics that learners can select from. It is wise to include a few lines for comments at the bottom, however, to allow for input about topics not on the list (Krisjanson & Scanlan, 1989). No matter how experienced the educator is, it is important to let others review the needs assessment tool to evaluate for validity and reliability. It is suggested that local agencies consider pooling resources such as needs assessment tools, adapting them to be organization-specific.

A needs assessment is also a good mechanism to solicit volunteers to work on an education committee and gain information about learning methods preferred by respondents (Green, 1994). Although everyone cannot learn using the method they prefer for every topic, most learners can at least feel they have some control. Green's model needs assessment (1994) phrased the question by asking, "Which learning methods are you willing to try?" placing lines for check marks next to each method.

All components of a needs assessment must be clear to the learner. Two blank lines can be utilized under each system to fill in other skills or diagnoses. This format should be updated and modified on a regular basis. The learner can be asked to rate his or her knowledge and abilities as novice, advanced beginner, competent, proficient, or expert in each of the components (Benner, 1984). The difficulties about using a multi-level assessment tool are that staff may under- or overestimate their abilities based on confidence issues, or they may not understand the various levels' definitions. Secondly, there is potential that low self-ratings may further perpetuate feelings of low self-worth. Staff need to be motivated at every level and encouraged to strive for the next level, including all the responsibilities and work that accompany it. Furthermore, Benner (1984), referring to nurses, states that all do not process at the same rate from novice to expert. It is hopeful that comparisons will not be made among those who "started employment at the same time." It is important to mention that Benner described the novice as one who had no experience in the setting. She equated the new graduate with the advanced beginner level (Benner, 1984). Creating a needs assessment is similar to creating a skills checklist (Appendix B). In some organizations, the same tool that is initiated at orientation may be used as the needs assessment tool, updating as needed. A sample needs assessment is included in Exhibit 5–1.

Because the staff time is limited, the needs assessment should be brief yet as thorough as possible (Almquist & Bookbinder, 1990). Emphasis should be placed on assessment of those skills and knowledge that are most crucial to job performance and patient safety. It is important to construct a needs assessment with a reinforcement for completing it. Motivators include food, prize drawings, or other positive reinforcement.

Feedback is important to adult learners (Beeken, 1997). Immediately after the survey is administered, summarize the results and post them for the participants. Copies of the summary should be forwarded to administration and managers as well. Inservices based on needs assessments that are 6 months old offer little hope to the learner that their input was valid (Abruzzese, 1996). Another important caution about needs assessment data is that they need to be used before the information becomes outdated. Depending on the home care organization, the staff turnover may be such that a needs assessment done 6 months to 1 year ago is no longer appropriate. Client populations and organizational procedures also may have changed in the interim (Krisjanson & Scanlan, 1989). After the needs assessment has been administered, returned, and the results tabulated and distributed, the educational program should be initiated as soon as possible.

PROGRAM DEVELOPMENT

Planning an inservice is time consuming. Educators can expect to spend anywhere from 8 to 24 hours preparing a 1-hour presentation, depending on previous knowledge of the topic, the number of teaching aids developed such as handouts and overheads, and the format of the intended presentation. For example, a presentation that is strictly lecture may require more preparation time than educational games or use of pre-printed materials. The educator should consult with publishers to determine what materials have already been developed.

Objectives

Based on the results of the needs assessment, the educational plan can be developed. It is important that the educator does not impose his or her values on the data interpretation (Krisjanson & Scanlan, 1989). Specific objectives should be developed from the needs list to provide direction for teaching and evaluation (Krisjanson & Scanlan, 1989). Objectives seek a desired outcome or change in behavior of a learner and should be written using the cognitive, affective, and psychomotor domains (Marciniak, 1997). Originally created by Benjamin Bloom in 1956, each domain has subcategories that range from the simple to the highest levels of domain per-

Exhibit 5–1 Needs Assessment

Rate your overall knowledge of these topics. Circle *the number* that best corresponds to your knowledge and skill level.

	0 Very poor	1	2	3	4	5	6	7 Excellent
1. Diseases of the Circulatory System (e.g., rheumatic heart disease, hypertension, angina pectoris, congestive heart failure, cerebral vascular accident)								
A. Pathophysiology of disease process	0	1	2	3	4	5	6	7
B. Pharmacology	0	1	2	3	4	5	6	7
C. Screening/diagnostic tests	0	1	2	3	4	5	6	7
D. Assessment (physical)	0	1	2	3	4	5	6	7
E. Interventions (skilled nursing interventions such as teaching, skilled procedures, medication administration)	0	1	2	3	4	5	6	7
F. Evaluation	0	1	2	3	4	5	6	7
2. Injury and Poisoning (e.g., fractures, dislocation, internal injury, amputation, burns, toxic effects)								
A. Pathophysiology of illness/injury	0	1	2	3	4	5	6	7
B. Pharmacology	0	1	2	3	4	5	6	7
C. Screening/diagnostic tests	0	1	2	3	4	5	6	7
D. Assessment (physical)	0	1	2	3	4	5	6	7
E. Interventions (skilled nursing interventions such as teaching, skilled procedures, medication administration)	0	1	2	3	4	5	6	7
F. Evaluation	0	1	2	3	4	5	6	7
3. Infections and Parasitic Diseases (e.g., TB, septicemia, herpes, measles)								
A. Pathophysiology of disease process	0	1	2	3	4	5	6	7
B. Pharmacology	0	1	2	3	4	5	6	7
C. Screening/diagnostic tests	0	1	2	3	4	5	6	7
D. Assessment (physical)	0	1	2	3	4	5	6	7
E. Interventions (skilled nursing interventions such as teaching, skilled procedures, medication administration)	0	1	2	3	4	5	6	7
F. Evaluation	0	1	2	3	4	5	6	7

4. Diseases of the Musculoskeletal System and Connective Tissue (e.g., arthritis, rheumatism, disc disorders, acquired deformities, neuralgia, neuritis)

A. Pathophysiology of disease process	0	1	2	3	4	5	6	7
B. Pharmacology	0	1	2	3	4	5	6	7
C. Screening/diagnostic tests	0	1	2	3	4	5	6	7
D. Assessment (physical)	0	1	2	3	4	5	6	7
E. Interventions (skilled nursing interventions such as teaching, skilled procedures, medication administration)	0	1	2	3	4	5	6	7
F. Evaluation	0	1	2	3	4	5	6	7

5. Diseases of the Respiratory System (e.g., pneumonia, bronchitis, emphysema, asthma, pneumoconiosis)

A. Pathophysiology of disease process	0	1	2	3	4	5	6	7
B. Pharmacology	0	1	2	3	4	5	6	7
C. Screening/diagnostic tests	0	1	2	3	4	5	6	7
D. Assessment (physical)	0	1	2	3	4	5	6	7
E. Interventions (skilled nursing interventions such as teaching, skilled procedures, medication administration)	0	1	2	3	4	5	6	7
F. Evaluation	0	1	2	3	4	5	6	7

Courtesy of Visiting Nurse Association, Lancaster, Pennsylvania.

formance (Dyche, 1988). The advantages to having objectives are many. Objectives provide a guide for teaching, ensure focus, guide in material selection, provide standards for measurement, enhance communication between the educator and the learner, give the learner advanced notice of expectations, increase educator accountability, and, most importantly, draw the learner into organized thoughts and efforts toward meeting objectives (Dyche, 1988). Learning objectives are the link between the learner and the desired outcomes. They must state what the learner will be able to do, under what conditions, and define the acceptable level of performance or criteria (Dyche, 1988). Objectives should be learner-oriented, deal with output rather than input, and be realistic to achieve (Dyche, 1988).

Research

To begin research of a particular topic, the educator can begin the phase the writer calls "presearch." Presearch involves talking to experts in the field of interest about the topic. This important step, which serves as a precursor to reviewing the literature, helps the educator focus on the priorities, "cutting through" the nonessential information available. In addition, after talking with a few people who are knowledgeable on the topic, the educator can get a quick, effective review of the vocabulary and basic principles that are involved in the "real world" aspect of the topic, increasing comprehension as he or she reads the literature about the topic.

Next, a thorough search of the literature is essential. Educators can perpetuate the need for research-based practice in home care and should also keep current with the research relevant to activities of their job and those of all other clinical staff. Unfortunately, publication is not synonymous with research validity. Although anecdotal reports of what one educator did or qualitative research can be interesting and informative, to be considered empirical data, it must meet certain criteria. For basic guidelines to evaluating research, refer to a research text. Research should be empirically sound, with appropriate research design, sample size, and control of external variables. Reliability and validity should be demonstrated if a questionnaire or some form of survey tool was utilized to collect data (Burns & Grove, 1995). Validity is the extent to which a measurement actually measures what it claims to measure (Burns & Grove, 1995). Reliability means that the same test would consistently get the same results no matter how many times it is utilized. Most educators in the home care setting have had at least an undergraduate course in nursing research; if not, it is important they do so.

Reviewing at least three current sources is necessary for a short presentation (Burke, 1996). Most libraries have user-friendly computer workstations with access to CINAHL, MEDline, and even the Internet. You should use sources that are no more than 4 to 5 years old, unless you are referring to seminal work done on a subject that has not been replicated since (Burke, 1996). It is important to review the selected publications thoroughly. Retaining interesting bits of little-known trivia related to the topic can be used as your "hook" to spark interest (Burke, 1996).

Reality Check

Once a literature review has been completed, conflicts may emerge between current policies and procedures used in the home care organization and what current practice is as reflected in the literature. Home care agencies that have a clinical practice committee can allow the educator to present his or her research findings at meetings, and decisions can be made to alter policies to reflect current practice. Should the organization not choose to do so, the educator must teach the procedures as written, assuming there is not an extreme case where patient safety is violated or regulatory bodies have warned otherwise.

In any health care organization, it is not uncommon to have educators and clinicians in a mutual misunderstanding. Educators can potentially lose sight of what is practical and realistic for the organization; to be successful, an educator needs one foot planted in research and the other embedded in the real world. Home care administrators and managers are focused on productivity and can lose sight of the time that is required to maintain a well-run competency program. It is important that both sides work together. It is the responsibility of the educator to be sure that the educational calendar is approved by management and will be supported; for it is ineffective if no one attends.

As an educator gains experience, mistakes will be made. A particular issue that comes to mind took place when I was employed at a home care organization as an educator. One person requested an inservice on personal safety/protective equipment. I consulted with the managers, booked the room, obtained qualified speakers from the local police department, and publicized it. Everything went smoothly except only three people attended, including myself. The person who had been so adamant about the need for the inservice was not in attendance. The organization had many more significant needs at the time, and I should have rescheduled the inservice for another date. This example reinforces one of the greatest challenges of the staff development educator in home care. Educational needs revealed through assessments should result in program development and presentation as soon as possible; yet, when scheduling inservices, the educator has no way of predicting that the very staff who requested it will be able to attend.

Scheduling an Inservice

Depending on the format selected, the dates and times should be selected well enough in advance so that staff have enough notice so they can plan their caseloads on that day, but not so far in advance that many unforeseen calamities can prevent staff from attending. As mentioned in the ongoing competency chapter, staff should be consulted regarding their preferences for dates and times, and it is best to avoid presenting inservices during the holiday or peak vacation seasons or times when the weather is unpredictable. Selecting a time that everyone will agree on can seem like walking through land mines for the educator. After making the decision, a room, and possibly special equipment, needs to be reserved. If requested in advance, it is possible to have at least one manager attend on the day of the inservice, increasing credibility and acceptance of educational inservices among the staff. It is best to offer the inservice at a choice of times. Usual program length is between 45 minutes and 1 hour (Burke, 1996); longer programs would be extremely difficult for most home care staff to attend, and possibly decrease attentiveness.

Preparation of audiovisual aids is usually worth the investment of time and resources. Audiovisual aids help focus the learner on key points and can be posters, outlines, overheads, audio tapes, or any other medium. Always obtain permission before photocopying all or part of someone else's work, however (Burke, 1996). Handouts are excellent accompaniments to any presentation, for they pull the learner's background experience into the topic context, facilitating learning, and they can be used as a resource after the inservice. Some learners benefit by taking notes, but some find it too distracting and don't listen.

LEARNING STRATEGIES AND STYLES

Concepts are formed through sensory experiences (Marciniak, 1997). To learn, home care staff must remember the knowledge they have gained through disciplinary-specific education and experience. They must then apply what they have learned to clinical practice, allowing new behaviors to replace old. The inability to take what was learned and apply it clinically, a lack of clinical experience to use as a frame of reference, and a lack of desire for continual growth and advancement in the profession can decrease learning among home care staff. Generally, the more senses a learner brings to the learning experience, the more learning and retention of knowledge take place (Dyche, 1988).

Information processing is different for many learners (Colucciello, 1993). How they think and absorb information, connecting the new information with the old, is called their learning style. There are wide varieties of learning styles, so educators must adopt more than one method of teaching to reach as many staff as possible. Some are auditory learners, some are visual learners, and most are tactile, or learn best by hands-on application of what is learned (Spradley & Allender, 1996). According to Babcock and Miller (1994), there are three distinct types of learners. Adult learners can be goal-oriented, activity-oriented, or learning-oriented.

Goal-oriented learners accomplish clear objectives through episodic educational endeavors. This type of learner is more likely to pay to learn, to read current literature that is appropriate to a role, and to seek out learning opportunities (Babcock & Miller, 1994). Typically, the goal-oriented learner is the one who will continue his or her education, pursue certification in a specialty, and challenge practice that is not congruent with current literature. As with other certifications, the nurse certification through the National Association for Home Care requires continuing education.

Activity-oriented learners enjoy the social aspects of learning (Babcock & Miller, 1994). In home care, this type of learner will do everything possible to attend inservices just for the social interaction with peers. This type of learner will attend inservices that are not necessarily needed or relevant to job performance. In many home care agencies, the educator has to approve reimbursement for outside educational opportunities. Depending on the budget, some of the programs that the activity-oriented learner may wish to attend may not be regarded as the best use for educational funds. The best part about activity-oriented learners is their faithfulness in attending educational offerings.

Learning-oriented learners learn just to learn and report having been so since childhood (Babcock & Miller, 1994). They are inquisitive by nature and select activities that are educa-tional. This type of learner actually reads the owner's manual and instructions *before* assembling, checks consumer reports before a purchase, and reads about a foreign land before traveling there. This type of learner in the home care setting makes an excellent performance improvement nurse! They are motivated by self-esteem and the pleasure that learning gives them (Babcock & Miller, 1994).

Learning styles have implications for educators. When planning educational programs, the principles of adult learning and learning styles should be considered. Attempts should be made to provide reinforcement that would be appealing to all types of learners; education should have a clearly defined purpose to improve role performance, should be self-directed, should boost self-esteem, and should meet social needs of its participants. It is important to meet the needs of all who attend inservices, because in home care it takes considerable effort to be able to attend.

Adult Learning Principles Applied to Home Care

Adults have special learning needs and principles that should govern educational planning decisions. For learning to take place, an educator must earn respect and acceptance from the home care staff. Adults have unique learning principles (Knowles, 1984). Adult learning principles can be customized to the unique setting of home care (Table 5–1). Readiness is also necessary for adults to want to attend educational opportunities. Staff who are new to home care may be so overwhelmed learning their new role that they may regard other opportunities as trivial. In addition, new caregivers may very well have less time to spend pursuing education, for they have not yet developed the time management skills that come with practice. What affects the learning readiness of adults includes the life stage they are currently in, their goals, and self-expectations (Babcock & Miller, 1994). Adult learners can be dealing with developmental tasks, such as caring for aging parents, facing the empty nest syndrome, and other responsibilities.

Table 5–1 Adult Learning Principles Applied to Home Care Workers

Adult Learning Principle	*Application to Home Care Workers*
Adults need to know why they need to know something.	They learn more when they perceive that it will directly improve their ability to provide home care. Education should be specific to topics as related to home care and provide opportunities for hands-on practice.
Adults must be ready to learn.	Home care staff may not have the time in their schedules to attend an inservice or the emotional energy left to concentrate on a topic. With the unpredictable nature of home care, only the flexible survive. This should also apply to the educator, who should not take it personally if an unpredictable event affects inservice attendance. Home care staff should have input into educational planning about topics and scheduling of inservices.
Adult learners like to get credit for previous experience.	Adults are defined by their experiences (Babcock & Miller, 1994). Many make excellent teachers, mentors, and presenters. It is frequent for experienced nurses new to home care to have difficulty adjusting to feeling like novices again. One way to help them build confidence is to continue to remind them of all that they know in other specialties and pull that knowledge toward application in the home care setting. Recognize expertise and use peer mediation.
Adult learners enjoy an informal atmosphere for learning.	Home care staff don't get many opportunities to socialize among other members of the health care team. Build camaraderie through the use of interactive and fun learning experiences.
Adults are motivated through enhanced self-esteem, quality of life, and job satisfaction.	Educators need to know the hearts of the home care staff. Education should be planned opportunities for staff to further their knowledge, help their career, and build confidence. Learning should be a positive experience.
Adults benefit from collaborative learning more than authoritative teaching.	Teaching should allow for interaction between all present. In home care, the educator may have more home care experience or experience in education, but the strengths and accomplishments of the staff should also be acknowledged. It is presumptuous and almost impossible for any educator to be the consummate expert in every area, and he or she should not pretend to know everything, but rather, where to find it.

Source: Data from M. Knowles, *The Adult Learner: A Neglected Species,* © 1984, Gulf Publishing Company.

The environment must be conducive to learning as well. The learner should be comfortable, free from distractions, and able to hear and see a presentation clearly. Lighting, temperature, ventilation, space, and time of day are important considerations affecting learners (Marciniak, 1997). The attitude toward learning at an organization is also considered an environmental factor. Do management, administration, and the budget support staff attendance at internal and external educational programs? Are staff encouraged to go, given positive reinforcement, and allowed to share what they learned at staff meetings? A good indicator of the "environmental climate" of an organization is the number of staff participating in outside education, certification, and inservices. Many organizations that do not have the funds to send staff to conferences can encourage staff in other ways, helping staff realize their personal responsibility to be educated, even if it means at their own expense.

There are also specific implications for learning that correspond to each level of expertise. If the learner has rated his or her skills or knowledge in a specific area as "novice," typical needs include heavy emphasis on "how to" instruction. Advanced beginners need to learn how to take the basics and adapt them to the real world. Typically, they have a routine that is difficult for them to modify appropriately as needed, being unable to judge relative importance (Benner, 1984). The competent nurse, generally one who has been in home care 2 to 3 years, benefits from decision-making and problem-solving games and simulations that provide practice "in planning and coordinating multiple complex patient care demands." Proficient performers are best taught with case studies and being asked to provide clinical examples for principles. These nurses have home care experience between 3 and 5 years, in most cases. The proficient and expert nurse will need to be challenged and motivated as much as any other level and benefit from a case study design (Benner, 1984).

Resistance to Learning

There are many variables that can affect participation in continuing education programs in home care. Barriers or deterrents can be institutional, educator-based, or situational. Institutional barriers occur when the expectations of the organization are not realistic: for example, if a therapist is given so many patients to see that he or she is unable to make it back for an inservice or the staff member was not informed in sufficient time about the educational opportunity (Ozcan & Shukla, 1993). In this case, the organization is at fault and not the therapist. The cultural influence of the agency may not encourage attendance. If there is no reinforcement for staff attendance, no consequence of not attending, or no acknowledgment of participants and encouragement to apply knowledge to real situations, there will be decreased motivation for learning. The educator may have done a poor job at assessing the needs of the learner, and the learner does not find the topic to be relevant to his or her needs (Krisjanson & Scanlan, 1989; Ozcan & Shukla, 1993). Two studies supported that, in the case of nurses, hands-on aspects of nursing care were the most popular continuing education offerings (Krisjanson & Scanlan, 1989). An example of a situational barrier to attendance at educational programs is an unexpected turn of events in the caregiver schedule, such as unanticipated car problems, extended visits due to emergencies, etc. These cannot be avoided, but, when possible, it is helpful to anticipate some unusual situations to occur and to prepare by perhaps increased staffing that day, even if there are just a few staff members placed "on call." Caution must be used to keep a clearly defined picture of what constitutes a need for extra support for staff.

Although numerous studies have been conducted to correlate variables such as age, educational background, and years of experience with participation in continuing education offerings, there are conflicting findings. This conflict is perhaps due to methodological weakness or perhaps a wide variance between staff in different geographical locations (Krisjanson & Scanlan, 1989). In addition, some use the terms "continuing education" and "inservice education" interchangeably, making application of some findings difficult. Motivational factors are multidimensional and interact to influence participation in educational programs (Krisjanson & Scanlan, 1989). Other possible barriers to participation in educational programs are learning difficulties, lack of confidence, illiteracy, emotional stress, and physical illness.

TEACHING STRATEGIES

Education should build on preexisting knowledge (Garland, 1996). This concept is called "conceptual bridging." If basic prerequisite knowledge is not present prior to teaching, it will lead to frustration, much like the child who is taught subtraction before he or she has mastered number recognition. As mentioned previously, creativity is essential, for the adult learner decides if and when he or she is interested in learning (Spradley & Allender, 1996). The home care nurse, therapist, and social worker offer an extra challenge to the educator, because some teaching strategies work better than others in the home care setting (Table 5–2). As anyone knows, home care staff are more difficult to assemble for educational offerings, because their caseloads take them in any number of directions away from the agency. In some cases, the staff may not even need to check in at the agency unless supplies are low. The principal methods of instruction requiring staff to be at the organization at a specific date and time are lecture, demonstration and coaching, simulation, role play/case studies, gaming, tutoring, or self-learning activities (Dyche, 1988).

Lecture is the most widely used teaching method. The technique is strengthened when an interactive component is added, such as discussion, role play, or choral responding. Choral responding (Harris & Sipay, 1985) is a technique that is used in reading instruction with children, but can also be effective with adults. It involves asking questions and everyone calling out the answer. This technique keeps the learners focused and reviews key facts throughout the presentation. More knowledgeable staff model for those who do not know the material. Basic guidelines to giving lectures are to be well-prepared and know the subject well, test equipment

prior to the presentation, dress professionally and free from distractions, avoid mannerisms that detract from what you are saying, and have an awareness of whether or not your audience is "tuned in." Be sensitive to signs of boredom, such as lack of eye contact, doodling, or other activities. A colleague once reported that she knew she was in trouble when she spied someone balancing her checkbook!

Demonstration and coaching can be done on an individual basis or in a group. At the beginning, the instructor is performing the procedure. The learner gradually assumes the responsibility until the instructor is only "coaching" the learner. The learner then performs the procedure without coaching. One popular phrase among educators is "see one, do one, teach one." There is some merit to this philosophy. By teaching someone else to perform a skill, usually, the teacher learns as much as the student, and the skill becomes more automatic. This may not be appropriate to every situation, however.

Simulation, role play, and case studies all strive to imitate the job environment. This enables staff to practice and demonstrate critical thinking, decision making, and problem solving in a multidimensional way. As mentioned previously, sometimes learners are good "test takers" but don't have a good ability to apply knowledge directly to clinical practice. Simulations and scenarios help sharpen critical thinking skills. It is important to note that, as with the skills lab, specific criteria must be developed to determine "pass vs. fail" performances in the scenarios or case studies. A subjective opinion of the evaluator is not sufficient.

Critical thinking applied to the home care setting requires imagination, reason, and consideration of the patient's needs emotionally, spiritually, economically, socially, and physically. It is way beyond the basic thinking that typifies the novice. Comparison and synthesis of known scientific facts combined with assessment findings help the home care staff meet the needs of the patient. College nursing programs examine curricula to make sure that critical thinking is woven in throughout, for although some are critical thinkers without a course, education is helpful to

Table 5–2 Comparison of Some Teaching Methods Used for Competency

Teaching Method	Advantages	Limitations
Lecture	Meets learner time limit constraints.	Can be boring, over-used, non-interactive, passive learning; difficult to match to adult individualized learning needs. Offers no choice of times unless offered more than once. Sequencing of information controlled by educator.
Self-learning: CAI, audiocassette	Gives adult learner control of pace, ability to review difficult areas, and scheduling. Various strategies for learning can be utilized. Computer-assisted instruction can save money in the long run. When audiocassettes are used, they may be played numerous times to increase learning.	At times, no resource is readily available to answer questions. Requires a motivated learner, will require updating on a regular basis for reuse. CAI has a high initial expense. Audiocassettes must be developed. All self-learning modules may become outdated and need updating.
Gaming	Provides an enjoyable learning mechanism. Involves active learning. Usually provides immediate reinforcement of correct answers. Educator can identify outcomes of educational process.	May cause staff not to take information seriously. May provide uneven participation; perhaps everyone cannot play, depending on group size.
Visuals: Bulletin boards, flyers, newsletters	Easy to document what was done, update, and reuse as needed. Usually not expensive, can improve morale and uplift. Maintains supportive stance of staff development. Can be tailored to meet specific needs.	Little room for learner input. Unless a post-test is attached, there is no way of knowing whether the reader learned anything, much less read it. Some do not learn well using a visual input. Design is essential, or the information can seem cluttered, overwhelming, and distracted. Some educators may feel unable to create visuals.
Journal Club	Each group is assigned to review one periodical monthly and summarize a pertinent article as assigned. This way staff have to read only one article a month and get the benefits of reading all journals. Using library copies saves the staff money. Empowers staff to read with an inquiring mind. May help them appreciate organizational policies and staff development. May be directed toward specific topics that are relevant to the organization at the time.	Difficult to get staff together for meetings. May lose journals by allowing them to leave the library. Requires commitment to work well, or members may resent reading articles without any benefit. Difficult to measure outcomes unless a pre-test or post-test is utilized and PI data are recorded.

assist all health care staff in developing critical thinking skills, so that they may go beyond the routine and minimal care.

Gaming is a popular method of teaching, although there are some potential dangers. When educational games are used to teach and assess, it is challenging to be sure that all the material is discussed and that everyone gets an equal opportunity to participate. It is also important to make sure that no one is made to feel silly, put down, or stupid. Usually, there are roles for those who do not wish to play, such as scorekeeper, host, etc. Almost any board game can be adapted to home care, substituting the dice or spinner with a question about home care or any specific topic. If the question asks learners to list three signs of congestive heart failure, for example, they move one if they can only list one, two if they can list two, and so on. Game shows that are on television can be adapted with hilarious results. Gaming can be the method that gets even the most uninvolved staff excited.

Independent Teaching Strategies

There are many strategies that are more appropriate than others when educating home care staff. Some of these include self-learning programs such as audiocassettes, modules, computer-assisted instruction, reading folders, brown bag "lunch and learns," and tutoring (Green, 1994). This is not to say that the standard lecture format doesn't have its place from time to time, but there needs to be a structured opportunity for alternatives on those many days when staff cannot meet for a group learning activity.

Audiocassette Program

One obvious suggestion that would meet some home care caregivers' learning needs is an audiocassette module program. Developing audiocassette modules can be relatively low cost when compared to sending staff to outside educational opportunities. Because home care staff spend a great deal of time in the car, if they own a cassette player and can learn in an auditory

manner, the possibilities are limitless. Certainly, the topic should not require so much concentration that driver safety could be compromised, but entertaining and enjoyable tapes could provide the repetition and review that some nurses need in certain cognitive and affective areas of competency. If you have ever heard a powerful and inspiring presentation on meeting the special needs of the geriatric client, for example, you know that even a tape recording of the presentation would certainly meet affective learning needs. There are commercial tapes available of review of cardiopulmonary resuscitation skills, advanced cardiac life support, and many other topics. Some publishers merely sell the master tape so that the educator can copy it for each appropriate staff member within the organization. This is an excellent opportunity to utilize time appropriately for education. The educator can prepare a post-test for each tape, give recognition to the progress through the audio library, and provide reinforcement by sharing the participant list with the managers.

Cognitive Testing

Another teaching strategy that works well for home care staff is the cognitive test. Usually associated with measurement alone, a test can also be used as a teaching tool if the answer key provided explains rationale for correct answers. Although an overuse of criterion-referenced tests could result in an unbalanced competency assessment and education program, frequently, the cognitive competency in a certain topic is prerequisite to competent skill demonstration or appropriate role function. An appropriate use of a criterion-referenced test is a pharmacological test for nurses. Scoring well on a test is no guarantee that the staff will administer medications correctly, do proper patient education, or document in the correct manner. However, it is the prerequisite to being able to do those things. Examples of criterion-referenced tests include multiple choice, fill-in-the-blank, essay, and short answer. There are advantages and disadvantages of each type of cognitive test (Exhibit 5–2). Re-

Exhibit 5–2 Questions Matched to Cognitive Objectives

Questions to ascertain knowledge

- When should you wash your hands when giving patient care?
- What is the next step in this procedure?
- Identify the chambers of the heart.

Additional questioning words that can be used to ascertain knowledge are *name, define, describe, who, what,* and *how.*

Questions to ascertain comprehension

- Compare two methods of protective room isolation.
- Explain the rationale for flushing a central venous device with heparin.
- Why would serum calcium levels increase in an immobilized patient?

Additional questioning words that can be used to ascertain comprehension are *contrast, predict, explain, illustrate, which,* and *why.*

Questions to ascertain synthesis

- Develop a patient care plan for Mrs. A, a patient who has undergone open heart surgery.

- Formulate a plan for responding to an angry family member.
- How would you as a preceptor provide support and direction to a new graduate who is repeatedly making the same mistakes?

Additional questioning words that can be used to ascertain synthesis are *suggest, create, synthesize,* and *derive.*

Questions to ascertain judgment

- Select the most appropriate way to teach a patient how to change an ostomy pouch.
- Defend your method for intervening with a child who will not eat.
- What is the most appropriate way to develop a self-learning module?

Additional phrases or words that can be used to ascertain judgment are *select on the basis of, decide,* and *judge.*

Source: Reprinted with permission from R.S. Abruzzese and B. Quinn O'Neill, Orientation for General and Specialty Areas, in *Nursing Staff Development: Strategies for Success,* R.S. Abruzzese, ed., p. 231, © 1996, St. Louis, Mosby-Year Book, Inc.

gardless, criterion-referenced tests have their place in education of home care staff, for they provide the flexibility that adult learners need (Yoder Wise, 1996). Tests allow staff members to select an optimal time for completion, giving them control of their day. All that is needed is a proctor, who need not be the educator. Some organizations give their staff the answer key location, to self-correct when completed, using an honor system. This is up to the discretion of the organization.

Tests frequently supplement other teaching modalities, such as videos, programmed instruction, or lectures. Videos or programmed learning with a post-test can be just as effective a teach-

ing method as lecture and may be more compatible with the unique time constraints of the home care provider (Flynn, Wolf, McGoldrick, Jablonski, Dean, & McKee, 1996) (Table 5–3).

Self-Learning or Programmed Instruction Modules

Self-learning modules are a boon to the home care educator and have been proven to be as effective as the lecture method of teaching (Schmidt & Fisher, 1992; Grant, 1993; Flynn et al., 1996). Programmed instruction modules, a type of self-learning module, frequently have questions with answers throughout the module,

Table 5–3 Criteria for Test and Measurement Construction

Criteria	How To Construct Test To Meet Criteria
Reliability—able to measure knowledge consistently	Structure tests so that the answer is either wrong or right, not a judgment call on the part of the evaluator. Pilot the test with peers to see if it is clearly understood. Perform an error-analysis when all have completed the test and use to eliminate "bad" questions.
Construct validity—degree to which test accurately measures competency	Design the test to simulate the home care job setting as much as possible. Is the question applicable to "operations" or the "real world"? If someone does well on the test, is it more likely that he or she capably performs those elements evaluated by the test? Avoid "giving away the answer" within the question. Select the best test to measure the content. For example, if you wish to assess cognitive competency about medications, a matching test or fill-in-the-blank test would be appropriate. Assessment of effective aspects of giving care can best be assessed by using an essay test or direct observation in the home using a performance checklist. Assessment of competency in a specific skill can be measured by direct observation of performance or simulation in a skills lab setting. The test designer should be more interested in accurate measurement, rather than determining if someone is good at taking tests. Be fair.
Content validity—does the question contain all the most important elements?	The content of the test should not be superficial. It should contain the most important aspects of the data it is attempting to measure. Emphasis should be placed on knowledge that is most essential for giving care within the organization and most commonly seen. Within the topic, measure those facts that are essential for competency first, followed by those that are less essential.
Adequate length	Do not attempt to measure too large a body of material at one sitting. After too long, retention of material will be affected. Eliminate questions that are the "trivial pursuit" type, that no one cares about or that may not ever affect care to the patient.
Objectives	Always list objectives prior to test development to stay focused.
General guidelines	Have extra questions in case you need them. Listen to those who appeal an answer; they may give good input for future test design.
Feedback	Always return tests immediately to enhance learning. Be sure to include good comments as well as bad. Thank them for participating, even if it wasn't an option.

directing the learner to the appropriate page should he or she select an incorrect answer. This is called a feedback mechanism and takes the place of the instructor in reinforcement throughout learning (Schmidt & Fisher, 1992). Although programmed modules are more work to develop, they catch errors earlier than the simpler modules, which have the questions at the end. Another advantage to programmed modules is that they almost force the learner to get it right by the end of the module. If the module is just information with a post-test, staff may just wish to complete the obligation and may not bother checking why answers were incorrect.

After module development, the educator is free to do other work, unless staff have questions about the topic (Schlomer, Anderson, & Shaw, 1997). Unlike one-time lecture presentations, staff who are hired after the original presentation date or are absent can readily complete their educational requirement. Learners can complete self-learning modules at their own pace and review material when they realize they do not understand it (Schlomer et al., 1997). Self-learning modules offer the learner an opportunity to control when and, in some cases, even where he or she will learn. When modules are prepared using specific guidelines, they can challenge and motivate staff to enhance their performance. The module can be placed on a tri-fold board or assembled in booklet form for ease of transportation.

To truly measure outcomes of a module, a pretest and posttest can be utilized. Pretests can reveal that the learner does not need to do the module, can serve to justify the need for the module in the mind of the learner, or can measure efficacy of a module (Schmidt & Fisher, 1992). Staff may demonstrate knowledge on a test and application of that knowledge in the home without utilizing the available module. It is up to the discretion of the educator whether or not a more advanced module can be developed for that staff or that the competency level is sufficient for all staff. Certainly, if staff frequently perform well on pretests, the educator should consider whether programs have been developed based on real needs.

What are the criteria for selecting the self-learning module method? First of all, the content should be appropriate for a self-learning module. Abstract or other skills requiring validation do not lend themselves well to the self-learning format (Schlomer et al., 1997). Content appropriate for a module is usually that from the cognitive domain. Although education of skills included in the affective domain is more frequently appropriate in a group setting (Ellis, 1992), if questions are worded carefully, the affective domain can be assessed as well to some degree. Questions must be created require the learners to input their own values and beliefs. Problem solving of simulated scenarios where staff are forced to make judgments based on cognitive and affective learning can be of great benefit. In addition, a psychomotor assessment can be accomplished with the addition of a demonstration-return demonstration component (Schmidt & Fisher, 1992). The educator must also consider learner preference. Those with less formal education may prefer the classroom setting (Schlomer et al., 1997). There may be others who, for other reasons, prefer another teaching method. Educators need to vary teaching methods to avoid staff boredom (Grant, 1993).

One limitation of self-learning modules is that they may be more time consuming to prepare than lectures, because it can be difficult limiting the information to the size of the module. If the module will not be used by many staff members, it may not be worth the time that is required to prepare it (Schmidt & Fisher, 1992). Also, if the topic will quickly become outdated, it will take too much time to update (Schmidt & Fisher, 1992).

The first page of the module should list the learning objectives. Initially, the module should be instructionally heavy, necessitating only light participation on the part of the learner. Gradually, prompts should fade, increasing the part the learner has in the module. In general, information should be broken down into "bite-sized pieces." This way, the learner will not feel overwhelmed. The module should use a variety of techniques to keep the learner's interest. For example, reading passages that teach about breath sounds followed by questions can then direct the learner to an audiocassette to review the sounds. After facts have been taught, it is important to assess the learner in a patient case study or another type of measurement as a follow-up, because recitation of facts is not all there is to learning. Critical thinking requires the knowledge of the subject and the ability to synthesize and make good judgments (Schmidt & Fisher, 1992; Stark, 1995). Because people learn in different ways, it is important to teach and measure learning from different approaches (Schmidt & Fisher, 1992).

The type of language used in self-learning modules should be conversational, and the most important and interesting facts that the learner needs to know should be repeated frequently (Schmidt & Fisher, 1992). Pictures, diagrams, and other illustrations help clarify information to the reader and may keep his or her interest. Other resources should be provided near the module, should the learner wish to know more than is in the module (Schlomer et al., 1997). After modules have been developed, they should be piloted using a small sample. The input gained from the pilot should influence any revisions. The self-learning module is then ready for implementation. Following implementation, modules must be updated as needed to reflect current practice and revised as evaluations from staff yield valid suggestions for improvement.

Computer-Assisted Instruction

Another type of instruction that is also considered programmed instruction is computer-assisted instruction. Many companies have produced educational software for home care agencies, and some are better than others. Usually, the companies offer a choice of CD-ROM, DOS, or Windows programs, to name a few. The hardware requirements are clearly explained so there is no danger of an organization purchasing software that will not be compatible.

One company that custom develops home care-specific software is the Williams and Wilkins company in Baltimore. Currently, they offer all of the Joint Commission and Occupational Safety and Health Administration-mandatory topics such as infection control, back safety, cardiopulmonary resuscitation, or others utilizing a system called de'Medici. This system was reviewed by Criddle (1995), and she found it saved her hospital money after the initial outlay costs. Computer-assisted instruction has several advantages and disadvantages. The main advantage is learner flexibility. Learners can sign up for a time to complete educational requirements at a time convenient to them. Also, computer-assisted instruction offers a standardized test and an educational tracking component, freeing the educator to develop other programs. When employees first log on to the system, the software asks them to enter their occupation. This way, specialists in every discipline receive information specific to their job. Lastly, employees in Criddle's facility reported that using computer-assisted instruction was "fun." Also, some of the educational products are fully approved for use to meet certification requirements. Although one might be concerned about the materials becoming outdated, there is just a small fee for updating data as needed (Criddle, 1995). Considering the expense of such an initial outlay, organizations need to check out the many software packages available. The main limitation to computer-assisted instruction is that some staff may not be competent in using a computer. It is then the job of the educator to assist them (Coffman, 1996), for initial negative experiences with a computer can undermine future competency efforts. To realistically calculate the costs of implementing this learning method, the time to educate staff including the educator should also be included. Some staff will require more education than others, for some of the older working population had no previous exposure to computers (Coffman, 1996). Other limitations to computer-assisted instruction are that only one staff member can complete requirements at a time, some learners may not enjoy it, it requires a computer with a lot of memory because it stores educational records as well as several versions of each module, and the initial expense. However, considering the costs of paper, recordkeeping, program development, distribution/collection time of educational records, and annual time needed to update materials, computer-assisted instruction is worth exploring.

Reading Folders

Background experience can help learners learn, and this background experience comes not only from life's lessons, but can be accelerated by reading. One of the first and best things an educator can do for staff in the home care setting is help link them to the health care literature specific to their discipline and the others they work with. After gaining permission from publishers, articles can be reproduced for educational purposes. Each employee can have a colored folder in his or her mailbox at the home care organization. This folder can serve as an information channel between the educator and the employee. If the employee is having a specific need for literature about a certain topic, the educator can place helpful articles in the folder. Enclosed in the folder is a reading log, which can be maintained for the employee and can be entered into the employee's file periodically, having implications for evaluation and promotion, as well as disciplinary action. Another use of reading folders is that the staff can receive interesting updates on what is new in their field of practice. The term "reading folders" was obtained from an article by Green (1994), although the thoughts about what they should contain are the author's.

Lunch and Learn

Depending on the geographical location of home care staff, a lunch and learn can also be utilized. Staff can bring a bag lunch, or the educator can seek a donation from a pharmaceutical representative or other source. Lunch and learns are almost always enjoyable and offer the caregiver a chance to gain group support prior to completing the day's tasks. Furthermore, many times, it is a luxury to eat lunch when you are not in a moving car. Organizations need to acknowledge that employees should be paid for this time because they are attending an inservice, even if it is overtime.

Tutoring

Many staff seek out or are referred for extra help with specific deficiencies. Staff who do so should be commended. Sometimes new staff during a busy orientation never understood a basic part of home care documentation, for example. Peer tutoring or getting help from the educator is an excellent opportunity to prevent further discouragement and losses of productivity. Collegiality can motivate and encourage staff to seek tutoring help; a problem arises if the tutor who is selected is also weak in the topic. Managers need to be sensitive to this possibility and channel the staff to the right people who can help them.

CREATIVITY IN EDUCATION

The reason that advertisers use unusual techniques in commercials is that they know you won't easily forget their product. The educator must employ creative techniques to compete with other thoughts trying to keep the learner's attention. Creative presentations can be unforgettable, enhancing retention of material as well. Certainly, no educator has intended to develop a dull inservice, but there are some reasons inservices can lack creativity. The main reasons involve time, money, and energy.

Putting a creative spin on a presentation, workshop, or module requires extra time beyond the time it already took to do the essentials, such as needs assessment, literature review, and program development. Creativity often requires taking one or more components of the outline and making an analogy. For example, one home health agency decided to dress up each speaker and give her a name appropriate to the topic she would be presenting. "Vicious VRE" and others in the "cast" made their appearances and talked from a disease perspective (Harris & Yuan, 1997). Certainly, no one will forget that inservice for some time.

Some educators may think, "I'm not creative; that is not my style," but everyone can learn to change to do a job more effectively. This is not to imply that professional educators shouldn't be polished, well-prepared, and well-groomed. But there are times in any home care agency when a good dose of "comic relief" goes a long way. A sense of humor is definitely an asset in home care for educators and clinical staff! Some other uses of humor besides the use of role playing include comics, skits, sound effects, and humorous anecdotes. It never hurts to start a presentation with something humorous to break the ice. Of course, good taste is expected.

Creative ways of presenting material are endless. One hospital in which the author worked used to put a weekly rhythm strip in the bathrooms with the saying, "Can you name this arrhythmia?" Placing a very brief tidbit of information in with the paychecks is another way to disseminate information. Flashcards with little known facts about frequently used medications can be used on an alternating basis by placing them in the employees' mailboxes and asking them to rotate them to the mailbox below the following week. Having regular staff challenges, either written or scenario-based, at frequent intervals encourage learning. Staff will readily respond to opportunities to grow taking small steps. Sometimes attending an inservice seems like the impossible dream to busy home care staff, and it is up to the educator to provide frequent opportunities for education that are of short duration.

Another way to be creative is through newsletters and bulletin boards. Clip art is a great, easy, budget-friendly way to get pictures. Bulletin boards can take some of the common sayings of the day and apply them to something important in home care. A current saying that is commonly heard in this region when someone doesn't understand something is, "What's up with that?" A bulletin board with a balloon saying "What's up with . . ." could be recycled all year by just making big letters that spell out the topic each time. Post-tests can be provided on bulletin board topics complete with an envelope to place completed tests in for inservice credit.

Newsletters can encourage staff by acknowledging who is going to school, who attended a special inservice, who are newly trained preceptors, etc. Part of the newsletter could present important information essential to home care. There could also be a post-test on the topic discussed in the previous newsletter. Newsletters should contain information that can be read in one sitting, in most cases.

Themes are always fun and help the educator tie the program together. Some basic themes include western, 50s, holidays, sports, luau, and so on. There can also be health-related themes such as Nurse's Week, National Physical Therapy Week, and so forth, but be sure not to leave any specialties out! Topical themes, such as wound care, infection control, and wellness, can also be used. After a theme has been selected, try to think of a song or songs that can be played during the introduction. Tapes are available from television themes, which can prove very useful. Themes from shows such as *The Twilight Zone*, *Mission Impossible*, *Leave it to Beaver*, and other old hits can instantly bring associations that can be used to the educator's advantage. For example, imagine teaching an inservice on documentation using the "Zone" theme, or one on a particularly challenging aspect of home care calling it "Mission Possible."

Snacks can be served that go with the theme, if desired. Remember that "everything doesn't have to match," or the idea will get old. Advertisement for the inservice can contain a logo that is related to the theme. Usually, subtle things that trigger the learner to see that there is a theme are better than obvious attempts. People cringe when things are overdone.

There is a fine line between being "campy" and using themes in a highly effective manner. It really depends on the topic, the audience, the educator, and the philosophies of the agency. Themes should be used sparingly, or they cease to be creative. There is also the incredible temptation to "over-pun" when doing a presentation. Let enough be enough, and be sure the actual presentation is taken seriously. Just remember that a well-timed burst of creativity will keep your audience talking about your inservices and encourage them to return. They will also probably influence someone else to make the effort to attend.

EVALUATION OF LEARNERS

There are definite guidelines about how tests should be constructed to best evaluate the learner. This section will briefly outline these guidelines and apply them to the home care learner. Criterion-referenced tests are designed to have only one correct answer for each question, and the learner is compared to or "referenced" against that standard (Exhibit 5–3). A commonly used criterion-referenced test is when staff are asked to perform a skill, and it is either performed correctly or it isn't. Norm-referenced tests are tests that use data to benchmark scores against the scores of a national average or other groups of similar learners. An example of a norm-referenced test is the National League for Nursing exam. Most of the tests used by home care educators are criterion-referenced, with the criteria being derived from professional standards, policies, and procedures. A good test helps the educator and learner focus on where more work is needed and thus saves time (Blank, 1982). Informal self-assessments are seldom enough to plan to meet educational needs; with a cognitive test, learning needs become clearer.

Constructing test questions for a written criterion-referenced test determines whether or not the test will be reliable, valid, interesting, and effective. It is possible for multiple-choice questions to tap higher level critical thinking and clinical reasoning skills and be a valid measure of knowledge (Salvatori, 1996). Multiple-choice questions are usually easiest to grade. When writing multiple-choice questions, write alternatives to the correct answer with some degree of truth so that the answer is not obvious. However, be sure to include something in the wrong answers that makes them "good and wrong." If a learner spends too much time decoding what the evaluator meant by a question, the question is not worded clearly.

Matching is another form of multiple choice, only the learner must select from a larger answer pool to start with. It can be difficult to keep only one answer for one question; be sure not to confuse learners with more than one possible match to each item, unless you intend them to match column A with more than one selection from column B. Clarify to the learner what is expected. Matching questions are generally viewed as "fun" and challenging.

Long or short essay questions are a good opportunity to get an idea what the learner knows about the topic (and sometimes more than an idea!). The advantages of essay questions are that there are no clues prompting the learner, some learners enjoy writing, and the test takes less time to prepare. However, grading can be a real problem and takes much longer than multiple choice. Also, there is a subjective component to grading the essay. Some learners may take it personally if you criticize something they wrote, for they "own" it far more than they did the response they put on a multiple-choice test.

What are some ways to be sure that evaluation is not a negative, destructive process? Many educators get the red ink flying and don't realize that the last thing they should want to do is have staff associate inservice education with every negative thought they ever associated with learning in the formal educational setting. Being a positive evaluator takes more than switching to green ink to correct post-tests. Each learner should be treated with respect and dignity. When placed in a learning environment, participants may feel especially vulnerable to criticism, possibly thinking that the evaluator is questioning overall job competency. Always approach the learner with a positive attitude and mention the strengths you have observed, as well as the areas that require further work. Consider possible causes for poor performance during assessment including nervousness, anxiety associated with test-taking, emotional difficulties at home, pain, or other causes. However, if participants attribute poor performance to one of these causes, it is important to ask them if their performance in the home is also affected. Some participants may

Exhibit 5–3 Sample Criterion-Referenced Examination for Clinical Professional Staff

---

a 1. One reason that an assessment of the patient's home safety is completed upon admission is that
   a. a baseline is established as a means of comparison during subsequent visits.
   b. it dictates the repairs that the patient will make to continue service.
   c. home safety is the complete responsibility of the home care organization.
   d. you are responsible to correct all the safety deficits you find in the home.

d 2. Should exposure to blood-borne pathogens take place, the *first* thing the clinician should do is
   a. contact the appropriate supervisor, and instruct the patient to wash all soiled linens with bleach.
   b. initiate strict respiratory isolation procedures with all patients having airborne diseases.
   c. remove gloves and wash hands.
   d. clean up all spills by use of 5% alcohol solution, blotting up excess with paper towels.

a 3. What is your best line of defense against blood-borne pathogens while employed in home care?
   a. Barrier protection—intact skin, gloves, personal protective equipment as per agency policy.
   b. Instituting a full risk assessment for potential pathogens prior to admission.
   c. Ask the patient what diseases he or she has.
   d. Wear a mask into every home and double glove.

c 4. What type of patients are *most commonly* immunocompromised?
   a. Thin, wiry patients of Carribean descent
   b. "Generation-Xers"
   c. Elderly, pediatric clients
   d. All of the above

b 5. Based on your knowledge of Medicare guidelines and the following information, which patient would be considered homebound?
   a. Mr. Smith; CHF, oxygen-dependent, lives alone, transported by neighbor 5 × week for evening meal at Senior Center. Able to walk when using oxygen. No supporting family nearby.
   b. Mrs. Spiffy; S/P Total Knee Replacement with infected wound, attends church in wheelchair once a week, gets hair done once every two weeks.
   c. Miss Hernandez; newly diagnosed IDDM, lives with parents, continues to attend classes at a nearby community college, checking in daily at college infirmary.
   d. Mr. Guleccio; S/P MI 6 mos. ago, coumadin therapy. Bowls twice a week in bowling league. Visits his doctor every month. Volunteers at local cardiac rehabilitation program three days/week.

d 6. Another name for medical plan of care that is approved by the physician and reviewed every 60–62 days for Medicare patients is:
   a. The nursing care map
   b. Medicare care and uptake sheet
   c. Physician referral form
   d. The 485

d 7. Only three disciplines can "stand alone" when ordered by a physician, according to Medicare:
   a. Skilled nursing, nurse's aide care, social work
   b. Dietary consults, physical therapy, occupational therapy
   c. Occupational therapy, skilled nursing, physical therapy
   d. Physical therapy, speech therapy, skilled nursing

continues

Exhibit 5–3 Sample Criterion-Referenced Examination for Clinical Professional Staff

_b_ 8. Of the following, which of these can stay on the case if all other disciplines have met their goals?
   a. social work
   b. occupational therapy
   c. respiratory therapy
   d. speech therapy

_d_ 9. Documentation should include the following:
   a. subjective data, reference to chronicity of condition, current information and orders
   b. record of all assessments, interventions, the patient's response to interventions, and homebound status

   c. the teaching done to the patient, any procedures, and charting against both the 485, care plan, and clinical plan if one is used
   d. b and c

_a_ 10. When documenting abuse or neglect, the home care employee must realize that
   a. the client's best interest comes first.
   b. chart what you think is going on.
   c. use the words "seems" and "appears" to justify your suspicions.
   d. if you think better of what you wrote on the previous list, the best thing to do is just cross it out and write the word "ERROR" above it.

Match the service this organization offers with the indicators for a *possible* referral. Indicators may be used more than once.

_e_ 11. Private duty nursing
_a,d_ 12. Occupational therapy
_b_ 13. Hospice
_d,g_ 14. Home Care Aide
_c,f_ 15. Speech therapy
_c,f,g_ 16. Dietary consultation
_c,h,j_ 17. Social work
_b,h,j_ 18. Psychiatric services
_i_ 19. Cardiac/cardiac rehabilitation
_a,d_ 20. Sports medicine/physical therapy

a. Unsteady gait
b. Terminal diagnosis
c. Inability to swallow
d. Decreased range of motion, unable to do ADL's
e. S/P Total Hip, progressing well but confused
f. Failure to thrive, develop normally (child)
g. Poor hygiene related to extreme obesity
h. Family conflict, suspected abuse
i. S/P MI, PTCA
j. Withdrawn behavior as reported by family, financial difficulties

find that an in-home evaluation is better, or they need to utilize stress-reduction techniques.

It is different to tailor an educational program to meet specific educational needs. For example, if a social worker has difficulty learning visually due to a learning disability, perhaps someone could read the material and the exam to the person with the difficulty. Then, one has to question how the social worker is able to find the homes on the map. There are also times when members of the staff have other difficulties with learning. It is important for the educator to filter the program and make sure that those staff members learn only the essential information. For the most part, modifying an evaluation method for

the learning impaired is rare. Because the job requires a certain level of capability, there are usually not many learners who experience profound learning difficulties.

One of the most important aspects of ongoing competency is the encouragement and motivation it can spark in participants as they feel validated. Even well-meaning administrators and managers get too busy to give a physical therapist or other staff member a word of encouragement when it is needed. If evaluations are handled tactfully and strengths are emphasized, learners will leave the experience feeling like the caring and skilled professionals that they are (Table 5–4).

Table 5–4 Comparison of Two Testing Alternatives

Type of Test	Advantages	Disadvantages
Selection-type: Multiple choice, matching	• Scoring is quick and easy. • Higher scorer reliability. • Can test a large amount of content. • Can reduce bluffing. • Easier for educator to target specific facts.	• Learners may guess correctly. • Take longer to construct since more items are included. • Require educator determination of level of difficulty prior to administration. • No room for creativity on the part of the learner.
Supply-type: Fill in the blank, essay, short answer	• Less time to construct. • Reduce guessing to a minimum. • Fill in the blank questions do not take too much time to score. • Essay questions allow learner to use self-expression and justify answers. • Essays can measure critical thinking by asking learner to compare, contrast, explain, describe, and summarize. • More likely to give educator serendipitous information that could prove useful in educating learners.	• Lengthy to grade. • More time consuming to take, so may be more likely to affect productivity. • More subjective to evaluate. • Can become tedious quickly for the learner. • Those having reading comprehension problems may find multiple choice easier to understand because there are options that may trigger the correct response.

REFERENCES

Abruzzese, R.S. (1996). Evaluation in nursing staff development. In R.S. Abruzzese (Ed.), *Nursing staff development: Strategies for success* (2nd ed.) (pp. 242–258). St. Louis, MO: Mosby-Year Book, Inc.

Albrecht, M.N. (1990). The Albrecht nursing model for home health care: Implications for research, practice, and education. *Public Health Nursing, 7*(2), 118–126.

Almquist, G., & Bookbinder, M. (1990). Developing an educational needs assessment. *Journal of Nursing Staff Development, 6*(5), 246–249.

Astarita, T., Materna, G., & Savage, C. (In press). Perceived knowledge level among home health nurses: A descriptive study. *Home Health Care Management and Practice.*

Atwood, H.M., & Ellis, J. (1971). The concept of need: An analysis for adult education. *Adult Leadership, 19,* 210–212, 244.

Babcock, D.E., and Miller, M.A. (1994). *Client education:*

Theory and practice. St. Louis, MO: Mosby-Year Book, Inc.

Beeken, J. (1997). The relationship between critical thinking and self-concept in staff nurses and the influence of these characteristics on nursing practice. *Journal of Nursing Staff Development, 13*(5), 272–278.

Benner, P. (1984). *From novice to expert: Excellence and power in clinical nursing practice.* Menlo Park, CA: Addison-Wesley.

Blank, W.E. (1982). *Handbook for developing competency-based training programs.* Englewood Cliffs, NJ: Prentice-Hall.

Burke, R. (1996). Yes, you can give an inservice—with ease. *RN, 59*(6), 17–22.

Burns, N., & Grove, S.K. (1995). *Understanding nursing research: Conduct, critique, and utilization.* Philadelphia: W.B. Saunders.

Coffman, S. (1996). Applying adult education principles to computer education. *Journal of Nursing Staff Development, 12*(5), 260–263.

Colucciello, M.L. (1993). Learning styles and instructional processes for home healthcare providers. *Home Healthcare Nurse, 11*(2), 43–50.

Criddle, L.M. (1995). Computer-assisted instruction. A successful approach to mandatory annual review education. *Journal of Nursing Staff Development, 11*(4), 219–225.

Dyche, J. (1988). *Educational program development for employees in health care agencies.* Murfreesboro, TN: Tri-Oak.

Ellis, C. (1992). Incorporating the affective domain into staff development programs. *Journal of Nursing Staff Development, 8*(3), 127–130.

Flynn, E.R., Wolf, Z.R., McGoldrick, T.B., Jablonski, R.A., Dean, L.M., & McKee, E.P. (1996). Effect of three teaching methods on a nursing staff's knowledge of medication error risk reduction strategies. *Journal of Nursing Staff Development, 12*(1), 19–25.

Garland, G.A. (1996). Self report of competence: A tool for the staff development specialist. *Journal of Nursing Staff Development, 12*(4), 191–197.

Grant, P. (1993). Formative evaluation of a nursing orientation program: Self-paced vs. lecture-discussion. *Journal of Continuing Education in Nursing, 24*(6), 245–248.

Green, P.H. (1994). Meeting the learning needs of home health nurses. *Journal of Home Health Care Practice, 6*(4), 25–32.

Harris, A., & Sipay, E. (1985). *How to increase reading ability* (8th ed.) (p. 112). White Plains, NY: Longman.

Harris, M.D., & Yuan, J. (1997). Creative inservices to meet mandatory requirements. *Home Healthcare Nurse, 15*(8), 573–579.

Joint Commission on Accreditation of Healthcare Organizations. (1996). *1997–98 Accreditation standards for home health care education and training.* Oakbrook Terrace, IL: Author.

Knowles, M.S. (1984). *The adult learner: A neglected species.* Houston, TX: Gulf Publishing Company.

Kobs, A. (1996). Competence: The shot heard around the nursing world. *Nursing Management, 28*(2), 10–13.

Krisjanson, L.J., & Scanlan, J.M. (1989). Assessment of continuing nursing education needs: A literature review. *Journal of Continuing Education in Nursing, 20*(3), 118–123.

Marciniak, C.J. (1997). A systematic plan for nurse educator development. *Journal of Nursing Staff Development, 13*(2), 99–108.

McAnnally, R., & Barnett, J. (1997). Reorganizing competency programs. *Nursing Management, 28*(9), 33.

National Nursing Staff Development Organization. (1994). *Getting started in nursing staff development.* Pensacola, FL: Author.

Ozcan, Y.A., & Shukla, R.K. (1993). The effect of a competency-based targeted staff development program on nursing productivity. *Journal of Nursing Staff Development, 9*(2), 78–84.

Puetz, B.E. (1987). *Contemporary strategies for continuing education in nursing.* Gaithersburg, MD: Aspen.

Radke, K.J., & McArt, E. (1993). Perceptions and responsibilities of clinical nurse specialists as educators. *Journal of Nursing Education, 32*(3), 115–120.

Salvatori, P. (1996). Clinical competence: A review of the health care literature with a focus on occupational therapy. *Canadian Journal of Occupational Therapy, 63*(4), 260–271.

Schlomer, R.S., Anderson, M.A., & Shaw, R. (1997). Teaching strategies and knowledge retention. *Journal of Nursing Staff Development, 13*(5), 249–253.

Schmidt, K.L., & Fisher, J.C. (1992). Effective development and utilization of self-learning modules. *Journal of Continuing Education in Nursing, 23*(2), 54–59.

Spradley, B.W., & Allender, J.A. (1996). *Community health nursing: Concepts and practice* (4th ed). Philadelphia: Lippincott-Raven.

Stark, J. (1995). Critical thinking: Taking the road less traveled. *Nursing, 25*(11), 52–56.

Wheeler, L.A. (1994). How do older nurses perceive their clinical competence and the effects of age? *Journal of Continuing Education in Nursing, 25*(5), 230–236.

Yoder Wise, P.S. (1996). Learning needs assessment. In R.S. Abruzzese (Ed.), *Nursing staff development: Strategies for success* (2nd ed.) (pp. 188–208). St. Louis, MO: Mosby-Year Book, Inc.

CHAPTER 6

Frameworks and Models for Competency Program Development

FRAMEWORKS

Frameworks serve to design and structure educational planning and competency measurement for staff development. They provide a grounded reference and home-base effect, providing direction and disposition. Frameworks for competency program development in home care can be modeled after professional literature, customized to meet organizational needs, based upon care maps, or a combination of all. The research–based literature contains limited reference to the specialty of home care competency program framework development. The available literature can be divided into three categories of competency frameworks: Dreyfus Skill Acquisition Model applied to nursing (Robinson & Barberis-Ryan, 1995; Gavin, Haas, Pendleton, Street, & Wormald, 1996), Scrima theoretical framework (Scrima, 1987; McGregor, 1990; O'Grady & O'Brien, 1992; O'Shea, 1994), and other various independent frameworks (del Bueno, Barker & Christmyer, 1981; Kelly & Matlin, 1993; Belanus & Hunt, 1994; Humphrey & Milone-Nuzzo, 1994; Meyer, 1997). The majority of this literature is based upon frameworks from the acute care setting with only approximately 40% being unique to the practice setting of home care. In addition, some of the literature cited encompasses the subject of competency-based orientation (CBO). The subject of CBO will be expanded upon in upcoming sections and is only utilized here to explore frameworks for development of competency programs in general. A brief review of the literature related to competency frameworks will be provided. In addition, the use of care maps and the Outcome and Assessment Information Set (OASIS) for framework development will be examined.

The Dreyfus Skill Acquisition Model was applied to nursing practice and utilized to develop competency assessment in home care by Robinson and Barberis-Ryan (1995) and Gavin et al. (1996). This model describes five levels of clinical performance observable in actual practice. In addition to using the Dreyfus Model, Robinson and Barberis-Ryan (1995) also utilized del Bueno's Dimension of Nursing Competency (1987), which contains the technical, interpersonal, and critical thinking aspects of care delivery. Gavin et al. (1996) applied the Dreyfus Model to new graduates who were entering home care. The authors operationalized a framework that is research based in the acute care setting and applied it to the auspices of the home care setting.

Two frameworks that are similar to Scrima's Theoretical Framework (1987) were identified. The Scrima framework provides a consistent, structured method of documenting selected clinical proficiencies and facilitates the achievement of individual learning needs in an acute care setting. The Scrima framework follows a systematic approach to program development. The sequence for competency program development includes the interview, performance standards, remedial study, maintenance of competence, and external accreditation or certification. O'Grady and O'Brien (1992) get a little bit more specific starting with assessing the environment, developing the plan, defining the competencies, designing evaluation tools, preparing preceptors, and piloting the program, whereas McGregor (1990) begins with developing standards and skill lists, assessing learning needs, planning educational programs, evaluating learning outcomes, and cognitive testing and skills achievement. The pattern identified by both sources is one of intense planning prior to program implementation and is highly structured and patterned.

The independent frameworks found within the literature are varied in their structure and provide insight into the unique and creative ways organizations are building their competency programs. A classic representation of competency program development is that of del Bueno, Barker, and Christmyer (1981). They recommend the use of a competency-based model that has the following characteristics: "(1) an emphasis on outcomes or achievement of performance expectations, (2) use of self-directed learning activities, (3) flexibility and time allowed for achievement of outcome, (4) use of the teacher as a facilitator, (5) assessment of previous learning, and (6) assessment of learning styles" (p. 24). Their program also embraced planning stages that included administrative and supervisory personnel in the process of development. Belanus and Hunt (1994) describe a framework adapted from Maslow's hierarchy of needs for home care nurses who have completed orientation but have been in the role less than 1 year. They identified needs that appear after orientation and addressed these needs through the use of Maslow's hierarchy. Meyer (1997) describes a continuing education program that prepares experienced nurses to transition to home care. A coalition of many organizations developed a 12-credit-hour college program to help develop a successful transition. They utilized the nursing process to guide the curriculum. The Omaha Taxonomy (1992), which is divided into four major domains, was utilized as the organizing framework. Humphrey and Milone-Nuzzo (1994) developed a Nursing Practice Model for home care orientation. The model is educationally based and reality focused and incorporates Benner's novice to expert premises. This model demonstrates that orientation should be seen as the foundation of nursing practice in home care. Lastly, Kelly and Matlin (1993) describe the use of a conceptual framework in planning and implementing an orientation program. The authors indicate that a customized conceptual framework was developed based upon current practice within the organization. Six key elements provide the framework: (1) customer and caregiver expectations, and professional, regulatory, and legal constraints; (2) philosophy of nursing; (3) standards of practice; (4) standards of care; (5) unifying elements used to integrate standards of practice and standards of care; and (6) results of nurse performance and patient outcomes (p. 175). This framework provides a logical and comprehensive approach to program development.

No discussion on frameworks would be complete without addressing the Albrecht Model of Home Health Care (Albrecht, 1990). Although not seen in the competency-related literature, the model deserves attention because it is feasible that a competency program could utilize Albrecht as a framework. The model facilitates predicting those variables that promote self-care capability in the client at home. The model addresses nursing practice needs as well as need for inservice programs and can also assist in identifying educational content for undergraduate and graduate-level programs. The Albrecht model can also be used as a framework for nursing research, measuring nursing practice outcomes, health status outcome in working adults (Albrecht & Nelson, 1993), and client satisfaction with a self-care intervention program (Albrecht, Goeppinger, Anderson, Boutaugh, Macnee, & Stewart, 1993).

Frameworks as evidenced by the literature presented provide structure and guide the development and maintenance of a competency program. Home care organizations should first embark on the development of a framework that best meets their mission and vision and can demonstrate measurable outcomes. Existing frameworks can be easily adapted to meet the unique needs of any organization. The literature presented demonstrates that a need exists for scholarly inquiry into the types of frameworks that are functional for the home care setting. In addition, inquiry to identify whether there are differences between frameworks of various specialty settings and disciplines is also needed.

CARE MAPS

In the quest to identify a framework that best fits a home care organization, the concept of care maps (also called clinical maps or critical maps) should not be overlooked as a potential framework for competency program development. The structure and process of care maps can function as a significant dimension to the design of a competency program. Care maps or critical paths are a delivery model of care that originated in the acute care setting and only recently began to appear in the home care setting, first as an appendage to the end of the acute care map but now more and more as a primary model of care delivery. Corbett and Androwich (1994) relate that home care in the past really did not have an impetus to define and structure care in this model primarily because of Medicare's retrospective pay system. However, today, the impetus does exist due to the advent of managed care, preauthorization, and the drive to cut costs and demonstrate measurable outcomes in home care. Care maps in home care serve a multitude of functions, which are beyond the scope of this discussion. In general, they serve to improve patient care, provide consistent patient education, plan care delivery, predict resources, and integrate care by all disciplines. From a competency framework perspective, care maps serve educators well in that they are an excellent learning mechanism for nurses who are new to home care. A competency program framework could combine care maps and one of the aforemen-

tioned frameworks to demonstrate a comprehensive system for competency achievement. Care maps provide a complete picture of standards of care, defining how care is to be delivered, in what time frame, and with what outcomes. They serve to identify patient needs, particularly delineating patient teaching standards (Corbett & Androwich, 1994). Their use by educators can be multifaceted with an array of teaching-learning opportunities and competency-assessment strategies. Care maps can function as an organization's standards of care and can help to teach care expectations and outcomes of such care. In addition, care maps help to organize care and, thereby, can teach how to organize care delivery. Because the nature of home care lends itself to being unstructured and uncoordinated, care maps can certainly assist the novice home care nurse to conceptualize care delivery in this unique setting, which in the past has been hard to attain. If care maps are utilized by a home care organization, educators should utilize them as part of the foundation for competency program development.

OASIS

The Health Care Financing Administration's (HCFA) new National Medicare Quality Improvement Demonstration Project has proposed for purposes of outcome-based quality improvement the OASIS. OASIS will be the vehicle by which home care providers reach outcomes-based performance improvement (Koch, 1997). It is proposed that all Medicare-certified agencies will be mandated to implement OASIS. The expectation is that OASIS will provide reliable and valid outcome data on adult home health patients. These data will help organizations to "determine the most cost-effective case management practices and appropriate utilization levels, demonstrate quality to consumers and payers, and identify the impact of restrictions on home care service utilization. In addition, organizations will use the data to determine a patient's classification under a prospective payment system for Medicare home health organizations"

(National Association for Home Care, 1997, p. 15). To date, 50 home care organizations have been participating in the HCFA demonstration on outcomes-based performance improvement for more than 1 year.

OASIS data have allowed organizations to look at the care that is provided and to see its impact on patients, provided consistency in assessment, and helped to analyze patient needs in a more global perspective (Koch, 1997). It has provided many other benefits that are applicable to an administrative perspective. However, the benefits just mentioned are of primary interest to educators in home health. OASIS will change the way competency programs are designed and the way clinical staff are oriented to the specialty of home care. One can only speculate at how beneficial OASIS will be in helping define and conceptualize the practice of home care. It will be the infrastructure for documentation and will define the approach to care plan development and the provision of care. OASIS will be a part of an intimate part of an organization's orientation program and,

therefore, should be a substantial part of the competency program.

It is obvious from the content provided that competency programs can be derived from the foundations of many different frameworks and models, not just the few that have been identified in the literature. Alspach (1996) relates that "there is no right or best organizing framework to use in identifying competency. Rather, the framework selected to organize competency areas should be one that is appropriate for the role and setting, meaningful to those developing the program and as easy and expedient to use as possible" (p. 41). It is important to be visionary and to anticipate how gross changes in the home care environment will impact the nature and structure of the competency program, such as with OASIS.

Staff development personnel, in collaboration with administrative personnel, need to identify which model or models best suit the needs of the organization prior to program development and then must stay abreast of industry or organizational changes that will impact upon the way the program is implemented.

REFERENCES

Albrecht, M.N. (1990). The Albrecht nursing model for home health care: Implications for research, practice and education. *Public Health Nursing, 7*(2), 118–126.

Albrecht, M.N., Goeppinger, J., Anderson, M.K., Boutaugh, M., Macnee, C., Stewart, K. (1993). The Albrecht nursing model for home healthcare: Predictors of satisfaction with a self-care intervention program. *Journal of Nursing Administration, 23*(1), 51–54.

Albrecht, M.N., & Nelson, T.E. (1993). The Albrecht nursing model for home healthcare: Predictors of health status outcomes in working adults. *Journal of Nursing Administration, 23*(3), 44–48.

Alspach, G. (1996). *Designing competency assessment programs: A handbook for nurses and health-related professionals.* Pensacola, FL: National Nursing Staff Development Organization.

Belanus, A., & Hunt, P. (1994). When orientation is not enough: A group approach for new home healthcare nurses. *Home Healthcare Nurse, 10*(6), 36–40.

Corbett, C.F., & Androwich, I.M. (1994). Critical paths: Implications for improving practice. *Home Healthcare Nurse, 12*(6), 27–41.

del Bueno, D., Barker, F., & Christmyer, C. (1981). Implementing a competency-based orientation program. *Journal of Nursing Administration, 11*(2), 24–29.

Gavin, M.J., Haas, L.J., Pendleton, P.B., Street, J.W., & Wormald, A. (1996). Orienting a new graduate nurse to home healthcare. *Home Healthcare Nurse, 14*(5), 381–387.

Humphrey, C.J., & Milone-Nuzzo, P. (1994) Homecare nursing orientation model: Justification and structure. *Home Healthcare Nurse, 10*(3), 18–25.

Kelly, M.M., & Matlin, C.S. (1993). Use of a conceptual framework in planning and implementing an orientation program. *Journal of Nursing Staff Development, 9*(4), 174–178.

Koch, L.A. (1997). Using OASIS to reach OBQI. *Caring, 16*(8), 34–46.

McGregor, R.J. (1990). A framework for developing staff competencies. *Journal of Nursing Staff Development, 6*(2), 79–84.

Meyer, K. (1997). An education program to prepare acute care nurses for a transition to home health care nursing. *Journal of Continuing Education in Nursing, 28*(3), 124–129.

National Association for Home Care (1997, May). OASIS and data set designed for use by case-mix research study participants. *Homecare News, 12,* 15.

O'Grady, T., & O'Brien, A. (1992). A guide to competency-based orientation: Develop your own program. *Journal of Nursing Staff Development, 8*(3), 128–133.

O'Shea, A.M. (1994). Transition professional nurses into home care: A 6-month mentorship program. *Journal of Home Health Care Practice*, 6(4), 67–72.

Robinson, S.M., & Barberis-Ryan, C. (1995). Competency assessment: A systematic approach. *Nursing Management, 26*(2), 40–44.

Scrima, D.A. (1987). Assessing staff competency. *Journal of Nursing Administration, 17*(2), 41–45.

CHAPTER 7

A Blueprint for Design of a Competency Program

"All great things are simple."
—Winston Churchill

Competency: the thought of the word brings chills and monstrous headaches to clinicians, management, and staff development regardless of the practice setting. However, with proper planning, utilizing regulatory, industry, and organizational specific standards, you can develop a streamlined yet value-packed competency-assessment program that is operationalized to fit the organization.

Competency assessment is important to perform upon hire and is ongoing. This should be a priority for home care organizations: first, because of Joint Commission on Accreditation of Healthcare Organizations standards for home health care; second, due to the expanding scope of practice for all clinical roles, particularly the aide staff; and lastly, because of the risk management issues associated with not doing it. And, of course, we should be doing it because ethically it is a good thing and we want to ensure safe patient care in a setting that is largely unsupervised.

Benner (1984) has been referred to within this text as providing a definition of competency. She defines it best as "the ability to perform the task with desirable outcomes under varied circumstances in the real world" (p. 304). Real world is the key in this definition and particularly so within the home health arena. Training and assessment for minimal competency parameters can occur in a lab setting; however, primary competency assessment should occur in the home setting on a live patient. This is especially important when dealing with home care aides.

How do you begin to build your blueprint for design of a competency program? Assuming that you have assessed your position as far as the pre-development considerations and all is well, then you are ready to begin drafting your program. Following these key steps will put you on the road to building a successful program (Exhibit 7–1). A summary of each will be provided.

ASSIGN RESPONSIBILITY AND ACHIEVE SUPPORT AND BUY-IN FROM ADMINISTRATION

As discussed in Chapter 2, it is essential that the organization assign one role to the development of and accountability for the competency program. The most logical role is that of staff development. In addition, administration should be included from day one of planning. They should be provided with a proposal for program implementation and periodic updates of progression. Chances are, the program in its entirety will meet less resistance if administration is included in every aspect of development and decision making. In doing so, the program will be a true reflection of the organization's beliefs, values, and mission.

DEVELOP POLICIES

After acceptance of the proposal for competency program implementation, the next step is that of policy development. Policies that reflect

Exhibit 7–1 Blueprint for Design of a Competency Program

1. Assign responsibility
2. Develop policies
3. Select a framework
4. Review standards of practice
5. Design and implement needs assessment
6. Establish competency statements
7. Establish performance criteria
8. Provide education
9. Assess competency
10. Document competency
11. Evaluate competency

the responsibilities, process, and evaluative mechanisms of the competency program need to be drafted. Policies can take many forms and include many aspects of program functioning. The policies should match what it is that you will be doing. The policies should include the following components: the individual who is accountable for the program, how the competency program is organized and how it operates, what constitutes competency assessment, how needs are identified, how competency assessment is carried out for each discipline and the frequency of evaluation, how the program is evaluated including performance improvement activities, what is documented, where competency evaluations are housed, and remediation techniques (Exhibit 7–2). In addition, aspects that are related to competency should also have policies drafted specifically in regard to continuing education and inservice education. Policy development forces one to be visionary about the program that is going to be implemented and should function as a road map, helping to direct activities in an organized, intellectual way. Policies also serve as reference tools for those not intimately involved with the program and function to announce the expectations of staff in competency evaluation.

SELECT/DESIGN A FRAMEWORK

As discussed in Chapter 6, frameworks serve to design and structure educational planning and competency assessment. Framework develop-

ment should be the first part of the competency program proposal so that input can be obtained from others within the organization. The framework will assist in guiding the core beliefs and ethics of the program and is the foundation from which development occurs (Table 7–1).

REVIEW STANDARDS OF PRACTICE AND JOB DESCRIPTIONS

This is an essential step in order to precisely and comprehensively develop discipline-specific competency elements. To gather a full understanding of a discipline and what constitutes expected care delivery, standards of practice need to be examined. Standards of practice can be obtained from the discipline's professional organization. Review of job descriptions can further individualize the competency requirements to the organization. In collaboration with this review, one would also incorporate all the determinants of competency as discussed in Chapter 4.

DESIGN AND IMPLEMENT NEEDS ASSESSMENTS

It is of great importance that discipline-specific needs assessments be developed and employed as the starting block for the development of competencies. The information obtained from the needs assessment is then viewed as part of a larger picture that incorporates many aspects of need identification within an organization: to name a few, performance improvement (formerly called quality assurance/quality improvement results, new procedures and equipment, high-risk low-volume procedures, customer concerns, and results of performance reviews. The best way to approach all this information is to take the results of the needs assessments to administration where a collaborative approach can be undertaken to discuss and analyze the needs of the organization and what would be in the best interest of the disciplines being discussed, the organization as a whole, and the consumers. This multidisciplinary approach should result in the formulation of a template identify-

Exhibit 7–2 Clinical Competency Policy

Clinical Competency Policy

Policy 1234

Applicable to

_X_ LPN	_X_ HCA
_X_ RN	_X_ OT
_X_ PT	_X_ SW
	_X_ ST
	_X_ Dietitian

Policy:

Direct care providers will have their clinical competency assessed at predetermined intervals as determined by the organization's staff development program.

Purpose:

Measure and evaluate the competency of direct care providers

Improve and/or expand individual performance and quality of care

Develop, maintain, or improve competency

Ensure safe provision of care

Ensure care delivery reflects organization standards of care

Comply with regulatory and accreditation standards

Procedure:

1. Prehire competency assessment will be verified by way of the following:
   – interview
   – references
   – verification of education, licensure, and certification

2. Upon hire and prior to completion of orientation, discipline-specific competency will be assessed using a combination of direct observation of clinical practice, performance within a simulated lab, self-assessment, and cognitive testing.

3. Ongoing competency assessment will be performed at predetermined intervals as prescribed by staff development.

4. Identification, implementation, and evaluation of ongoing competencies are the responsibility of staff development and are based upon the following indicators:
   – results of performance improvement initiatives, including customer concerns, incident reports, and utilization review
   – staff self-assessment summaries
   – identification of low-volume, high-risk clinical skills
   – implementation of new procedures, equipment, or patient populations
   – managerial or administrative concerns based on data collection or supervisory visits

5. Competency documentation will be filed in the individual's personnel file and will include the following:
   – clinical skills assessed and how assessed (lab, direct observation in practice)
   – verification of demonstration of competency
   – date of assessment
   – signature of evaluator
   – plan for remediation if required

6. Clinical competency program evaluation will occur after every competency endeavor.

7. Staff development will maintain up-to-date descriptions of the following:
   – organization-specific competency evaluation program
   – discipline-specific competency plans
   – staff development conceptual model
   – staff development performance improvement plan
   – educational design principles

---

ing exactly what competencies need to be assessed for an identified time period.

ESTABLISH COMPETENCIES

As noted above, the needs assessment lends itself directly to the identification of competencies. Competencies should be specific to the role being identified, be measurable, and be beneficial to the employee, the organization, and its customers. Competency identification may not only be the performance of skills but the evaluation of critical thinking skills, judgment, and attitudes. The discipline being analyzed should

Table 7–1 Home Care RN Competency Framework

Standards	Competency Statements
Theory	Applies theoretical concepts as a basis for decisions in practice
Data Collection	Collects and records data that are comprehensive, accurate, and systematic
Diagnosis	Utilizes health assessment data to determine nursing diagnosis
Planning	Develops care plans that establish goals: Is based upon nursing diagnoses and incorporates therapeutic, preventative, and rehabilitative nursing actions
Intervention	Intervenes to provide comfort; to restore, improve, and promote health; to prevent complications and sequelae of illness; and to affect rehabilitation
Evaluation	Evaluates clients' and families' responses to interventions in order to determine progress toward goal attainment and to revise the database, nursing diagnoses, and plan of care
Continuity of Care	Provides appropriate and uninterrupted care along the health care continuum, utilizing discharge planning, case management, and coordination of resources
Interdisciplinary Collaboration	Initiates and maintains a liaison relationship with all appropriate health care providers to ensure that all efforts effectively complement one another
Ethics	Utilizes code for nurses established by the ANA as a guide for ethical decision making in practice
Structure and Process of Home Care Organization	Demonstrates professional responsibility in the RN home care role

Source: Adapted with permission from *Standards of Home Health Nursing Practice,* © 1997, American Nurses Association.

also partake in the decision-making process, providing input into what competencies would be realistic, would be useful, and would encourage learning and growth.

DESIGN TOOLS

Two different categories of tools need to be designed. First are tools that will help to organize competency program information. These tools are used to not only organize program information but also to allow easy filing and retrieval of competency records (Appendix B). Second are tools that are used to direct and measure competency. These tools include skills or performance checklists and/or paper and pencil examinations (Exhibits 5–3 and 7–3). The performance checklists should depict industry standards of care and organizational policies and procedures. They should serve to direct practice by defining the ideal way a skill is to be performed or carried out. They are best applied in the home setting; however, they can also be exercised in simulated situations, such as a skills lab. Before implementing such a tool, it is vital that the tool be reviewed by multiple individuals, including administration, to determine its application to practice and reflection of standards of care. Whereas paper and pencil tests are best used to assess a cognitive aspect, paper and pencil tests have limited primary usefulness in competency assessment. They are best used as an adjunct to competency assessment; for example, they could be employed to identify critical thinking ability and problem-solving ability when used in conjunction with clinical case studies. Cognitive measurement is further discussed in Chapter 5.

DESIGN A PLAN FOR REMEDIATION AND RETESTING

This should be easy to undertake because this aspect should have been addressed in step three,

---

Exhibit 7–3 Sample Procedural Performance Checklist

Name: _____   Title: <u>Home Care Aide</u>   Date of Hire: _____

Simple Dressing Change
Competency: Demonstrates dressing change technique by performing the following steps:

Step	Competency Met/Date	Evaluative Method Used
1. Review procedure		
2. Review RN instructions		
3. Gather equipment		
4. Explain procedure to patient		
5. Wash hands		
6. Prepare supplies		
7. Open dressing packages, maintaining sterility		
8. Don clean gloves		
9. Gently remove old dressing, observing drainage color, odor, consistency, and size of wound		
10. Discard dressing and gloves appropriately		
11. Don clean gloves and apply new dressing		
12. Wash hands		
13. Document procedure		
14. Notify RN of changes: color, odor, amount of drainage, swelling, pain, redness, fever.		

continues

Exhibit 7–3 continued

Name: _____   Title: <u>Licensed Practical Nurse</u>   Date of Hire _____

Phlebotomy

Competency: Demonstrates phlebotomy by performing the following steps:

Step	Competency Met/Date	Evaluative Method Used
1. Review procedure		
2. Review RN instructions		
3. Gather equipment		
4. Explain procedure to patient		
5. Wash hands		
6. Prepare supplies and assess sites		
7. Apply tourniquet to arm selected, keeping on no more than 2 minutes		
8. Don clean gloves		
9. Insert needle bevel up		
10. Troubleshoot failure to obtain specimen		
11. Collect specimens as appropriate for tests ordered		
12. Invert specimens gently 3-4 times upon collection		
13. When collection is completed, release tourniquet and vacuum in vacutainer		
14. Smoothly withdraw needle, and place gauze on site, instructing patient to apply pressure		
15. Label and place specimens in biohazard bag, then insulated container as per policy		
16. Wash hands		
17. Document procedure		

developing policies. At least in theory, there should be a plan; however, at this point, the plan needs to be operationalized. It is also at this point that thresholds for successful achievement of competency are set. For example, on the skills checklist, a threshold might be set that all performance criteria need to be met, whereas on a paper and pencil exam, a threshold of 90% may be set for successful achievement. The remediation and retesting techniques should be designed to meet the type of competency being assessed. The policy in step three should also speak to the unfortunate situation where, after repeated attempts, an individual cannot successfully achieve the competency. The individual's manager, if not already informed, needs to be made aware of the situation so that appropriate actions can be undertaken.

ESTABLISH COMPETENCY STATEMENTS

Competency statements are important in that they describe the competency area that is to be measured and define what it is that the employee needs to achieve. They are written broadly and in a way that is measurable, clarifying the intended outcome.

ESTABLISH PERFORMANCE CRITERIA

Performance criteria basically define what an individual needs to accomplish in order to be deemed competent based upon a specific competency statement. Table 7–2 provides examples of registered nurse performance criteria. In essence, performance criteria are expectations for performance of a specific competency. They define the performance behaviors that are necessary for an identified competency. Performance statements are fundamentally behavioral objectives and should begin with a verb. In addition, they should be appropriate to the cognitive, affective, and psychomotor domains defined by Bloom (1956).

PROVIDE EDUCATION

Now that the essential steps of the blueprint have been developed, the next step is to inform and educate key individuals. These individuals include internal customers, such as clinical staff, managers, senior administrators, quality assurance personnel, and human resources. The blueprint in its entirety should be explained to these individuals. In addition, the need for competency assessment and the process by which it will be achieved need to be explained. It is at this point that training is provided to staff who have evaluation responsibilities for other disciplines, such as in the case of the registered nursing staff assessing competency of home care aides in the home setting.

ASSESS COMPETENCY

This is the fun step, the step everyone has been anticipating and should be the easiest step. This step is pretty much self-explanatory. The only point to highlight is that, as discussed in Chapter 4, the evaluators of competency should meet the identified criteria, and, secondly, a remediation plan should be in order in the event that incompetency needs to be addressed.

DOCUMENT COMPETENCY

This is probably the most important step. The old saying stands true, "if you didn't document it, you didn't do it." There are many computer-automated programs available for both staff development and human resources that provide streamlined, easily accessible records. But with any system, it is only as good as the one who enters the data. Many may still rely upon the laborious hand-filing system. The bottom line is that the mechanism that works best for your organization should be used. Disciplines will most likely have many competencies assessed over a short time period, producing many pieces of paper, all of which should not be placed in their human resources file. Instead, it is recommended that a competency template be developed that lists all the competencies assessed with the identification of successful job performance and the signature of the evaluator. Exhibit 7–4 lists the advantages of a competency template. The template should then be filed in human resources in the individual's personnel file. This mechanism works extremely well, particularly at survey time. The surveyor will be happy to find all documents relating to an employee all in one place. The template then only needs to be updated annually. Because home care organizations are generally not as large as hospitals, maintaining this information within a central location such as human resources is probably best; however, the information could also be stored within the auspices of staff development or another convenient location. However, the human

Table 7–2 RN Orientation Competency Performance Criteria (Samples)

Standard—Interdisciplinary Collaboration

Competency Statement	Performance Criteria
Initiates and maintains a liaison relationship with all appropriate health care providers to ensure that all efforts effectively complement one another	• Initiates referrals when appropriate • Documents evidence of interdisciplinary collaboration

Standard—Ethics

Competency Statement	Performance Criteria
Utilizes code for nurse established by the ANA as a guide for ethical decision making in practice	• Provides an example of an ethical dilemma encountered in home care practice • Verbalizes the chain of command to be used when encountering an ethical dilemma

resources files are only a reliable source of competency documentation if there is an efficient and accurate system for filing. It is essential that there be a mechanism for documentation and filing. This mechanism should be spelled out within a policy and should be very functional and useful to those intimately involved. Competency documents such as pretests or posttests, lengthy procedural skills checklists, or evaluations of educational programs should be filed in a location other than the human resources files. Documentation of competency should lie with the individual responsible for the program whether it is initial or annual competency assessment. This individual should also be accountable for making sure that records are up to date and easily accessible and retrievable. Chapter 9 refers comprehensively to competency documentation requirements.

EVALUATION OF THE COMPETENCY PROGRAM

In order to ensure a quality product, the competency program must be evaluated at predetermined intervals. The general items to be evaluated include cost, savings, impact upon care delivery, risk management, and customer satisfaction. The evaluation should demonstrate measurable outcomes. The program can be evaluated by the individual who is responsible for the program or by individuals such as performance-improvement personnel. Exhibit 2–4 represents an example of a program evaluation tool. Chapter 10 refers extensively to performance-improvement initiatives.

The blueprint for competency program development presented can be changed to meet the individual needs of the organization. The sequencing can be transformed as well as the approach to each step. The information provided is only a blueprint, but certainly should not be overlooked as encompassing the essence of program development within a home care setting.

Exhibit 7–4 Advantages of a Competency Template

- Decreases number of competency-related or staff-development documents in human resource file
- Consolidates competency information into one tool
- Provides centralized, accessible competency information
- Utilizes one format for all disciplines

REFERENCES

Benner, P. (1984). *From novice to expert: Excellence and power in clinical nursing practice.* Menlo Park, CA: Addison-Wesley.

Bloom, B.S. (1956). *Cognitive domain, taxonomy of educational objectives. Handbook 1.* New York: David McKay.

CHAPTER 8

Competency-Based Orientation

"Either do not attempt at all or go through with it."
—Ovid

Transitioning professionals and paraprofessionals into the specialty of home care can be a challenging, time-consuming, and costly undertaking for home care organizations (Astarita, 1996). Professionals enter home care with a variety of educational and experiential backgrounds. For the professional entering the home care environment for the first time, the transition can produce culture shock, particularly for those leaving a highly specialized setting. For the paraprofessional, home care may be seen as a vastly unpredictable and unstructured beast, a setting that is probably unlike any that they have ever been exposed to or associated with in the past. Both professionals and paraprofessionals may experience myriad feelings during the orientation process to home care ranging from anxiety, ambivalence, and feeling overwhelmed to feeling more or less challenged psychomotorly and cognitively. Home care organizations have a unique challenge when it comes to orienting individuals to their specialty, primarily because home care is unlike any other health care specialty. The autonomous, unsupervised nature coupled with the knowledge and skill base required to manage payers, a caseload of patients, and a complex documentation system requires a creative approach to learning. In addition, the new paradigm concerning physical and environmental assessments, safety, driving, productivity, and communication mechanisms commonly needs to be employed. The orientation experience needs to be realistic, rewarding,

and measurable. In addition, in this day of cost containment, measures to ensure less financial risk to organizations, such as the costs associated with orientation and turnover, must be closely examined. In doing so, the home care organization will reap the benefits of cost savings and of staff who are confident in their career change and prepared to practice as competent and productive individuals (Astarita, 1996). For the sake of simplicity, this chapter will focus on the professional nurse as the template for competency-based orientation (CBO) development. However, other disciplines will be referred to throughout this chapter, and Appendix C will be referenced as containing examples of CBO for each discipline. The foundation surrounding CBO in home care will first be explored in order to provide a deeper meaning and understanding of this important aspect of competency.

UNIQUENESS OF THE ORIENTATION PROCESS IN HOME CARE

Home health care, as we know, is a rapidly transforming and evolving specialty. From the late 1980s until today, home health care has undergone dramatic alterations in its scope and complexity of services delivered from its traditional roots, with the primary influential forces being both societal and political. Societal factors include forces such as the aging population, frail elderly, the increasing number of women who work outside the home, the increasing mobility of society, and the growing numbers of single-parent families. Political factors include health care entitlement programs and prospective payment systems. Nothing, however, has impacted home care as greatly as managed care. Managed care has caused many changes in the home care setting. Of primary importance is the impact it has had upon the delivery of care for both professional and paraprofessional clinicians. Of all the clinical roles in home care, none has changed as dramatically as nursing. Home care nursing encompasses components and competencies of many different professions. To ensure effective care delivery, home care nurses have had to broaden their clinical repertoire to encompass the skills of a higher-level generalist as well as the knowledge and skill of a social worker, financial counselor, dietitian, teacher, case manager, housing inspector, supervisor, and coordinator. In light of this, the ideal nursing candidate for home care should possess the capability of the aforementioned as well as proficiency in medical-surgical and critical care skills, possess excellent interpersonal communication skills, be able to practice independently, be self-directed, and be computer literate. Additionally, strong decision-making skills, good driving skill, thorough working knowledge of reimbursement and community resources, teaching ability, and the ability to independently manage the complex physical, psychosocial, and environmental needs of individuals of all ages, races, educational levels, socioeconomic, and religious status are required (Astarita, 1996). Once oriented, home care nurses need to develop an understanding of the business of nursing, from managed care contracts and compliance with regulations to how their clinical interventions and judgment have an impact on the organization's bottom line. Humphrey and Milone-Nuzzo (1996) indicate that it is most important that home care nurses possess an up-to-date understanding of the entire health care delivery system, not just the clinical components, in order to provide the best possible care for clients. In spite of the fact that home care nurses embrace all these characteristics and skills, less than desired perceptions of home care

nursing still haunt the specialty today. The perceptions are changing for the positive but needlessly still exist. Some perceive that home care employment is low tech, low stress, and dull; but perceptions vary (Astarita, 1996). Surprisingly, with this perception also comes a curiosity. Other hospital-based disciplines are signing up as contract staff for home care organizations. Non-home care nurses are hearing and reading that home care is the place to be and are experiencing firsthand that care is being transferred to the home earlier and earlier and with greater acuity. These nurses are curious to learn why home care is the place to be. The answers to this include job security, the formation of managed care alliances, the scope and complexity of service delivery, and professional perks.

The formation of managed care alliances is impacting on the job security of nurses within acute care facilities. Downsizing, rightsizing, reengineering, or whatever term is favored, has eliminated nursing positions, prompting nurses to explore other options for employment. Scope and complexity of service delivery refers to the technology and depth of care delivery that is being provided in the home. Home care is now providing the skills and coordinating the services that were once only provided in the acute care setting. The last factor influencing the transition is professional perks. Professional perks are those things that attract nurses into the specialty of home care. For the most part, they include autonomy, the rewards of true case management, hours of work, salary, benefits, and the paradigm shift just mentioned regarding the scope and complexity of service delivery.

Providing an outcome-focused orientation experience for staff who are novices to the specialty of home care is a challenge to most home care agencies. The exponential growth of the home care industry and the rapid expansion of nursing specialty programs within home care have created a demand for agencies to provide orientation programs that are standardized but individualized, quality based but cost effective, and that demonstrate learning outcomes (Astarita, 1996). A solid, outcome-oriented orientation program is not an option. Payers and regulatory and accrediting bodies are requiring it and, to some extent, so are the consumers of the service. The literature reveals that positive outcomes can be achieved through orientation programs such as recruitment and retention of skilled professional nursing staff, delivery of quality patient care, reduced liability, improved job satisfaction, decreased cost of turnover, enhanced agency image, more efficient use of time, regulatory compliance, and improved performance-evaluation process (Snow, Hefty, Kenyon, Bell, & Martaus, 1992; Kenyon, Smith, Hefty, Bell, McNeil, & Martaus, 1990; Brent 1994; Twardon, Gartner, & Cherry 1993; Humphrey & Milone-Nuzzo, 1996).

The orientation process is pivotal to the success of the individual and the organization (O'Shea, 1994). With this in mind, it is essential to recognize that home care agencies are faced with a number of challenges regarding orientation. The challenge that can have the greatest impact is the ability to recruit professional nurses who demonstrate the aforementioned characteristics and skill and then thoroughly screen the candidates regarding their perceptions of the specialty of home care nursing and their career goals. All of these are crucial factors that can be very costly to an organization if overlooked or if not comprehensively investigated. If a true picture is not painted of the job expectations and the uniqueness of home care nursing during the interview process, the organization faces the risk of losing valuable and costly resources should the orientee choose to leave within the first 6 months to 1 year of hire. The small dedication of time in screening and finding the right match may save the organization a significant amount of resources long-term (Astarita, 1996).

Historically, home care orientation was provided by the agency director or an identified nurse manager, consisted of a few hours of one-on-one instruction and a few days in the field orienting with a visit nurse, and was carried out in a nonstructured, nonmeasurable format. After 4 to 5 days, the nurse was set free and was ex-

pected to begin to manage a group of patients. Today, if nurses undergo this type of orientation, they should run as fast as they can away from the organization and never look back. Home care organizations can no longer afford to provide a poor orientation to home care, particularly in today's health care environment. Professionals should not tolerate a poor-quality orientation program to home care; from a risk management and job-satisfaction perspective, it is to their benefit that they do not. During the interview process, professionals contemplating entering the specialty of home care should question the organization about the type of orientation that is provided including its content, length, and expected outcomes. In actuality, all clinical disciplines should be given their specific CBO to peruse during the interview process. This is beneficial to the organization in that it demonstrates to candidates what they will be learning and what is expected of them upon completion of CBO. There is no hidden agenda, and everything is spelled out upfront. The potential candidate is, in essence, getting a global look at a new specialty, the standard of care expectations, and performance expectations associated with the new role.

Entering the home care environment is a challenging endeavor for both professionals and paraprofessionals. Difficulties in making a smooth transition to a new role in the home care setting are not limited to the discipline of nursing. Nursing must coordinate all services, increasing challenges for the educator. In other nursing specialties, nurses are not required to know the inner workings of so many other disciplines as thoroughly as they must in home care. Paraprofessionals may also find home care a difficult environment within which to function, particularly if the individual is a novice to the role as well. Overall, home care is a unique specialty that brings with it distinctive characteristics to each clinical role. All of this posts a huge challenge to staff development in the development of CBOs that are standardized to the setting, yet unique to the role and the individual.

THE ORIENTATION EXPERIENCE

Comprehensive and outcome-focused orientation to a new role or position for any vocation is cardinal to the success of not only the new orientee but also the organization. It is during this time period that both are sizing up one another, deciding if the match is right. The organization is in a position to gain or lose a lot during this transitional period. It can gain the continued employment of an exemplary candidate, a one-of-a-kind individual who is the best match for the position. The benefits of this match long-term are intangible. If the match is not right from the perspective of the organization, the organization basically seeks to lose out on the cost of the hiring process and time lost to finding a better match. However, if the match is not right from the perspective of the orientee, the organization seeks to lose in many regards that can affect it fiscally, organizationally, and socially. It is during this time period that both seek to sell themselves, and it is during this time that the organization has the best opportunity to assist the individual in developing the competencies needed for optimal job performance. If this window of opportunity is not taken by the organization to present a colorful picture of itself and to affect behavior on the part of the new orientee, it stands to lose an imperceptible amount. Probably the worst case scenario is one where a good match is found by the organization, the organization provides a low-quality orientation, and the orientee chooses to stick it out in spite of the poor orientation. Both the orientee and the organization lose in this respect. The orientee is at risk of providing unsafe care, placing both at legal risk; the orientee may not be as productive as possible, costing the organization fiscally; and the orientee may produce minor mistakes on a day-to-day basis that, when compiled, are also costly. There are probably many other intangible losses as well. On the contrary, if the orientee decides to leave within the first year of hire because the skills to function in the role have not been provided, the organization once again stands to lose fiscally. Turnover during this time

period is expensive to organizations and is one aspect that can be diminished dramatically through a solid orientation program. Next to having a good hiring process, the most important aspect is the orientation program. The orientation program should be designed not only to assist orientees to become competent in their new roles but it should also serve to allow the organization to identify red flags; that is, behaviors both clinically and interpersonally that would indicate incompetence and or the ineffectiveness to perform to the standards of the role. The orientation package presented is ultimately a reflection of the educational beliefs of the organization. It is the wrapping on the present that, when removed, reveals if the contents or, in this situation, the job itself is capable of being performed competently based upon the knowledge and skills that were provided during the orientation period. Orientation must be a positive experience and is important because it influences subsequent attitudes toward the entire organization (Abruzzese, 1996). If an individual chooses to leave because of the poor quality of the orientation program, the organization is at risk of negative publicity, which can come back to haunt it with the quality of its applicants, its referral base, its consumer market, or in a number of other ways that can have lasting effects. It is demoralizing to current staff, who perhaps already have low morale from working without enough staff. Abruzzese (1996) relates that "the orientation experience should make staff feel welcome, safe, valued, and excited about learning opportunities." The preceptor-orientee relationship should never be taken lightly, for through the orientation process the preceptor can once again review the organization's good and bad points, as seen through the eyes of the orientee. The preceptor, in turn, may be so negative about the specialty or the organization that the orientee's first and lasting impression of both leads to his or her demise.

In addition to the information provided, one may ask why orientation in home care is so essential. The answers to this are multifaceted and include in part the (1) autonomous nature of home care, (2) unpredictable environment, (3) vast amount of information specific to payers and community resources, (4) interdisciplinary nature of home care, (5) responsibility of care transfer from provider to patient and or family, (6) relationship between documentation and reimbursement, and (7) safety as a new paradigm. These major reasons will be explored briefly.

Clinical personnel in home care work independently. Personnel cannot stick their heads out into the hall and ask for help or a second opinion. They are on their own. Of course, they can always telephone someone, but it is not the same as having another individual present to auscultate breath or heart sounds or to assess a wound. Warner and Albert (1997) indicate that practicing independently in the community environment without the benefit of on-site, readily available resources presents its own challenge. Home care clinical personnel work in an unpredictable environment; one could argue that other traditional health care settings are also unpredictable, but for the purposes of this discussion unpredictable refers to the setting or environment, not the patient. Personnel never know what they will be walking into. The environment can be an immaculate home; a drug-, bug-, and dirt-infested home; or possibly a box under a bridge.

Knowledge base of payers and community resources is necessary for the professional staff, primarily nursing. In order to effectively and legally correctly care for patients, a comprehensive knowledge base is necessary. Traditionally, baccalaureate nursing programs may stress this information but only in a global nature, and in the acute care setting, nursing has had no need to concern itself with this information. Payer and reimbursement information is dramatically different based upon the geographical location and client population being served. Therefore, working knowledge of the local community resources and payers is needed.

In settings other than home care, disciplines such as occupational therapy, physical therapy, speech therapy, dietary, and social work, are interdepartmental, whereas in this setting there are no walls of impediment. Consequently, all clinical personnel need to have a working knowledge of the role functions and care delivery aspects of all disciplines. The disciplines present a cohesive approach to care delivery in the home health care setting and rely on one another more so than in any other setting.

The patient and family are in charge of their care, not the health care provider. The health care provider is on the patients' "turf" and, therefore, needs to display respect and direct interactions based upon this premise.

Reimbursement is based upon documentation. This may sound elementary and implausible; however, the traditional Medicare model reflects this premise. This is starting to change with prospective payment systems but in general is still the norm.

Safety takes on a new meaning for home care providers. Driving skill may need to be refined, and considerations in the event of adverse weather conditions need to be taken into account. Personal safety becomes paramount. Working alone in all types of communities day and night poses significant safety risks. Furthermore, safety of the patient in his or her home environment becomes the home care worker's business. Fall, fire, electrical, and medication safety are of prime importance. Lastly, the skills required of all clinical staff need to be refined and expanded upon, namely physical assessment and patient teaching skills. Because personnel work autonomously, assessment skills become paramount in their skill repertoire. Patient education is probably the number one skilled service in home care; hence, personnel need to be equipped with tools to assist them to become patient educators, educators who are able to measure the effectiveness of their teaching interventions.

Making the Transition from Other Settings

Most recently, the literature speaks to the provision of home care education programs that are marketed to nurses primarily for cross-training purposes or for making oneself more marketable in the employment arena (Reid, 1997; Meyer, 1997). More and more nurses are finding that partaking of an elective home care course is valuable for future employment, and many assist in their current practice by better understanding the global issues associated with the provision of health care services in general.

Reid (1997) discusses the implementation of a transition to home care course offered by a hospital-based home health agency. The purpose of the course was to assist the hospital with decreasing patient census and home care with its increasing census. The course allowed hospital staff to explore home care as a future alternative and provided home care executives the opportunity to expand the pool of nurses who have exposure to the practice of home health care nursing. The course provided 14 hours of lecture and 24 hours of clinical experience and covered topics such as the history of home care, licensing, reimbursement and accreditation, referral process, documentation, and case management. The benefits of the transition to home care course listed by Reid (1997) are multifaceted. Similarly, Meyer (1997) provides an example of a college-based certificate program developed to teach home health nursing skills to registered nurses with acute care experience. The program was developed out of concern that nurses employed in the acute care setting may lose the type of knowledge and skills learned at the baccalaureate level. Additionally, nurses from Associate Degree or Diploma programs may never have been exposed to the concepts of home health nursing. The program is a 12-credit hour, two-semester college program consisting of 8 hours of theory and 4 hours of clinical practicum and is based upon the Omaha Taxonomy. Meyer (1997) relates that the program was developed to maintain the economic welfare of nurses in an era of hospital layoffs, to promote professional development, and to enhance the transition of nurses to home health nursing.

Clearly, Reid (1997) and Meyer (1997) provide examples of creative approaches to meeting the needs of nurses as well as the needs of the ever-increasing alliances between hospitals and home care organizations. For organizations that cannot financially afford to provide an educator to transition nurses into home care, perhaps a feasible option would be to rally with local educational institutions, other home care organizations, and health care facilities to develop a program that would be mutually rewarding to all. It cannot be stressed enough that even if an individual comes to the organization with previous home care experience or a certificate from a home care course or program, it does not negate the fact that the individual still needs an orientation to home care. In theory, the individual still needs to venture through an organization's CBO program.

OVERVIEW OF CBO

CBO can be defined as "a system of orienting one to a role while building on previous knowledge and skill" (O'Grady & O'Brien, 1992). Del Bueno, Barker, and Christmyer (1981) relate that CBO should focus on (1) the outcomes or achievement of performance expectations, (2) use of self-directed learning activities, (3) flexibility and time allowed for achievement of outcomes, (4) use of teacher as facilitator or resource, and (5) assessment of previous learning and learning styles. They also state that a CBO should be individualized to the orientee based on previous experience. A competency model by Alspach (1984) indicates that competency-based curricula should (1) contain clearly articulated competency statements based on the real world, (2) be directed at a specific role in a specific setting, (3) be derived from and validated by expert practitioners, and (4) include criterion-referenced evaluations. Competency curricula utilize adult learning principles, thereby encouraging learning at one's own pace. Of course, in order to be successful, one needs to be internally motivated to learn. Abruzzese (1996) defines CBO as being practice oriented and emphasizes the performance of tasks and not necessarily the acquisition of knowledge. CBO provides structure with learning activities clearly identified. Staab, Granneman, and Page-Reahr (1996) indicate that in CBO, the orientee is given the freedom to individually meet the expectations of the organization because the focus is shifted from the process of instruction to the process of learning. CBO encourages self-learning and is less structured than traditional programs. Traditional orientation is lecture-discussion, whereas CBO focuses on (1) assessment of previous mastery, (2) utilization of self-learning modules or packages, and (3) what the individual can do at the end of orientation. Grant (1993) surveyed nurses to identify their preferred learning method based on their education background and found that, regardless of their educational background, most preferred self-learning. CBO provides an effective, efficient, practical, and cost-effective approach to orientation. It also provides increased quality control by providing consistent information to each new orientee. It is a nontraditional, outcome-focused, educational method that is responsive to adult development needs and learner readiness (Redus, 1994). The advantages of CBO as stated by Ward Norstrand, Rzucidlo, and Culang Levine (1995) include (1) there is a well-defined mechanism to document the basic competencies of a newly hired nurse, (2) management is provided with a comprehensive structure to evaluate performance, (3) the organization is provided with an orientation program that decreases orientation hours and promotes high-quality patient care as a result of clinically competent nursing staff, and (4) if used in conjunction with a preceptor program, recruitment and retention are enhanced by support of the orientee and professional growth of the preceptor.

CBO is not without limitations. Limitations to CBO include the cost of development, time required for performance review, and the requirement that the learner be self-motivated or self-directed. There is no question that CBO, if done properly, will consume organizational resources in the development phase but, over time, should reduce expenditures by defining entry-level practice, providing validation mechanisms for the nurses' practice level, providing preceptors with a clear guide for directing clinical experiences, and providing immediate feedback to orientees regarding their skill level (Redus, 1994). It is, therefore, to the organization's benefit to dedicate resources in advance to the development of CBO. Flewellyn and Gosnell (1987) compared the costs of a CBO program with a traditional program and found that the CBO was double the cost of the traditional program. However, the CBO costs were consistent with preparatory time in the development of the program, acting as a facilitator of learning and in-office activities.

Considerable time for the orientee and preceptor or nurse manager is needed to review performance within a CBO program. A key aspect of a successful CBO program is the selection and training of preceptors. Preceptors are generally thought of as experienced, competent role models who have a good understanding of the organization's mission, philosophy, culture, and operations. They should possess sound interpersonal skill, supervisory capability, and an understanding of the unique experience and characteristics that orientees bring with them. Most importantly, they must have a fondness for teaching. O'Shea (1994) describes that a preceptor's role is to foster growth, independent functioning, and adult learning and to enhance socialization of an orientee. As most can probably attest to, a preceptor can help to make or break a new orientee. How are preceptors chosen? In reality, they should not be chosen, nor should they be made to precept. Instead, an individual should express desire to become a preceptor. At this point, staff development, in collaboration with the individual's manager, should further identify whether the individual meets the prerequisite requirements. Preceptors should be required to attend a preceptor workshop, which should cover learning styles inventories, principles of adult learning, preceptor and orientee rights and responsibilities, conflict resolution, and role modeling as well as the components of the organization's CBO and designated preceptor responsibilities. To retain excellent preceptors, they should be rewarded either financially or through some other organizational mechanism, or they will not feel appreciated and may choose not to precept or may exhibit less than satisfactory performance as a preceptor. Furthermore, evaluation of their performance and the preceptor program should be ongoing. Preceptors and precepting are expanded upon in Chapter 3.

Considerable paperwork may need to be completed in a CBO program. This, of course, depends upon how the CBO program is structured and how simplified the documentation requirements are made. The last limitation of a CBO program is that the learner may not be motivated or self-directed (del Bueno, 1978). The basic premise of CBO is that of self-learning and self-study. Therefore, if the orientee is not motivated or self-directed in his or her learning, then CBO will not be successful for the individual. In summary, the literature surrounding CBO greatly supports its use as a fine method for orientation, despite the minor disadvantages noted (Abruzzese, 1996; Gaffney, Anselmi-Majoros, & Vitello-Cicciu, 1989; Voorhees, 1996; Lassiter, Kearney, & Fell, 1985; O'Grady & O'Brien, 1992; Alspach, 1996).

O'Grady and O'Brien (1992) offer steps in the development of a CBO program. These steps are similar to the ones provided in the blueprint for design of a competency program in Chapter 7. The concepts from both are similar, and the reader is referred to these as resources for CBO development.

The research-based literature regarding CBO in home care is nonexistent. The literature referenced thus far is acute care based. Thus, there is a grand opportunity for nursing scholars to make inquiry into this meaningful area for the home care industry and educators alike. The writers, from their practice in staff development, have found many benefits of CBO in home care. CBO provides a uniform knowledge base, provides a standardized evaluation mechanism, identifies early on if an orientee is not going to succeed in the home care setting, provides expectations upfront of the job requirements for knowledge and skill acquisition, examines and defines home health care practice, improves morale of nurses involved in a preceptor program, im-

proves documentation of staff competency, can be used by managers as an evaluative mechanism during probation, and produces clinical staff who are comfortable and confident in their roles.

CBO FORMAT

The format for CBO can be varied, but generally there are assessment tools utilized to assess the orientee's skill and knowledge level. In addition, there is some type of format that lists all the components of competency validation. Stewart and Vitello-Cicciu (1989) provide three essential components of a CBO program. They include competency statements, critical behaviors, and learning options or resources. Additionally, a time frame or target date for accomplishment should also be addressed. Alspach (1996) utilizes competency statements and performance criteria in the development of competency programs. She identified five essential characteristics of competency statements (Exhibit 8–1) and seven essential characteristics of performance criteria (Exhibit 8–2). Alspach (1996) first identifies the competency areas, then develops competency statements, which are then followed by the development of performance criteria that define what staff must be able to demonstrate as evidence that they are competent in that area. She also does a fine job delineating the differences between instructional objectives and performance criteria (Table 8–1), highlighting that traditional instructional objectives emphasize knowing, whereas performance criteria emphasize doing. Four essential components for constructing a competency have been proposed by Gurvis and Grey (1995). They include the competency statement, critical behavior or criteria, learning option, and evaluation method, all of which provide for a clear, measurable expectation of competence for the learner and the validator. The three references cited provide similar themes for constructing a competency. Establishing explicit and correct content of a competency validation tool that meets the intended needs of the orientation or ongoing competency assessment program is one

Exhibit 8–1 Essential Characteristics of a Competency Statement

- Describes a general category of behavior or performance
- Describes employee behavior
- Describes behavior that is observable and measurable
- Includes no conditions imposed on performance
- Is validated by practitioners in a designated role and setting

Source: Reprinted from *Designing Competency Assessment Programs: A Handbook for Nursing and Health-related Professions* with the permission of the National Nursing Staff Development Organization, © 1996.

Exhibit 8–2 Essential Characteristics of Performance Criteria

- Describe employee behavior
- Describe behavior that is observable and measurable
- Are limited to a single behavior
- Include sufficient description of the behavior
- Include desired conditions imposed on performance
- Include a performance standard
- Include only essential aspects of performance

Source: Reprinted from *Designing Competency Assessment Programs: A Handbook for Nursing and Health-related Professions* with the permission of the National Nursing Staff Development Organization, © 1996.

of the most important aspects of competency program development.

Of interest is the recommendation of Goodman (1997) to structure hospital nursing orientation as a critical pathway that is integrated with case-teaching methods. The orientation is based on a case-management model and functions to provide a consistent structure for orientation, streamline the orientation process, and enhance the development of orientees to competent levels of nursing practice. Goodman (1997) further relates that the critical path for orientation describes the course of events for orientation and delineates specific orientation activities that occur during segments of the orientation period. It provides clear communication of performance and progress expectations. This is a creative approach to orientation-program structuring, is based upon adult learning principles, and contains a few components of a competency-based program. The author provides yet another approach to teaching new orientees that can be utilized as the format for orientation presentation and development.

Use of a competency-based model for design of an orientation program in home care is advantageous. In light of the uniqueness of the home health care setting, it seems only natural to utilize an approach that, in actuality, fits the design and structure of home care like a hand and glove.

Identification of Orientation Competencies

Orientation competencies are derived from accrediting and regulatory bodies, standards of care (Appendixes A and B), and organizational specific standards as well as the literature. The Joint Commission lists the minimum orientation topics that must be included in orientation (Exhibit 8–3). Likewise, Medicare Conditions of Participation list the competencies for hiring of aide staff (see Appendix A). One cannot go wrong by using these topics as the framework for the orientation program and then building upon them according to the other components mentioned.

Once again, insufficient research-based literature is available regarding the specific orientation needs and competency evaluation methods of clinical home care staff in general. The avail-

Table 8–1 Comparison of Instructional Objectives and Performance Criteria

Feature	Instructional Objectives	Performance Criteria
Behavioral emphasis	Knowing	Doing
Means of evaluation	Written test	Performance checklist
Location of evaluation	Classroom	Work setting*
Relationship to job	Indirect and limited; relate only to knowledge about job	Direct and full; represent essential aspects of competent job performance

*or a simulation of the actual work setting

Source: Reprinted from *Designing Competency Assessment Programs: A Handbook for Nursing and Health-related Professions* with the permission of the National Nursing Staff Development Organization, © 1996.

able literature speaks strictly to the specialty of nursing and is not consistent in its documentation of findings. The rationale of this is perhaps because nursing has not empirically defined what home health nursing practice is. Daley and Miller (1996) are the only published authors who have sought scholarly inquiry into the actual practice of home health care nursing. The available literature can be divided into three categories: (1) research-related literature, (2) content for inclusion in the orientation programs, and (3) individual and organizational descriptions of home care orientation programs.

The first category is reflective of the work by Daley and Miller (1996). Daley and Miller (1996) conducted a qualitative interpretivist study to analyze the characteristics of nursing practice in home health care using Benner's (1984) framework. The purpose was to move away from the current surveys and assessments that make up the knowledge base in home health care nursing and instead study the practice of nursing. Twenty-one registered nurses with home health care experience ranging from 1 month to 25 years were purposively sampled from one home health agency. Data were collected in the form of exemplars or clinical narratives. They found that home health care practice develops along a continuum of levels within do-

mains. Four major domains of practice in home health care were identified. They include assessing and using physiologic and pathophysiologic data; initiating and monitoring therapeutic interventions; assessing and using family and environmental data; and integrating data, interventions, and context. Daley and Miller (1996) indicate that

> the findings suggest that home health care nurses need a broad comprehensive educational base along with staff development and continuing educational programs that upgrade and enhance their knowledge, skills and abilities. The authors further propose that the levels be used to develop orientation programs that include content on the environment and home management, use of community resources and collaborative practice, and the analysis of expert exemplars of home health care nursing practice for the purpose of understanding the complexity of integrating data, interventions and context.

The second category encompasses the content that is recommended for inclusion in a home

Exhibit 8–3 Minimum Orientation Topics

- Organization's mission, vision, and goals
- Types of care or services provided
- The organization's policies and procedures, including those for advance directives and death and dying
- Confidentiality of patient information
- Home safety, including bathroom, fire, environmental, and electrical safety
- Safety issues in the home care organization, including fire prevention and security
- Emergency preparedness
- Appropriate action in unsafe situations
- Infection prevention and control, including personal hygiene; aseptic procedures; communicable infections; precautions; and cleaning, disinfection, and sterilization of equipment and supplies
- Storing, handling, and accessing of supplies, medical gases, and drugs
- Equipment management, including safe and appropriate use of equipment
- Identifying, handling, and disposing of hazardous or infectious materials and wastes in a safe and sanitary manner and according to law and regulation
- Tests to be performed by the staff
- Screening for abuse and neglect
- Referral guidelines, including guidelines for timeliness
- Care or services provided by other staff members to facilitate coordination and appropriate patient referral
- Community resources
- Care or service responsibilities
- Other patient care responsibilities

Source: Data from *Comprehensive Accreditation Manual for Home Care*, p. 391, © 1996, Joint Commission on Accreditation of Healthcare Organizations.

care orientation program. Humphrey and Milone-Nuzzo (1994) identify key content areas that should be addressed in a home care orientation program. They include the structure and specialty of home care, strategies for effective clinical management, supervision, documentation, quality assurance, legal aspects, the home visit, infection control, the Medicare home care benefit, client teaching, and home care nursing strategies for success. These authors relate that orientation is the beginning of a home care nurse's practice and demonstrate this through the use of a nursing practice model (1996). They also state that regardless of previous clinical experience, all nurses entering home care do so as novice practitioners (1996). Benefield (1996) indicates that a home care orientation plan should include content that reflects the elements of productive practice. These elements reflect 35 areas of knowledge and abilities and represent critical job categories for home care. Lastly, American

Health Consultants (1996) suggest that the following be provided: education on home care documentation, infection control, and safety; ensuring that nurses can read maps; and explanation of physician communication procedures. They also recommend providing instruction from specialists to broaden the narrow focus. Hefty, Kenyon, Martaus, Bell, and Snow (1992), Kenyon et al. (1990), and Snow et al. (1992) are often quoted in the home care literature in terms of their recommendations for content inclusion in a community health orientation. However, because their focus is community health and not home health, exploration of their recommendations will not be undertaken. The third category contains literature that represents individual or organizational depiction of home care orientation structure and development (Astarita, 1996; Leighton, Davis, & Anderson, 1990; O'Shea, 1994; Twardon et al., 1993; Green, 1994; Harris & Yuan, 1991; Belanus & Hunt, 1994). This literature reflects orientation programs that range from very basic to complex. Some are based upon conceptual frameworks, and some reflect the auspices of CBO. Taken in their entirety, they provide a functional home care orientation program but one that would not reflect the summation of this book.

The literature presented contains underlying themes that can be used to further develop and refine the content of a home care orientation program. In general, all disciplines should be subject to common core competencies that are specific to the character of home care and to the organization. Exhibit 4–3 provides a summation of some of the recommended common core competencies. It is recommended that staff development construct the core competencies and then seek out a multi-disciplinary review in order to ensure accurateness and completeness. In addition, it cannot be stressed enough how important it is to incorporate competencies that are unique and specific to the day-to-day functioning of the organization. Obviously, this material is difficult to portray in the context of this book because each educator needs to develop his or her own organization-specific competencies. The templates in Appendix B are reflective of professional standards, regulatory and accreditation standards, and recommendations from the literature. Combining these recommendations with organizational standards will lead to the development of orientation competencies that are specific to the discipline, are functional, are beneficial to the learner, and are reflective of the organization. Until additional inquiry into the orientation needs of home care personnel is sought, staff-development personnel will need to continue to design competencies that reflect the categories presented.

Essential Design Components

There are fundamental design components of a home care CBO program. They include an orientation schedule, modules, self-assessment tools, self-study guide, and an evaluation tool. An orientation schedule forces staff develop-

ment and other disciplines within the organization to get organized. Home care schedules are extremely important because the new orientee needs to be directed in this autonomous setting. Home care orientation schedules should be provided on the first day of employment to the orientee, maybe even before, and should encompass at least the first 4 weeks of employment (Exhibit 8–4). Orientees will find the schedule a godsend. This shows orientees that they were expected and planned for. Orientees will also perceive the organization as having its act together. The schedule should include the following: prescheduled appointments with identified individuals who partake in educating new employees, designated visit days, blocks of self-study time, and other scheduled experiences, such as competency assessment and classes. The schedule should also list pertinent information such as preceptor and manager name and phone number, location of appointments, and, if appropriate, a map of the organization.

Modules serve to divide orientation by time and to structure the learning process. They also serve to guide the orientee and provide a map of learning expectations. Modules can be formatted in many ways; nevertheless, they should include competency statements, critical behaviors, learning resources, and an area for competency signature validation (Appendix C). The modules demonstrate the outcome expectations of the orientation experience and can be utilized as an orientation performance tool by management. Modules need to be discipline specific and should be customized as such.

Self-assessment tools should be customized to meet the needs of the role and the organization. The self-assessment tools can be administered during the hiring process or during the orientation process. The tools can be used as screens, assisting staff development to better customize the unique orientation needs of the new orientee. They should be used only as a guide that indicates what the orientee feels he or she needs to learn or is well skilled or versed at. Appendix 8–A provides an example of a self-assessment tool.

Exhibit 8–4 Sample Orientation Schedule

Orientee Name _____ Date of Hire _____

Primary Preceptor _____ Secondary Preceptor _____

SAMPLE WEEK ONE OF PROPOSED SIX-WEEK ORIENTATION

Date/Time		Topic	Contact Person/Location
MON 1/5	8–5 PM	General Organizational Orientation	Staff Development/Multi-Purpose room
TUE 1/6	8–9 AM	Infection Control	Staff Development/Office
	9–10 AM	TB Fit Testing/Bag Technique	Staff Development/Office
	10–11 AM	Office Tour	Office Manager/Front Desk
	11–12 PM	Supply Acquisition	Medical Supply Clerk/First Floor
	12–1 PM	LUNCH	
	1–5 PM	Home Visits	Preceptor/Lobby
WED 1/7	8–10 AM	CLASS ONE: Medicare Overview	Staff Development/Office
	10–12 PM	Self-Study per assignment	Library
	12–1 PM	LUNCH	
	1–5 PM	Laptop Computer Class One	Computer Learning Center
THUR 1/8	8–10 AM	CLASS TWO: 485/486	Staff Development/Office
	10–12 PM	Discipline-specific class	Team Manager/Office
	12–1 PM	LUNCH	
	1–5 PM	Home Visits	Preceptor/Lobby
FRI 1/9	8–12 PM	Laptop Computer Class Two	Computer Learning Center
	12–1 PM	LUNCH	
	1–3 PM	Self-Study per assignment	Library
	3–5 PM	CLASS THREE: Risk Management	Staff Development/Office

Self-study is an essential characteristic of CBO. As indicated before, the orientee needs to be self-motivated to learn, or CBO will not be an effective orientation mechanism for the individual. It is beneficial for organizations to set aside a learning environment within their building. This can be a library or other assigned area. The area should be conducive to learning and include all the reference and resource materials needed for the orientation process. The learning area may contain primary and secondary references, computer-assisted instruction, videos, sample charts, Health Information Manual (HIM 11), Medicare Conditions of Participation, policy and procedure manuals, infection control materials, organization-specific documentation resources, and any other materials that are educational in nature. A form should be developed that lists assignments and directs the orientees' self-learning (Exhibit 8–5). Staff development should act as a resource for the self-study requirements, answering questions that the orientee may have and further clarifying learned material. When should self-study be offered throughout the orientation period and how much time should be allotted to this endeavor? These questions remain to be answered. Staff development will need to design what works best for the organization and reevaluate and plan according to the orientation evaluations.

Exhibit 8–5 Orientation Self-Study Checklist

Assignment	Date Completed	Orientee Initials	Evaluator Initials
Policy Manual (assigned policies per module)			
Procedure Manual (assigned per module)			
Infection Control Manual			
Laboratory Manual(s)			
Utilization Management Manual			
Medicare Conditions of Participation			
Chart Review (Medical Records)			
Health Care Financing Administration Publication–11 (Section 2, Revision 222)			
Videos: (examples)			
1. Protect Your Back			
2. Universal Precautions			
3. Fire Safety			
4. Home Safety			
5. Defensive Driving			
6. The Home Visit			
7. Aseptic Bag Technique			
8. Organizing Your Day			
Journal Articles: (list selected articles)			
Computer-Assisted Instruction: (examples)			
1. Protecting Patient and Resident Rights			
2. Patient Education			
3. Orientee Choice			
Self-Learning Modules: (list per discipline)			

Orientee Signature/Date _____

Source: Reprinted from Astarita, T.M., Competency Based Orientation in Home Care: One Agency's Approach, *Home Health Care Management and Practice,* Vol. 8, No. 4, p. 45, © Aspen Publishers, Inc.

Orientation evaluation tools are a must. Every orientee should have the ability to evaluate his or her orientation experience both in writing and verbally if he or she wishes. The evaluation tool should be provided at the beginning of orientation so that the orientee, if necessary, can provide ongoing feedback. The evaluation serves as a quality-monitoring activity, identifying what works and what areas are in need of improvement. Chapter 9 refers in more detail to the evaluation process.

A creative approach to handling the orientation paper trail is to develop an orientation manual. The manual can contain the essential orientation paper components just referenced, as well as reference and administrative materials (Exhibit 8–6). The possibilities are endless as far as the format of the manual. The manual can be referred to as the home care brain, a resource and learning guide that is utilized by the orientee during the orientation process and perhaps as a reference for months afterward. The orientee can

Exhibit 8–6 Contents of Generic Orientation Manual

Orientation schedule

Competency-based orientation module

Organizational Mission or Vision

Frequently utilized policies and procedures

Sample documentation

Laptop usage instructions

Organization-approved abbreviation list

Specialty program information

On-call guidelines

After hours visit guidelines

Time codes

Beeper numbers

Equipment directions

Payer source guidelines

Safety tips

Referral indicators for multiple disciplines

PPE guidelines

---

be encouraged to add to the manual any materials that he or she finds essential to the performance of the job, such as key policies and procedures, community resources, phone list, preauthorization guidelines, medical assistance specifics, equipment instruction booklets, laboratory drop-off locations, documentation guidelines, nursing diagnoses, coding tables, and so on. The manual can be carried in the automobile and used as a quick reference. Of course, there will be a cost associated with the development of such a manual; however, the benefits of having such a resource most likely outweigh the small financial investment. The cost per manual is only a few dollars. To help save on cost, the manuals could be recycled. The orientee could be instructed to keep the manual as long as necessary and, when he or she feels that the manual is no longer a necessity, would be instructed to return it for recycling for another orientee. It is important to note that the manuals should be updated on a regular basis in order to provide correct information to the orientee. A multidisciplinary approach in the development of the orientation manual is best. The manuals should contain core information pertinent to all disciplines and discipline-specific materials that would be added based on the role being oriented.

Participants

In order for a home care orientation to be successful, all departments of the organization must partake in responsibility. The uniqueness of the home care environment is such that many individuals are responsible for providing education to the new orientee. Clinical personnel rely heavily on the many roles within a home care organization in order to be able to provide effective care, hence, the importance of having role-specific representatives educate the orientee on the various components/positions within a home health care organization. Additionally, because home care clinical providers spend the majority of their day in the field having no face-to-face contact with representatives of the organization, it is so important that face-to-face contact does occur with key individuals during the orientation process. When a favor is needed or consultation is sought regarding a patient care issue, it is nice to be able to place a name to a face and to know that a relationship was established during this time period. The individuals and or departments that should be included in the orientation process are the chief executive officer, director, risk management/systems improvement, marketing, finance, human resources, staff development, infection control, specialty team representatives, intake/referral, discipline-specific personnel, medical records, medical supplies, utilization/insurance, scheduler, and, last but not least, payroll. The degree to which these individuals and/or departments participate in the orientation process is negotiable. Mutually agreed-upon learning objectives should first be developed between staff development and the individuals or departments prior to the educational endeavor. It should not be overlooked that these individuals and departments are staff development's customers and should be treated as such. These individuals can have a positive or negative impact upon the new orientee, helping to paint a picture of the organization as a whole.

New Graduates in Home Care

No discussion of orientation would be complete without addressing home care's industry practice pertaining to new graduate nurses. Once again, the literature is lacking rationale as to why new graduate nurses in home care are not utilized. One can transpose that the rationale generally has to do with the level of competency of the new graduate, the autonomous nature of the setting, and the risk management issues associated with the provision of care by individuals who lack qualitative clinical experience. Gavin, Haas, Pendleton, Street, and Wormald (1996) suggest that nursing education does not facilitate a direct transition from the undergraduate program to employment in home health care. In light of this, schools of nursing and home care organizations should demonstrate a collaborative effort in the provision of home health care education and the quality and quantity of clinical experience. The establishment and nurturing of such a relationship would be mutually rewarding. Currently, home care organizations that employ graduate nurses should, because of the varied entry into practice educational levels, ascertain from every candidate the content of home health care knowledge and clinical experience that was provided in their educational program. The acquisition of this information will allow the home care organizations to select the most qualified candidates out of the graduate pool and will also allow the educator to effectively provide an individualized orientation experience to the profession of home health care nursing. Historically, home care organizations as part of their RN credentialing required 1 year of acute care experience, namely medical-surgical experience, for employment in home care. Of interest is the fact that new graduate social workers and therapists are commonly utilized in the home care setting. Gavin et al. (1996) developed a pilot program to orient newly graduated RNs (AD or BSN) with no previous nursing experience in the home health care field. Benner's model skill list was utilized to identify performance characteristics and teaching and learning needs of new graduates. In addition, ANA standards for home health nursing practice were used as the outcome criteria, and a preceptor course was developed to prepare the preceptors for the new graduates. The program time frame was 13 weeks. At 6 weeks, it was identified that the new orientees needed increased exposure to clinical skills and were provided exposure to these skills within health care facilities. At program completion, it was determined that all outcome criteria were met. The authors showed that a well-organized and supported new graduate preceptor program is a feasible alternative in home health care. It is of the writer's opinion that new graduate nurses can be utilized in the home care setting; however, this should only occur if there is an established new graduate nurse orientation program that is of sufficient content and length to meet the needs of new graduates. The CBO would extend beyond the one presented to include such content as basic nursing skill competency, critical thinking, principles of pharmacology, state nurse practice act principles, ethics, confidentiality, time management, organization, and perhaps communication skills.

EXPECTED OUTCOMES

The ultimate expected outcome of a home care CBO program is that the orientee has successfully met all the orientation outcomes. Further, having successfully met the outcomes, it is hoped that the orientee is providing safe, effective care and feels that he or she can carry out the role requirements and feels comfortable doing so, at least momentarily. Belanus and Hunt (1994) indicate that orientation is not enough and, indeed, feel that orientees have new needs at 3 and 6 months. They relate that home care nurses have many educational needs during the first year of employment. Using Maslow's hierarchy of needs, they classified learning needs and formed a "Group" to help meet the needs of developing home care nurses. Home health care nursing, as with any other nursing specialty, is in need of ongoing support, needs assessment, and education of novice staff. This is also true of the other disciplines in the home health care setting. All this is needed in order to help successfully transition staff through the levels of competency development. It is also hoped that CBO will enable the early removal of those individuals who will not succeed in the home care arena, has met the orientation requirements of the regulatory and accrediting bodies, has demonstrated being a cost-effective mechanism for educating individuals new to home health care, has identified personal strengths and areas needing extra attention of the new orientee, has provided a documentation mechanism of basic competencies, has assisted in the personal and professional growth of the preceptors, and lastly has demonstrated having an impact upon recruitment and retention.

REFERENCES

Abruzzese, R.S. (1996). *Nursing staff development: Strategies for success* (2nd ed.). St. Louis, MO: Mosby-Year Book, Inc.

Alspach, G. (1984). Designing a competency-based orientation for critical care nurses. *Heart & Lung, 13*(6), 655–662.

Alspach, G. (1996). *Designing competency assessment programs: A handbook for nurses and health-related professionals.* Pensacola, FL: National Nursing Staff Development Organization.

American Health Consultants. (1996). Transitioning to home care: Follow these 6 tips to orient ex-hospital nurses. *Home Care Education Management, 1*(1), 1–3.

Astarita, T.M. (1996). Competency-based orientation in home health care: One agency's approach. *Home Health Care Management and Practice, 8*(4), 38–49.

Belanus, A., & Hunt, P. (1994). When orientation is not enough. *Home Healthcare Nurse, 10*(6), 36–40.

Benefield, L.E. (1996). Productivity in home healthcare: Assessing nurse effectiveness and efficiency. (Part 1). *Home Healthcare Nurse, 14*(9), 698–706.

Benner, P. (1984). *From novice to expert: Excellence and power in clinical nursing practice.* Menlo Park, CA: Addison-Wesley.

Brent, N.J. (1994). Orientation to home healthcare nursing is an essential ingredient of risk management and employee satisfaction. *Home Healthcare Nurse, 10*(2), 9–10.

Daley, B.J., & Miller, M. (1996). Defining home healthcare nursing: Implications for continuing nursing education. *Journal of Continuing Education in Nursing, 27*(5), 228–237.

del Bueno, D. (1978). Competency-based education. *Nurse Educator, 5*(3), 10–14.

del Bueno, D.J., Barker, F., & Christmyer, C. (1981). Implementing a competency-based orientation program. *Journal of Nursing Administration, 11*(5), 24–29.

Flewellyn, B., & Gosnell, D. (1987). Comparing two methods of hospital orientation for cost effectiveness. *Journal of Nursing Staff Development, 3*(1), 3–8.

Gaffney, T., Anselmi-Majoros, K., & Vitello-Cicciu, J. (1989). Competency-based education in thrombolytic therapy: A modular approach. *Journal of Cardiovascular Nursing, 4*(1), 57–61.

Gavin, M.J., Haas, L.J., Pendleton, P.B., Street, J.W., & Wormald, A. (1996). Orienting a new graduate nurse to home healthcare. *Home Healthcare Nurse, 14*(5), 381–387.

Goodman, D. (1997). Application of the critical pathway and integrated case teaching method to nursing orientation. *Journal of Continuing Education in Nursing, 28*(5), 205–210.

Grant, P. (1993). Formative evaluation of a nursing orientation program: Self-paced vs. lecture-discussion. *Journal of Continuing Education in Nursing, 24*(6), 245–248.

Green, P.H. (1994). Meeting the learning needs of home health nurses. *Journal of Home Health Care Practice, 6*(4), 25–32.

Gurvis, J.P., & Grey, M.T. (1995). The anatomy of a competency. *Journal of Nursing Staff Development, 11*(5), 247–252.

Harris, M.D., & Yuan, J. (1991). Educating and orienting nurses for home healthcare. *Home Healthcare Nurse, 9*(4), 9–14.

Hefty, L.V., Kenyon, V., Martaus, T., Bell, M.L., & Snow, L. (1992). A model skills list for orienting nurses to community health agencies. *Public Health Nursing, 9*(4), 228–233.

Humphrey, C.J., & Milone-Nuzzo, P. (1994). Homecare nursing orientation model: Justification and structure. *Home Healthcare Nurse, 10*(3), 18–25.

Humphrey, C.J., & Milone-Nuzzo, P. (1996). *Manual of home care nursing orientation.* Gaithersburg, MD: Aspen Publishers.

Kenyon, V., Smith, E., Hefty, L.V., Bell, M.L., McNeil, J., & Martaus, T. (1990). Clinical competencies for community health nursing. *Public Health Nursing, 7*(1), 33–39.

Lassiter, C., Kearney, M., & Fell, R. (1985). Competency-based orientation, an idea that works. *Journal of Nursing Staff Development, 1*(4), 68–73.

Leighton, E.M., Davis, R.H., & Anderson, L.J.W. (1990). An orientation program for high-technology home care nursing. *Pediatric Nursing, 16*(2), 182–185.

Meyer, K.A. (1997). An educational program to prepare acute care nurses for transition to home health care nursing. *Journal of Continuing Education in Nursing, 28*(3), 124–129.

O'Grady, T., & O'Brien, A. (1992). A guide to competency-based orientation: Develop your own program. *Journal of Nursing Staff Development, 8*(3), 128–133.

O'Shea, A.M. (1994). Transitioning professional nurses into home care: A 6-month mentorship program. *Journal of Home Health Care Practice, 6*(4), 67–72.

Redus, K.M. (1994). A literature review of competency-based orientation for nurses. *Journal of Nursing Staff Development, 10*(5), 239–243.

Reid, G.C. (1997). Transitioning nurses from hospital to home. *Home Health Care Management and Practice, 9*(4), 22–30.

Snow, L., Hefty, L.V., Kenyon, V., Bell, M.L., & Martaus, T. (1992). Making the fit: Orienting new employees to community health nursing agencies. *Public Health Nursing, 9*(1), 58–64.

Staab, S., Granneman, S., & Page-Reahr, T. (1996). Examining competency-based orientation implementation. *Journal of Nursing Staff Development, 12*(3), 139–143.

Stewart, S., & Vitello-Cicciu, J. (1989). Designing a competency-based orientation program for the care of cardiac surgical patients. *Journal of Cardiovascular Nursing, 3*(3), 34–40.

Twardon, C., Gartner, M., & Cherry, C. (1993). A competency achievement orientation program: Professional development of the home health nurse. *Journal of Nursing Administration, 23*(7/8), 20–25.

Voorhees, M. (1996). Using competency-based education in the perioperative setting. *Nursing Management, 27*(8), 35–38.

Ward Norstrand, P., Rzucidlo, S.E., & Culang Levine, T. (1995). Implementation of learning activities. In *Core curriculum for nursing staff development* (pp. 153–170). Pensacola, FL: National Nursing Staff Development Organization.

Warner, I., & Albert, R. (1997). Avoiding legal land mines in home healthcare nursing. *Home Health Care Management and Practice, 9*(6), 8–16.

RN Self-Assessment

Name _____ Date _____ Employee I.D. _____

Part I: Nursing Intervention Self-Assessment

Directions: Place a check in the box if a favorable response is warranted.

DIAGNOSIS	I can identify signs & symptoms	I can identify at least 3 nursing interventions
CARDIOPULMONARY		
Angina		
Aortic Aneurysm		
Arterial Occlusion		
Congestive Heart Failure		
Endocarditis		
Hypertension		
Hypovolemia		
Myocardial Infarction		
Pacemaker Malfunction		
Pericarditis		
Peripheral Vascular Disease		
Acute Respiratory Failure		
Asthma/Bronchospasm		
Bronchitis		
Chronic Obstructive Pulmonary Disease		
Hypoxia		
Mucus Plugging		
Obstructed Airway		
Pleural Effusion		
Pneumonia		
Pulmonary Edema		
Pulmonary Eboli		
GASTROINTESTINAL/GENITOURINARY		
Colitis/Diarrhea		
Constipation/Impaction		
Esophageal Reflux		

continues

131

DIAGNOSIS	I can identify signs & symptoms	I can identify at least 3 nursing interventions
Gastrointestinal Bleeding		
Paralytic Ileus		
Urinary Retention		
Urinary Tract Infection		
Renal Failure		
Pre/Post Prostatectomy		
Prostatitis		
NEUROLOGICAL/SKELETAL		
ALS/MS		
CNS infections		
CVA, Impending or Post		
Guillain Barré		
Paraplegia/Quadriplegia		
Post Head Injury		
Seizures		
Compartment Syndrome		
DVT		
Fractures/Dislocations/Cast Care		
Osteoporosis/Osteoarthritis		
Post-operative infections		
Total Joint Replacement		
ENDOCRINE		
Hypoglycemia		
Hyperglycemia		
Communicable Diseases		
AIDS/Compromised Immunity		
HBV		
MRSA/VRE		
TB		

Part II. Nursing Skills Self-Assessment

Directions: Place a check in the appropriate box.

SKILL	EXPERIENCE			
	None	Limited	Moderate	Extensive
RESPIRATORY				
Oxygen Therapy:				
Face Mask				
Tracheal Collar				
Transtracheal				
Metered Dose Inhalers				
Suctioning:				
Nasal				
Tracheal				
Tracheostomy:				
Site Care				
Inner Cannula Change				
GASTROINTESTINAL				
Gastric:				
Insertion				
Maintenance				
Colostomy:				
Maintenance				
Irrigation				
Ileostomy:				
Maintenance				
GENITOURINARY				
Catheterization:				
Insertion-Male				
Insertion-Female				
Irrigation				
Ureterostomy:				
Maintenance				
Nephrostomy:				
Maintenance				
Suprapubic catheter:				
Maintenance				
Biliary tube:				
Maintenance				

continues

SKILL	EXPERIENCE			
	None	Limited	Moderate	Extensive
Flushing				
INFECTIOUS DISEASE				
Culture collection:				
Throat				
Wound				
INTEGUMENTARY				
Application of Compression Bandage				
Suture/Staple removal				
Wound Irrigation				
Removal of JP drain				
EQUIPMENT				
Pulse oximeter:				
Application				
Set-up				
Troubleshooting				
Nebulizers:				
Application				
Administration				
Tracheal				
Troubleshooting				
Suction Machine:				
Set-up				
Operation				
Troubleshooting				
Enteral pumps:				
Set-up				
Operation				
Troubleshooting				
Intravenous pumps: (List all used by geographical region):				
Glucometers: (List all used by geographical region)				

Employee Signature _____

CHAPTER 9

Ongoing Competency Evaluation Program

"It is possible to fly without motors, but not without knowledge and skill."
—Wilbur Wright

SCOPE

As indicated by Alspach (1996), competency is not a static phenomenon and, therefore, needs to be envisioned as ongoing and ever-changing. Hence, competency is not a once-and-done event and will need to be assessed at predetermined intervals that are identified by staff development in collaboration with management. In general, competencies should be (1) dynamic, changing from year to year for established staff, (2) based upon the needs of the role or the needs of the organization including high-risk, low-volume tasks, (3) unique to the responsibilities of the role, and (4) in agreement with the organization's competency policy; you must do what you say you're going to do (Alspach, 1996).

Ongoing competency assessment can be made quite simple with adequate planning and by maintaining a pulse on the ever-changing skill requirements of clinical staff. Of the two, planning is the more considerable aspect. Planning for ongoing competency evaluation includes the following steps: (1) identification of the frequency with which competency assessment is to occur for each discipline, (2) determination of how new/critical competencies will be identified, and (3) development of an implementation, documentation, and evaluation format. Each of these will be explored further.

Identification of the frequency of competency assessment should, in reality, be primarily dependent upon the case mix of the organization's

patient population and disease processes, the fundamental foundation for ongoing competency assessment. In addition, there are secondary components, which include administration and quality issues. Administration and quality issues, to name a few, include performance issues, role changes, customer concerns, addition of new equipment, and changes in policy or procedure. In effect, there should be planned competency assessment that occurs on an annual basis. As an industry, home care tends to perform competency assessment on an annual basis. The nature of the home care setting, being autonomous and sparingly supervised, lends it to being more cautious and compulsive in regard to the annual assignment for competency assessment. Performance concerns, the addition of new equipment, customer concerns, and changes in policy lead to ongoing episodic competency assessment instead of waiting for the anniversary competency date to appear. These indicators are critical indicators and, if not taken action upon in a timely manner, could pose serious risk management issues for the organization. An example of an episodic or critical indicator of competency assessment would include a situation where the home care organization has developed a program to provide epidural-controlled analgesia for hospice patients in collaboration with the local hospital's pain management center. This scenario lends itself well to an episodic competency. The hospice nurses and any other nurses who would come in contact with this pain management modality, such as intravenous team nurses, would be educated on epidural management and perhaps could spend time in the acute care setting learning how to adequately manage epidural catheters and pain. Competency assessment could occur in the acute care setting or in the home in collaboration with a nurse from the pain center or hospital who is proficient to expert in the care and management of epidural catheters. Staff development's role in this situation would be to develop the standards of care for epidural management, assist in policy formulation, plan the educational program, and oversee the competency-assessment process, in addition to ensuring that proof of competency was obtained and documented. It cannot be stressed enough that staff cannot be thrown into a situation where there is a new competency without first being educated and having their competency assessed. In this age of new programs and early discharge, frequently, home care is faced with having a never seen before patient-management issue, delivery device, or other equipment with no forewarning. In this situation, planning is difficult to do; however, the issue to remember here is that patient safety may be at risk. Everyone needs to keep in mind that the autonomous nature of home care warrants pre-planning as much as possible to lower the home care agencies' risk. It is best if the home care organization can keep abreast of new programs, equipment, or unique patient care management situations occurring in their geographical area so that adequate competency planning and assessment can occur in advance of encounters with the unknown.

The home care competency program that is set on an annual schedule would include the development of a needs assessment, administration of the needs assessment, analysis of the results, and planning in collaboration with management for the annual ongoing/critical competencies. This process should occur 3 to 4 months prior to the date for actual assessment of competency. Enough time must be allowed for identification of the competencies as well as the planning and development of the skills lab, in-home competency assessment, or acute care setting assessment.

The determination of how new competencies are identified is based upon the aforementioned administration and quality issues in addition to the assessment of the need for knowledge and skill through the implementation of a needs assessment, which is also frequently referred to as a self-report of competence (Garland, 1996). The determination of home care nurses' knowledge needs has recently been addressed in the literature by Astarita, Materna, and Savage (in press); Ark and Nies (1996); and Caie-Lawrence, Peploski, and Russell (1995). Employing such studies as these can greatly assist staff development in the formulation of tools that will yield appropriate and useful data with which to plan an ongoing competency program.

Development of an implementation, documentation, and evaluation format for an ongoing competency program should be an easy undertaking by following the steps for competency-based orientation (CBO) development. The most fundamental aspect of the ongoing program as mentioned previously is the planning phase (Table 9–1). With adequate planning, flexibility, and support from management, ongoing competency assessment will seem effortless to implement.

There are few recent published studies about ongoing competency assessment in home care. Ongoing competency is discussed more frequently regarding critical care nurses or hospital nurses in general (Lohrman, 1992; Benedum, Kalup, & Freed, 1990; Kelly, 1992; Scrima, 1987; Leidy, 1990). Many of the findings can be adapted to home care, but more research-based writing about home care competency is needed.

MULTIDISCIPLINARY COMPETENCY

One challenge faced by today's home care organization is the emphasis on multidisciplinary support of the patient in the home (Blocker, 1992). It is no longer sufficient for those in staff development roles to concentrate competency measurement solely on nurses. The need for competency assessment is not limited to home care nurses, but rather "all patient care" staff

Table 9–1 Determining Inclusions for Ongoing Competency Assessment Programs

Source To Review	Competency Areas To Look for	Examples
Joint Commission standards OSHA standards	mandatory requirements	Joint Commission: HR .5.1 Organization provides ongoing education, including inservices, training, and other activities, to maintain and improve staff competence (Joint Commission, 1996). OSHA: Measures to protect against bloodborne pathogens
Initial competency assessment	high risk, low frequency	Managing anaphylactic reactions
Annual staff performance evaluations	staff performance deficiencies that occur frequently	Clinical plans not being initiated appropriately and updated
Peer review reports	staff performance deficiencies that occur frequently	Admissions not completed within 24 hours of referral as policy dictates
Performance improvement findings (was QA, QI, TQM)	staff performance deficiencies that occur frequently	Documentation of inter-disciplinary meetings lacking from charts
Risk management findings	adverse incidents related to problems in quality of staff performance	Rising incidence of urinary tract infections in patients with Foley catheters
Policy and procedure manual	new or recently modified policies or procedures	New or substantially changed equipment, procedures, treatments, therapies, medications, or services
Job descriptions	new or modified position duties or responsibilities	Expansion of maternal-child nurse's responsibilities to include care of adult infusion patients
Materials management reports; increases in equipment replacement or repairs	patterns of inappropriate use of equipment	Staff pulling or not properly securing wires on apnea monitors
Minutes from staff meetings	questions or problems related to staff performance	Physical therapists unsure how to dispose of soiled dressings in the home

Source: Reprinted from *Designing Competency Assessment Programs: A Handbook for Nursing and Health-related Professions* with the permission of the National Nursing Staff Development Organization, © 1996.

(Joint Commission, 1996). Considering the mergers and acquisitions that take place, a home care educator may find himself or herself responsible for the competency assessment of pharmacists or other health personnel not previously associated with home care organizations (Remington, 1995). An Internet inquiry to the Home Care Group, etc., about competency measurements addressed to the home health nursing list on 3/10/97 resulted in 10 responses from across the nation. Of those 10, only one implemented competency measurement for disciplines other than nursing. One stated that managers had to complete skills labs as well, and another stated that supervisors and directors had to complete an annual 65-question test regarding Medicare criteria and other information. Physical, occupational, or speech therapists and social workers have guidelines for home care practice (Appendix A). Utilizing the standards of practice for many disciplines, competency and demonstration of competency on an ongoing basis are essential. A review of current literature reveals very few articles about competency assessment among non-nursing clinical staff. A recent article by Salvatori (1996) refers to the need for a combination of evaluation methods when assessing competence of occupational therapists. Although the therapist has the responsibility of maintaining competence, each profession maintains the responsibility for establishment of minimum standards of practice (Salvatori, 1996). In the United Kingdom, there is competency testing required for all professions (O'Hagan, 1996). As with all disciplines, competence should also be assessed on an individual basis (Joint Commission, 1996).

CONTRACT STAFF

As of 1990, one-third of the United States work force is made up of temporary staff (Leidy, 1990). It is predicted that by the year 2000, there will be more contract staff utilized in nursing than full-time positions, at least in the hospital setting (Shaffer & Kobs, 1997). Employing contract staff is a cost-effective way to utilize staff, especially those with expertise in a specialty, as

needed on an irregular basis (Shaffer & Kobs, 1997). Typically, orientation of contract staff is shorter and may not even take place at all (Leidy, 1990). The use of contract staff can save an organization money in paying overtime (Shaffer & Kobs, 1997). While in some ways contract staffing can improve quality of care by reducing regular staff fatigue from overtime, agencies should be concerned about the liability of utilizing temporary staff who are not fully oriented or assessed for competency (Shaffer & Kobs, 1997; Leidy, 1990). However, competency measurement of these staff can be difficult related to scheduling and the urgency of the need for them (Shaffer & Kobs, 1997). Creative solutions are required (Friedman, 1996). It is essential that home care human resources and education departments are fully knowledgeable about which specific contract staff services are eligible for review by the Joint Commission on Accreditation of Healthcare Organizations (Friedman, 1997). There are some contract staff who are exempt from this survey although the actual service can be scrutinized. They include first-dose or stat-dose pharmacies, dispensing-only pharmacies, or compounding-only pharmacies, delivery services only, contracts for supplies, medical equipment maintenance only, reverse contracts, referral arrangements, or Medicaid waiver programs (Friedman, 1997). Contract staff who have not been utilized within the past 12 months (triennial survey) will not be subject to competency review. The most important implication of this for home care educators is that, frequently, problems can be avoided at survey time if other agencies with which the organization has contracts are also Joint Commission-accredited providers. This has no bearing on the need to have competency measurement for contract staff who are either independent contractors or whose competency has not been assessed elsewhere.

Unlike regularly employed patient care staff, contract staff are not necessarily evaluated for competence based on the title and job description of the role they are replacing, for sometimes contract staff are not asked to perform every task. Their contract should be a precise list of elements describing the nature, scope, and type of care provided and specific guidelines regarding exactly what the contract staff will and will not be expected to do (Friedman, 1997). Human resources must review the standard LD.7 to ensure that the organization not only clearly delineates the duties of the contract staff, but has reassurance from staff development that competency will be assessed upon hire and regularly thereafter. If there are any doubts, an organization may request a written determination from the Joint Commission to determine whether or not a specific contract will be subject to survey review (Friedman, 1997).

Another related competency issue is the competence of part-time staff. When staff are working very few hours, such as one weekend a month, it may be difficult for them to remain competent in some areas. Communication should remain open between the educator and the part-time employee to allow for review as needed. Furthermore, if staff perceive that there is a particular skill that produces anxiety in the staff and potential danger to the client, the client should be reassigned. There are many advantages to part-time staff, but an organization needs to balance its need to accommodate the scheduling needs of its staff with making sure they work enough hours to maintain competency.

BENEFITS OF ONGOING COMPETENCY ASSESSMENT

Many home care agencies are certified through Medicare and surveyed through the Joint Commission and/or the Community Health Accreditation Program (CHAP). These and other regulatory bodies want evidence that an organization is utilizing competent staff appropriately. Their standards are patient-focused and performance-based (Shaffer & Kobs, 1997). Home care aides, for example, are to be "closely supervised to ensure their competence in providing care" (Beacon Health Corporation, 1996). Every home care organization seeking accreditation from the Joint Commission must "assess, maintain, and improve staff competence

throughout their association with the organization" (Joint Commission, 1996). This refers to clinical staff, those who provide direct patient care (Joint Commission, 1996). Organizations must "routinely assess and update" professional skills and competencies for all disciplines (CHAP, 1993). Besides meeting regulatory requirements, the benefits from regular competency assessment can be classified as either quality-related, staff-related, or team-related.

Quality-Related Benefits

Quality-related benefits of ongoing competency measurement include a lower incidence of equipment misuse, potential for more appropriate staffing assignments, and performance improvement. As staff become more competent in a specific procedure, they will most likely decrease the time they take to perform it. Current practice levels can be validated and performance enhanced. Regularly scheduled competency exercises can serve to enforce quality of care standards, exposing and correcting undesirable practices (Alspach, 1992). Another aspect of performance improvement resulting from competency assessment/education is that specialties in home care utilizing clinical nurse specialists have been demonstrated to reduce costs for the patient, in some cases by decreasing the amount of time required in the hospital or decreasing the number of re-admissions into the hospital (Carney, 1997). This benefit is of great interest to managed care and other payers. Staff can also be made more competent in data collection so that outcomes can be measured more concisely. Integration of the required competencies into the unit quality assurance program is essential (McGregor, 1990).

Home care nursing attracts experienced nurses from many specialty areas. Home care requires many different cognitive, psychomotor, and critical thinking abilities other than those utilized in other specialty areas (Caie-Lawrence et al., 1995; Ark & Nies, 1996; Carr, 1991), yet requires a broad scope of general expertise. Even the home care organization fortunate enough to hire staff experienced in home care must help them achieve "organization competence," a clear understanding of how things are done at the new organization. Evaluating the competency of health care professionals in general can support organizational goals, such as profit, productivity, customer service, and quality of care (Vincent, 1996). Critical thinking skills are utilized when staff draw on clinical knowledge to solve a clinical mystery, which can make the difference between life and death for the patient (Stark, 1995).

Staff-Related Benefits

Staff-related benefits of regular competency assessment include increases in confidence, professional growth, and possibly prevention of employee "burnout." In one study, ongoing education was credited with enhancing "progressive role development" and "leadership skills" (Schwerin, Gaster, Krolikowski, & Sherman-Justice, 1994). As the staff learn to perform better, it is likely they will feel more confident and have more assurance of patient outcomes (McGregor, 1990). Job-related stress is great when staff do not feel competent (Kramer & Schmalenberg, 1988). When staff are encouraged to stretch beyond their usual levels of performance, they are empowered. Clients exhibiting greater satisfaction with care can serve to reinforce nurses in a positive manner (Ark & Nies, 1996). Staff needing new challenges may be encouraged to try another specialty area within the organization rather than to seek a job elsewhere. Often, an organization wishes to offer a specialty program but must cross-train staff due to the lack of available experts in the specialty area (McGregor, 1990). A report on a home health organization's program to cross-train nurses to infusion states, "The plan to train existing staff promised to be more cost effective than hiring new staff, and was the workable approach chosen" (Paglione, 1991). Learning needs revealed at orientation can be followed up through ongoing competency exercises.

If the staff are to progress into the next level of proficiency, critical thinking skills need to be developed. One of the best ways to increase mutual learning in this area is to have scenarios that require analytical skills, such as a game that gives clues and has the staff use knowledge and experience to problem solve (Stark, 1995). Critical thinkers have a wide scope and vision, use intuition, and ask "why?" Yet, they know when to seek experienced peers when needed (Stark, 1995).

Organization-Related Benefits

One of the greatest benefits of regular competency assessment is that it builds teamwork and expertise. Team building takes time, and it requires that staff stay in one place long enough to form a bond (Kramer & Schmalenberg, 1988). As job proficiency increases, "expert" staff learn to mentor new staff, and mutual respect can develop. Establishment of mentoring relationships in turn can increase staff retention (Schwerin et al., 1994). McGregor (1990) reports that implementation of competency assessment in one facility resulted in increased collegiality between educator and manager. In addition, she also reports that in her facility physicians expressed "greater satisfaction with the nursing staff's ability to solve and anticipate patient problems."

STRATEGIES TO ACHIEVE COMPETENCY

Do some agencies do more than is needed for competency assessment? According to Kobs (1997), director of standards for the Joint Commission, surveyors find "an overabundance of paperwork." Daily work having no errors is indicative of competency to some degree (Kobs, 1997). Another common mistake is to assess competency for basic skills that can be assumed with licensure (Kobs, 1997). It is important to mention that the more competency assessment strategies a home care organization uses, the more preparation, recordkeeping, and development of policies and procedures reflecting these strategies are needed (Table 9–2). Because competency assessment is relatively new in home

Table 9–2 Benner's Competency Framework Applied to Home Care Nursing (Sample—One of Nine Domains)

Levels of Practice	Domain	Indicators
Novice	Monitoring and ensuring the quality of health care practice	• Seeks appropriate and timely response from members of health care team • Informs patients/caregivers of rights and responsibilities and interacts with patients in matters that uphold the same • Portrays knowledge of and follows clinical care paths • Communicates patient concerns in an appropriate and timely fashion • Reports incidents in concise, appropriate, and timely fashion • Identifies and monitors actual or potential patient/home safety problems • Demonstrates sound decision-making capabilities
Advanced Beginner		• Consults colleagues on patient care issues to ensure quality patient care and established outcomes • Participates in organizational performance improvement endeavors • Recognizes variances to patient care delivery and identifies rationale • Solicits prompt responses from physicians and colleagues
Competent/ Proficient		• Participates in monitoring the quality of care delivery • Assesses what can be discontinued safely, changed, or added to patient care orders and communicates findings to interdisciplinary team • Evaluates with the patient, family, and other health care providers the effectiveness, comprehensiveness, and continuity of interventions • Assists in the development of clinical standards of practice • Recommends changes to current standards of practice and questions "why?" on an ongoing basis • Recognizes patient care trends, correlates trends to populations with same diagnoses, and intervenes appropriately
Expert		• Evaluates and revises nursing practice as appropriate for individual patients, specific patient populations, or the practice of nursing • Functions with a healthy skepticism and ongoing questioning of treatment plans; prepared to act on own judgment if necessary • Recommends performance improvement initiatives • Designs performance improvement monitors • Assists in revising and developing nursing policies and procedures in area of expertise

Source: Data from P. Benner, *From Novice to Expert: Excellence and Power in Clinical Nursing Practice.* © 1984, Addison-Wesley Publishing Company.

care, some agencies may overreact to standards just to "be sure." There is also the danger of underassessment of staff competency. Although the Joint Commission standards are not the only basis for making organization decisions about "how far to go" with competency measurement, the standards basically leave that interpretation up to the organization, but "if you say you're going to do it, you should do it" (Joint Commission, 1996). It is one of the goals of this book that a balanced and rational approach be considered.

Pre-Employment Evaluators of Competency

Achieving staff competence begins in the pre-employment phase for all clinical staff (Abruzzese, 1996). According to the Joint Commission, competency standards should be used as hiring criteria (Joint Commission, 1996). Expectations should be clearly defined for any position, beginning with the advertisement used for recruitment. For example, some agencies require home care aides to have completed the Medicare-approved class of 75 hours prior to hiring them, while others offer the training on site. From a competency standpoint, it is important to hire the "best and brightest" for home care. As appropriate, a job applicant should be able to produce a completed application, license, educational record, certification verification, updated resume, or curriculum vitae that reflects his or her experiences. References should be checked and job experience validated (Joint Commission, 1996). Thoroughly checking previous competency as much as possible provides valuable input to use for hiring decisions.

The Interview

Home care organizations can implement an interview tool that is forwarded to staff development after the applicant is hired (Exhibit 9–1). This tool, which addresses basic competency issues, will ensure that the new hire receives an individualized orientation. These data can also assist with selection of topics/skills for competency assessment for all staff. Having the interview tool completed prior to orientation helps make the orientation experience more mutually satisfying. The educator maximizes use of time by knowing specific educational needs.

It is important to note that many managers who perform interviews have had no training in this area (Vincent, 1996). The weakness of unstructured interviews is that they can be subjective. The outcomes are frequently based on appearance, eye contact, head nodding, and facial expressions. Interviewers can also be affected by whether or not the applicant is like them and whether or not the applicant has strong verbal skills (Vincent, 1996). Interviews remain more objective when they are structured, because the interviewer is more likely to be assessing the potential of the applicant (Gingerich & Ondeck, 1997; Sherman, Bohlander, & Snell, 1996; Vincent, 1996). When conducting more than one interview for the same position, it is more valid to ask everyone the same questions. One structured interview that is helpful in laying the groundwork for competence assessment is the Situational Interview, where an applicant is asked to problem solve when given hypothetical events based on the job analysis (Vincent, 1996). There are structured interview packages available, some of which can be tailored to a particular organization's needs. The individual assigned to select new staff is legally liable to complete a thorough assessment of the potential employee's previous experience, educational background, licensure, and work history (Brent, 1994).

Skills Assessment or Self-Assessment

Agencies can request that the potential employee perform certain duties in a real or simulated setting, producing a "work sample" (Wolf, 1996; del Bueno, Weeks, & Brown-Stewart, 1987). This concept is utilized in non-medical settings as well (Wolf, 1996). Although this may give the employer a chance to see what the applicant can do, it also has limitations. Assessing an applicant's performance must be based on standard performance criteria to be valid. As with any competence assessment, the findings may possibly not generalize to actual work the appli-

Exhibit 9–1 Staff Development Hiring Flowchart

TO BE COMPLETED BY THE POTENTIAL STAFF NURSE

Name _____ Date _____

Should you become an employee, this will assist the educator in planning your orientation. Following are some topics that your orientation will address. Circle those areas with which you have had recent experience.

General

Home Care   Computer documentation   Time management and organization

Skills

Phlebotomy   Ventilators   Intravenous infusion,   Central lines site care,
                                     site care, insertion   infusion

Specialty Areas

Medical-surgical   Psychiatric   Rehabilitation   Orthopedics   Cardiac   Hospice   Maternal/Child

Please identify unique learning needs: _____

_____

_____

_____

_____

TO BE COMPLETED BY THE INTERVIEWER

Your name_____

If hired, does this employee require any special arrangements or modification of orientation?
If so, explain.

_____

_____

_____

_____

_____

Tentative start date for new hire: _____ Preceptor preference_____

Please complete this form and submit to staff development immediately if interviewee is to be hired. Thank you.

cant will perform once hired. Also, the cost may be prohibitive depending on the number of applicants, and if using "real patients," the liability can be a deterrent (Wolf, 1996).

A skills self-assessment checklist helps the interviewer see how the potential employees perceive their own competency. Research done with a sample of 287 home care agencies demonstrated that 92% used a skills self-assessment as a screening measure (Kalnins, 1989). Although not specifically required by the Joint Commission, if used, their purpose and how they are implemented should be clear (Kobs, 1997). There is the possibility that applicants may overrate their abilities in their desire to be hired. For this reason, they should be used only as an adjunct instrument in the hiring process. Should the individual be offered a position and accept it, competency measurement has been initiated, and the new staff member will recognize that the organization places value on competency. Skills self-inventories may potentially alert an organization to staff who will require more than usual amounts of education, observation, and mentoring. A national group of home health care nurses helped construct a profile that identified the knowledge and skills of productive nurses in home care (Benefield, 1996). The profile can be used during the hiring process to assess the level of skill of the applicant (Benefield, 1996).

Pre-Employment Testing

Today, workplace competency assessments vary widely from informal observations to rigorous and costly sophisticated systems. These formal systems can include "psychometric tests and questionnaires, and assessment and development centers" (Vincent, 1996). According to Vincent (1996), a recent publication listing commercially available tests for the workplace demonstrates that there are 3,009 available. There are also various screening tests an organization can administer to applicants. Pre-employment tests have been used for more than 40 years, and have been used to focus on mental abilities and personality traits (Leidy, 1990). Some of the tests available include tests of aptitude or ability,

ranging from tests for "visual acuity, manual dexterity, to cognitive tests of verbal, numerical, and spatial ability" (Vincent, 1996). Recent research has questioned the content validity of such practices. However, "general ability tests show strong predictive powers across all job types" (Vincent, 1996). Unfortunately, the employer must make extra effort to ensure cultural diversity in the workplace, because the tests have also shown to be culturally biased (Vincent, 1996). After the Civil Rights Act, a greater focus was placed on measuring job-related behaviors (Leidy, 1990). Test results should never be the sole determinant for hiring decisions (Gingerich & Ondeck, 1997).

Pre-employment cognitive tests certainly do not guarantee safe practice, but they can alert the employer to major problems (Leidy, 1990). They may merely demonstrate an individual's test taking ability rather than predict competent behavior in the future, however (Kobs, 1997). Tests of home care knowledge administered before and after orientation cannot only serve to evaluate the effectiveness of orientation, but target continued learning needs that the employee has if he or she is to function optimally.

Specific Strategies for Contract Staff

Possible solutions to the competency dilemma when utilizing contract staff include selecting staff who maintain competence elsewhere, copies of contract staff self-skills assessments being kept by the scheduling personnel to ensure a "match," and having someone observe the contract staff perform in a real or simulated situation prior to being assigned independently (Friedman, 1996). It is also possible to contract with an outside organization to perform competency assessment or only utilize staff who come from an organization where competency is assessed regularly (Friedman, 1996). It is not necessary to repeat competency measurement if done by another employer, but copies of the documentation should be obtained (Shaffer & Kobs, 1997; Friedman, 1996). Ultimately, it is the home care organization's responsibility for the competency of all of its clinical staff, including temporary staff (Joint Commission, 1996).

After the appropriate staff have been hired, they should be given a CBO, as described in Chapter 8. When orientation is completed, the nurse must be supported individually to progress from novice to expert (Benner, 1984). Benner's framework can be adapted to home care and even utilized as a formalized clinical ladder by the home care organization (Table 9–3). One hospital in New York established a clinical career ladder that addressed the proficient and expert nurse, so that these levels were not included in their competency framework (Robinson & Barberris, 1995). In many cases, new employees underestimate the amount of time it will take and new information they must learn to achieve expertise in the specialty of home care (Carr, 1991). Continual encouragement, assessment, and follow-up are very important so that new staff will not miss the opportunity to grow in this exciting and challenging specialty area.

Written Tests

Written tests are frequently utilized to measure knowledge, because they are usually low-cost and adaptable to various organization procedures, policies, and goals. An example of an appropriate use of a written test is a medicinal calculations test (Alspach, 1996), or tests constructed to measure specific weaknesses when general deficits are revealed through needs assessments. Other skills having performance criteria that are mostly cognitive include arrhyth-mia recognition and knowledge of disease process and symptoms management (Alspach, 1996). Questions should be formulated to maximize the need for staff to use critical thinking skills (Alspach, 1996). Refer to the section on evaluation in Chapter 5 for specific guidelines about test construction. Written or oral tests should not be overused as competency measures, for high scores may not necessarily generalize toward good work performance (Alspach, 1996; Salvatori, 1996; Kobs, 1997). Home care requires knowledge of subjects such as Medicare coverage, documentation, and the philosophies of the organization and home care in general. Agencies may choose to utilize tests of home care knowledge, but patient simulations requiring critical thinking beyond the basic knowledge are better preparation for the home care role (del Bueno et al., 1987). When a staff development educator is available, it is his or her role to help staff make the transfer from knowledge to performance (Gurvis & Grey, 1995).

Performance Evaluations

Performance evaluations or supervisory visits are required by Medicare (Beacon Health Corporation, 1996). These can be costly and time-consuming. Although this is one way to assess for competency, it is very time-consuming to isolate specific skills and observe each staff member perform them in the home setting. It may be difficult to observe every physical therapist use continuous physical motion machines, for example, because only certain patients re-

Table 9–3 Preferred Modes of Competency Assessment

Order of Preference	Mode of Assessment	Rationale
1st (optional)	actual job performance	matches reality of job
2nd best	simulated job performance	attempts to replicate some aspects of actual work situation
3rd best	written test(s)	only relates to cognitive aspect of job competency

Source: Reprinted from *Designing Competency Assessment Programs: A Handbook for Nursing and Health-related Professions* with the permission of the National Nursing Staff Development Organization, © 1996.

quire them. Observing the infusion nurses use a new type of dressing technique for Peripherally Inserted Central Catheter lines would perhaps not be a problem from an availability standpoint, rather from a geographical one. It is not unusual for infusion patients to be distant from each other, so that travel for the supervisor can become costly and time-consuming. The performance appraisal framework assists with establishing and communicating job expectations, conducting employee evaluations, scheduling interviews, and addressing training needs related to performance (Benefield, 1996). Because performance evaluations are not going to go away, each organization must decide how they will be best accomplished.

Direct Observation

Observation of actual job performance is the most valid way to determine if staff are capable of doing their jobs (Alspach, 1996). The real scenario holds all the variables, contingencies, and problems that are encountered with daily work. It is impossible to include every variable that a home care nurse or therapist encounters in a given day when trying to simulate a patient scenario. Medicare's regulation regarding supervisory visits ensures that most staff will be observed at one time or another. Furthermore, observation of staff performance in the home is utilized to follow up on concerns that became evident from customer concerns, event reports, patient surveys, or peer reports.

Medicare Conditions of Participation (1997) state that the home care aide should be observed annually performing specified skills on a person, not a mannequin, before being deemed "independent." Rather than bring the staff member back for education, it may be easier at times to simply demonstrate the new skill or equipment on the patient involved and have the staff member return the demonstration. Granted, skills and patients must be judiciously selected in this case. In the case of the home care aide, the nurse who is also on the case could time his or her visit to overlap when the aide would also be there. Oth-

erwise, it would be unusual to assess competency this way alone, because there is not enough time or money to allow for one person to observe every staff member in the home. In an ideal world, the staff development educator could facilitate these observations; however, this is not a cost-effective way to utilize the educator's time (Abruzzese, 1996). Perhaps for certain cases requiring interventional teaching strategies, observations by the staff development educator are appropriate.

Peer Review

A peer review competence program has worked well in some agencies; however, it requires experienced competent staff to act as reviewers. With the constant emphasis on productivity, peer review in home care is difficult at best. Exceptions are when certain skills can be observed when following another staff member in the home. For example, if the skill to be observed is documentation, direct supervision is not always necessary. If a peer was to see the patient within days of the nurse being assessed, perhaps the skill of documentation could be reviewed using certain criteria. A hospital utilized a peer competency-assessment program effectively in an intensive care unit (Kobs, 1997). This could perhaps be replicated for home care, but scheduling issues could possibly prove to be difficult. Nurses taking an active part in deciding competency measurement criteria is an excellent idea, however. Closely related to peer review are the concepts of mentoring and preceptors. In all cases, pairing an inexperienced clinician with one less experienced can facilitate learning, especially if the mentor or preceptor is clinically competent (Bartz & Srsic-Stoehr, 1994) and has been educated regarding basic principles of mentoring (Revis, Thompson, Williams, Bezanson, & Cook, 1996; Alspach, 1996).

Performance Improvement

Performance improvement data, including patient surveys, outcomes reports, chart reviews, infection control surveillance summaries, or any combination, can also serve to assess competency, to some extent. Should any incidents or "customer concerns" occur, remediation should occur immediately, so that the staff member does not "learn" the mistake (McMillan, 1997). Home care agencies should have policies in place for how the employee is informed of quality concerns and how action plans for correction will be implemented. It is interesting to note that, according to a 1993 study, there is not sufficient time spent teaching quality assurance improvement in many nursing school programs (Finnick, Crosby, & Ventura, 1993). There are no published data pertaining to competency in quality assurance among non-nursing clinical staff.

Skills Labs

Advantages

Many agencies have been able to assess their staff for competency using the skills lab (Alspach, 1996; McGregor, 1990). Well-designed skills labs closely simulate the job and can be analogous to performance evaluations (del Bueno et al., 1987). Also referred to as practice labs, practicums, skills fairs, or clinical assessment centers, these areas provide hands-on opportunities to demonstrate and practice with simulated patients, equipment, and scenarios in a nonthreatening atmosphere (McGregor, 1990; Bradbury-Golas & Carson, 1994). They offer the advantage of assessing staff performance before a high-risk or infrequently done skill is performed directly on a patient (del Bueno et al., 1987). If a skill is rarely required as part of a job, it is best simulated in a skills lab setting to develop proficiency in the learner (Alspach, 1996). If practice/assessment on a live patient would place the patient at risk or embarrassment or if it could lead to learner embarrassment, it is also best assessed in the skills lab setting (Exhibit 9–2). Skills labs work well when you want to control environmental variables or standardize the amount of variables for all staff to be evalu-

ated (Alspach, 1996). Another advantage includes the ability to provide aggregate data to nursing schools if there are error patterns. A hospital in Houston utilizing a clinical assessment center reported a "20-35% reduction in non-productivity costs of competency development" (del Bueno et al., 1987). Clinical assessment centers can also be used to follow up inservice presentations to determine retention of knowledge and ability to apply cognitive learning to a given scenario (del Bueno et al., 1987). Skills labs can be interesting and fun. They can also be used to meet inservice requirements mandated by the Occupational Safety and Health Administration, Joint Commission, and the Centers for Disease Control and Prevention (Jeska, Fischer, & McClellan, 1992). It is important to note that any one method of educating and evaluating staff can lose its effectiveness with overuse. The concept of an annual skills lab could remain interesting, however, by varying the theme, music, scenarios, and other elements (del Bueno et al., 1987). Skills labs can be used for ongoing competency assessment or as a part of orientation to the organization (Revis et al., 1996).

Difficulties and Limitations

Some agencies, especially the smaller ones, may not feel they have adequate time and resources to develop a skills lab. Developing and revising a skills lab as necessary takes time, and in agencies where staff-development duties are decentralized, this is an important factor to consider. It can be very difficult to schedule staff in advance for skills lab attendance, because there is no guarantee of patient census on a given day. It is arguable that some types of adult learners will not perform as well at a skills lab as others and that adult learning principles dictate that the learner has a choice of how he or she learns (Knowles, 1984). It is for this reason that the skills lab case studies must mimic the "real world" as closely as possible, so that if the staff cannot perform in the skills lab, it is an indication they cannot perform on the job. Other difficulties related to scheduling occur if the organization undergoes a planned or unplanned major

Exhibit 9–2 Conditions for Using Simulated Job Performance for Competency Assessments

- When a particular work situation requires appraisal but does not occur frequently enough to ensure its occurrence during the time frame available or planned for competency assessment (example: management of blood transfusion reactions)
- When use of a real work situation might pose risks or hazards to patients, family members, or staff (example: troubleshooting malfunctioning electrical equipment)
- When the individual being assessed might experience embarrassment or censure if his/her initial performance were not acceptable (example: management of a true medical emergency)

- When assessment in the actual work setting causes undue crowding or unnecessary noise or interrupts home dynamics
- When program designers wish to standardize assessment in a particular competency area so that all staff are subjected to the same performance conditions, such as managing conflicts or working with "difficult patients"
- When program designers wish to control extraneous environmental variables such as frequent interruptions from telephone calls, beepers, families, or visit schedules, so that these do not interfere with the assessment process

Source: Reprinted from *Designing Competency Assessment Programs: A Handbook for Nursing and Health-related Professions* with the permission of the National Nursing Staff Development Organization, © 1996.

change in process flow at the same time a skills lab is scheduled. Examples of a planned change that could disrupt a skills lab are implementation of laptop computers for documentation or initiation of a new organizationwide program. Unplanned changes that can alter the success of a skills lab are a high rate of staff turnover, the weather, or a sudden increase in patient volume. After scheduling skills labs, the organization must decide what will be done with staff hired after skills lab dates. Although, with the many mergers and alliances, more home care agencies have access to educational equipment than in the past, not all agencies may have access to expensive mannequins or other equipment required for a skills lab.

Another limitation of the skills lab is that competency is only measured for that day, in that setting. Staff may perform in another manner entirely under different conditions (Benner, 1984). Also, all facets and levels of competency may not be best measured in scenario-based simulation. For example, a nurse who has performed phlebotomy for several years and has always obtained a sample, never had a customer concern or lab incident report, and feels compe-

tent should not necessarily have to demonstrate the skill in isolation as many times as new staff to be deemed competent. After demonstrating the skills for the educator, that nurse would be an excellent resource to help the newer nurses achieve competency. Changing the passing criteria for different skills levels and experience makes sense, but could get problematic. For this reason, each educator must decide the criteria for passing each station and whether any exceptions will be made.

Another potentially difficult aspect of skills labs is the wide range of educational needs of today's home care staff. With the increase in specialization and the number of procedures that are performed in the home, the larger home care agencies may find that there are few skills deficits shared by everyone. Each caregiver has a different level of experience and his or her own specific strengths and weaknesses. Educators must plan on sometimes several different skills labs to meet the needs of the entire staff, not just a select few.

Another difficulty is that regulatory bodies such as the Joint Commission have expectations for competency measurement of *all* patient care staff. Typically, if a home care organization even has a staff development educator, the main emphasis for education has been nurses. Few educators have a working knowledge of the basic skills required to be competent as a physical therapist or social worker. There are few articles available to assist the educator in determining the educational needs of a multidisciplinary team in home care. It is very time-consuming to obtain standards of practice for each of the disciplines in home care, and most agencies are more concerned with the needs of nurses because they are the predominant discipline.

Home health organizations may find the cost of skills labs prohibitive, and outcomes resulting from skills labs need to be published more frequently to justify the expense. In one educator's experience in 1994, it cost $270.20 for supplies and $2,970.00 in registered nurse (RN) wages to competency test 72 RNs on 13 skills. This cost includes skills lab development, implementation, and materials. Home health agencies need to take the extra time and perform qualitative and quantitative research based on outcomes of skills labs. Some propose that measurement of competency based on a one-time performance on a special day is not as important as measurement of "habitual everyday performance" (McGuire and Harwood, 1989). This can be understood when one considers the "typical" day in home care and all the many external variables. Few educational assessments can match true competency required on a day when a patient isn't home, equipment malfunctions, a patient becomes clinically unstable, a new admission speaks only Spanish, or an unplanned dressing change and road construction wreak havoc on a well-planned schedule. The time has come when educators must prove that what they are doing makes a difference, or they will never gain respect for the specialty. Although simulation of actual patient scenarios and observing staff perform skills in these scenarios is a logical way to assess competence, more research is needed to measure quality indicators before and after skills lab. Pre- and post-evaluations should include staff's perception of their own competence,

number of difficulties encountered with the skill(s), evaluation of the skills lab, and any other related data. This will ensure that any aspects of skills lab or any other competency measures will continually improve.

Management Support

Most importantly, there must be a team approach, and management must support the need for a skills lab (Abruzzese, 1996; McGregor, 1990). Without the support of management, a skills lab is doomed to failure. Management should be supplying input for skills labs from the onset of the planning stages and assist when possible. This conveys the message to all staff that the importance of competency assessment is a basic belief of the organization. Furthermore, participation in continuing education and skills labs should be one of the criteria used for performance evaluations. Lastly, policies and procedures should support both mandatory and other continuing education.

Planning the Skills Lab

There are many recommended steps for implementing an educational program according to Lockhart & Bryce (1996), McGregor (1990), Robinson and Barberris (1995), Gurvis and Grey (1995), and Wolf (1996). According to this proposed model, there are seven phases to planning a skills lab: (1) assignment of roles, (2) development of standards and framework, (3) development of skills lists, (4) data collection, (5) selection of skills, (6) attendance requirements/promotion, and (7) educational planning. A checklist for planning can be adapted to suit the individualized needs of the organization (Exhibit 9–3).

Role Assignments

Skills lab development and implementation require a program director, typically the staff-development educator if the organization has one employed. To run a skills lab well, it is necessary that educators understand the scope of practice in home health not only for nursing, but for many other disciplines as well (Salvatori,

Exhibit 9–3 Checklist for Planning Skills Labs

❏ Review literature about skills labs

❏ Develop working plan, as much as possible, to be prepared to present to management: How will staff attend and keep up with patient visits? About how much will it cost in materials? How many hours do you expect the skills lab to take to complete?

❏ Obtain support from management

❏ Administer Needs Assessment

❏ Gather other data to help determine focus of skills lab, such as performance improvement reports, manager input, infection control reports, patient survey data, etc.

❏ Determine focus of skills lab

❏ Recruit assistants

❏ Plan sources of equipment needed and confirm availability with source

❏ Review literature about focus topics

❏ Prepare promotion of skills lab and post sign-up sheets

❏ Plan materials needs, including snacks, and make plans for obtaining (seek donations, submit check request, etc.)

❏ Develop written expectations for staff so that they may prepare cognitively

❏ Set up the physical aspects of the skills lab at least 2 weeks prior to the first date for staff practice

❏ Implement skills lab; consider leaving a message to each participant prior to his or her day

❏ Distribute evaluations to participants, including managers, and ask for suggestions for future offerings

❏ Summarize skills lab results using performance improvement format: Number of participants, % passing, itemize skills addressed, pretest/posttest scores where applicable, final cost, hours paid to staff, your prep time, informal observations, summary of evaluations

❏ Share report with administration, development, and staff

❏ With assistance of performance improvement nurse, staff nurses, managers, and patient surveys, monitor application of addressed skills in the home care setting

❏ Review skills as necessary with those who are not performing them well

1996; Shaffer & Kobs, 1997; Brent, 1996). The educator must understand the organization's operation, mission, and vision thoroughly and have experience in program development. Educators must utilize skills of diplomacy, communication, resiliency, and creativity. Time management is essential, for the one who plans the skills lab must continue with other job requirements at the same time. Refer to the complete description of the role of the educator in Chapter 3.

The use of other staff to help proctor skills labs enhances their professional development (McGregor, 1990) and can "free" the educator to assume other job-related duties (Lockhart & Bryce, 1996). If a peer who works "alongside in the trenches" is visibly involved in the skills lab, it will increase the staff's perception of the validity and worth of the skills lab. There are times

it is helpful to utilize someone who is outspoken about, perhaps at times critical of, educational programs. Should they see the skills lab from an involved perspective, they may accept it more readily, and their outspokenness can be an asset. On the other hand, utilizing staff who are very positive can perhaps encourage them to be more verbal and involved. The most important consideration is expertise. It is important to use someone with experience and expertise in the areas being tested. Consider using staff who have recently attended a conference on certain topics to mentor or supervise others (Lockhart & Bryce, 1996), or look outside the organization to experts in areas identified.

Qualified staff members are needed to assess the individual's competency. A "qualified" individual is one with the same knowledge, training, and experience as the nurse who is being assessed. The same or higher licensure, education, and competence are required of the evaluator (Ondeck, 1997; Friedman, 1996). Observed and deemed competent, clinically competent supervisors or peers can be utilized. According to Medicare, those who assess the competency of home care aides should have at least 1 year of home care experience (Beacon Health Corporation, 1996). Some organizations contract for outside services to competency-assess their staff (Ondeck, 1997). Joint Commission (1996) HR standards state that if a supervisor does not have appropriate training and experience in a clinical specialty area, then a qualified individual is consulted.

Development of Standards and Framework

Home care organizations must identify in writing, perhaps in policy format, how staff competence is assessed during hire, before orientation, after orientation, and when new or updated technology, products, procedures, or services are introduced (Friedman, 1996). The organization must plan its work, then work its plan. Performance standards must include specific guidelines for how competency will be measured and documented.

Some home health agencies may already have professional standards in place. Standards are the heart of policies and procedures and clearly define what organization personnel can and cannot do. They should be based on professional standards and the scope of practice of each professional organization. In order to construct a skill checklist that incorporates knowledge, skills, and abilities, you must be able to define tasks performed by all (Caie-Lawrence et al., 1995). There are national associations for nursing, physical and occupational therapy, and social workers. Copies of the home care standards for various disciplines are included in the appendixes of this book, as well as the addresses for each professional organization. Professional standards for each discipline should be the basis for all job descriptions and should be consulted

when policies and procedures are developed. Some agencies purchase already-constructed policies and procedures; they should check to see that they are congruent with the standards of practice for the profession expected to perform the procedures. To be sure that a new program for home infusion complied with legal standards as well, one home health organization consulted with legal advisors (Paglione, 1991). An example of application of a professional standard is shown in Table 9–4. Agencies can develop a list of competency statements that are specific for each job and specialty (Abruzzese, 1996).

To reduce health care to a list of standards, policies, procedures, and skills is a simplistic view of what comprises a nurse, therapist, or social worker. Working as a nurse, therapist, or social worker in home care does offer many regulations, but some parts of the job might just not fit into the procedural template (Benner, 1984). The affective part, the "guts," the "instincts," the "heart" are all what "glues it all together." Probably every home care organization has employed someone who had the skills but lacked the "glue." Frameworks can ensure that no aspect of competency measurement is omitted. One framework that can be used is Benner's empirically based domains of nursing practice (1984). The domains listed can directly relate to home care, and some of the functional divisions can be adapted to categorize aspects of the roles of the physical, occupational, and speech therapist, and social work, as well. The domains are the helping role, the teaching-coaching function, the diagnostic and patient-monitoring function, effective management of rapidly changing situations, administering and monitoring therapeutic interventions and regimens, monitoring and ensuring the quality of health care practices, and organizational and work role competencies.

The competencies listed are applicable to the experienced nurse as well as the novice. Setting priorities, team building, contingency planning, anticipating work overload, maintaining a caring attitude, and maintaining flexibility toward patients, technology, and bureaucracy are all important competencies for home care nurses and

Table 9–4 Application of Performance Standards (Social Work Used for Sample)

Professional Standard	Applied to Organizational Policy	Applied to Competency Assessment Criteria

Standard 1. Social workers in home health setting shall have knowledge of chronic, acute, and terminal illnesses, physical disabilities, and the resultant age-specific impact.	I. Competency Policy
	A. Social Work
	  1. Upon hire, social workers must demonstrate knowledge of chronic, acute, and terminal illnesses, physical disabilities, and the resultant age-specific impact as measured by written test.
	  2. Should the newly hired social worker not meet the criteria to obtain a passing grade on the exam, remediation must occur. The social worker must achieve the desired score on the exam prior to providing any patient care.
	  3. Competency will be re-assessed on an ongoing basis.
		1. Social worker will achieve at least 80% on exam titled "Age-Specific Impact of Chronic, Acute, and Terminal Illness" before being permitted to care for patients.
		2. Social worker will demonstrate age-specific care to patients with chronic, acute, and terminal illnesses in simulated patient scenario during skills lab as assessed by another individual who is competent in social work.
		3. Social worker will demonstrate age-specific care to patients with chronic, acute, and terminal illnesses in the home, as evidenced through documentation, assessment by nurse and peers, and absence of customer survey data indicating otherwise.

Source: Data from *NASW Standards for Social Work in Health Care Settings*, p. 28, © 1995, National Association of Social Workers.

---

other disciplines. Increases in stress and job turnover can be attributed in part to a lack of competency in any of these areas. A perpetual turnover of staff contributes to increased costs for the organization, increased workload, decreased morale, and decreased opportunity for building expertise. It behooves agencies to retain staff, empower them to become excellent home care clinicians, and provide an atmosphere of nurturing and support. Although the research was related to the hospital setting, a study about "magnet hospitals" listed the criteria of an organization to retain nurses. One of the most important things to a nurse is that he or she can make a difference, have the opportunity to grow professionally, and be heard (Kramer &

Schmalenberg, 1988). Benner then went on to apply the Dreyfus model for skill acquisition to create a framework for nursing proficiency, with progressions ranging from the novice to the expert levels (1984). This model has successfully served as a predictive framework for the development of an acute care case manager orientation in one hospital (Strzelecki & Brobst, 1997). This concept potentially brings competency assessment to a whole new level. Why not design a competency template that allows for evaluation beyond "He performed a skill correctly"? As mentioned previously, competency measurement is still a somewhat new concept to some agencies. Competency assessment performed in this manner will challenge nurses who are at every level, rather than just the novice. The educational needs of the novice have a greater psychomotor emphasis, but expert nurses need to validate higher-level competencies (Gurvis & Grey, 1995). Few managers assess degree of skill among their nurses, and even fewer tell the nurse their findings (Benefield, 1996).

The advantages of using a multi-level model are many. Staff can aspire to advance and have their progress recorded. The form can be utilized by the employee to set professional goals and make a plan to achieve those goals. It can be used during annual employee performance evaluations to assist in making promotion decisions, and some agencies may wish to implement a clinical ladder system. It is also possible to utilize a clinical ladder program to determine annual wage increases. Strzelecki and Brobst performed a study of 385 RNs (1997) in which most nurses related job satisfaction with recognition for clinical practice. The disadvantages to using a multi-level assessment tool for staff competency is that there then needs to be set criteria for what behavior demonstrates what level. Measuring informal observations of work behavior is time-consuming and difficult to quantify objectively.

Miller and Daly (1996) proposed that there are four domains of home care practice: assessing and using physiological data, initiating and monitoring therapeutic interventions, assessing and using family/environmental data, and integrating data, interventions, and context. The literature repeatedly emphasizes the need for strong abilities in physical assessment, for, in the home, there are no colleagues to provide input. There are four distinct levels within each domain, ranging from level 1 (strictly following protocols) to level 4 (using inductive and deductive thought processes). This model may also prove useful as a framework on which to develop competency skills checklists.

Developing Skills Checklists

After gathering standards, job descriptions, and scopes of practice, where applicable, and even fundamentals textbooks, there must be a form that lists the main skills that the health care worker is expected to be able to perform. Other sources include fundamentals textbooks, current literature, and courses and field experts (Caie-Lawrence et al., 1995). Skills checklists are one way to keep an ongoing record of competency of individuals employed by the home care organization. Hefty, Kenyon, Martaus, Bell, and Snow (1992) isolated core skills for community health nursing. The list is intended to combine those skills needed by both home health and public health nurses. Skills are divided into two categories: nursing process or professional skills. Examples of nursing process skills include sociocultural assessment, environmental assessment, establishing a nursing diagnosis, assisting with mobility, and evaluating learning. Examples of professional skills include communication skills, coordination of care, ethical/legal considerations, and personal professional growth (Hefty et al., 1992). Another way to categorize job tasks is according to "nursing tasks," such as professional direct care, nonprofessional direct care, professional indirect care, or nonprofessional indirect care (Ozcan & Shukla, 1993). Ozcan and Shukla contend that all clinicians perform some aspect of each of these categories (1993). These categories can also be applied to skills performed by other disciplines. Agencies should develop their own role and setting-specific skills checklists, because the needs vary between agencies (Gurvis & Grey, 1995). Also, home health competency measurement tools should not be the same as community health, for there are many fundamental differences between the two roles (Caie-Lawrence et al., 1995). Regardless, implementing a checklist, updating as necessary, and utilizing the same list for initial assessment, education, and performance evaluation is cost-effective and benefits managers and staff (Snow, Hefty, Kenyon, Bell, & Martaus, 1992). Agencies should also consider using the skills checklists as the foundation for their needs assessment. If a home care organization chooses to utilize skills checklists, it is important that it omit the skills that can be assumed with licensure, unless they are skills that are high risk and low frequency (Kobs, 1997).

Home care agencies must demonstrate that they have assessed staff for competence in provision of age-specific care, particularly for the infant, child, adolescent, and elderly (Friedman, 1996; Kobs, 1997; Joint Commission, 1996), assuming those are populations they service. The proportion of patients aged 80 or older is "one out of every three" nationally (Van Ort & Woodtli, 1989). Staff must be competent in physical assessment, customer service, and the use of all equipment and monitoring devices (Friedman, 1997; Kobs, 1997; Joint Commission, 1996). When one hospital completed a needs analysis, even though most of the nursing staff were "competent and beyond" in most areas, interpersonal and critical thinking dimensions scored at a lower level (Robinson & Barberris, 1995). As nurse practice changes to accommodate changes in health care, systems and individual nurses' clinical practice must change in a "symbiotic manner" in order to advance clinical practice (Robinson & Barberris, 1995).

While it is valid to use skills checklists, other criterion-referenced assessment tools can be developed to determine competence during a skills lab (Alspach, 1996; del Bueno et al., 1987). Some form of performance checklists should be made for each staff member. It is not necessary to include any aspects of a skill that are already measured on a written test. The tool should be complete, clear, easy for both the evaluator and staff member to use, and uncluttered. There is no need for a rating scale; either the skill is done according to standards or it is not (Alspach, 1996). The skills should be listed, and there should be a column for the evaluator to sign and date. Be sure to include the date competency is demonstrated and the name of the person who verified it; this assigns accountability to the person signing the skill "off." Some like a comments section so they can keep ongoing notes. The form can be altered for both clinical supervisor and educator use. Completion generally must be at 100% because it either is done or isn't (Gurvis & Grey, 1995;

Alspach 1996). Performance criteria should be the basis of these tools. A literature review yielded little about how to develop and construct a well-written competency validation tool (Gurvis & Grey, 1995). Some agencies virtually take a procedure that describes the skill and reproduce it in a checklist format to assess competency, making more work than is actually needed. It is sufficient to state that "per organization procedure # 2045 the above named nurse demonstrated competency in the following." The skills lab participant should have had access to the procedure before the assessment, and the evaluator should use the procedure as they assess the performance of the participant. As ongoing competency validation takes place, the competency template that was initiated upon hire should be updated (Appendix B).

Data Collection

Krisjanson and Scanlan (1989) studied 132 articles and books about skills labs. They reported there are many different methods an organization can utilize when conducting needs assessments. Adult learning principles reinforce the need for the participants to be able to identify their own learning needs (Strzelecki & Brobst, 1997). A needs assessment is one excellent source of data that should assist in this decision, but staff must be honest as they examine their competence and expertise. Some hospitals report giving the needs assessment to the clinical coordinators, while others report gathering data only from the caregivers themselves (Bradbury-Golas & Carson, 1994). The purpose of a needs assessment should be not only to determine skills in which the staff do not feel competent, but to also evaluate which skills they feel are most important to know (Caie-Lawrence et al., 1995). The individual assigned to conduct the needs assessment is responsible for clarifying and defining the construct "need" (Krisjanson & Scanlan, 1989). Unless staff are given some decision making about their own learning, the skills lab will not be as effective (McGregor, 1990). Refer to the section on needs assessment for specific guidelines for designing needs assessments.

Data informally or formally collected through use of competency strategies mentioned previously can be further evaluated in a skills lab setting. Skills self-assessments from the orientees hired within the previous 6 months could also provide insight regarding needs. Also, if there were significant customer complaints about the inability of nurses to correctly perform a specific procedure and the skills lab was to take place within a short period of time, review and assessment of that procedure would be appropriate. Obviously, if a situation develops where competency is needed immediately, it would not be appropriate to wait for skills lab to educate and reassess the nurses involved. Some skills that are necessary to perform a job lend themselves better to the simulation setting of a skills lab than others. The closer the conditions of the simulation mimic reality, the better indications of competence they are (Alspach, 1996). Reviews of patient records, minutes of team meetings, marketing reports, statistical reports of most common diagnoses served by the organization, and infection control reports can all help assess learning needs (Yoder Wise, 1996). When interpreting data, it is important for the educator to focus on learning needs, not administrative changes that need to be made, for this will distract from the job at hand.

Selection of Skills

Each organization is responsible for determining which skills must be observed, remembering that it is impossible to evaluate every skill (Friedman, 1996). There are many general categories of skills. This section will mention several of them. In general, there are three realms of competence: psychomotor, cognitive, and affective (Kobs, 1997; Bradbury-Golas & Carson, 1994). This is referred to as "Bloom's Taxonomy of Educational Objectives" (Bloom, 1956). Psychomotor skills are knowledge-based physical tasks. Knowledge, or the "cognitive domain," involves the ability to plan and act based on knowledge or perception. Affective-interper-

sonal skills include customer service, working as a team, and provision of care interdependently with other members of the team (Bloom, 1956). Affective domain competency is less frequently measured than the other domains. Perhaps this is because it is a challenge to measure and also receives less attention from litigious clients. In this competitive health care system, staff must demonstrate caring and the ability to support and meet the needs of patients (Ellis, 1992). Staff should learn and have an opportunity to demonstrate understanding of powerlessness, ethical dilemmas, emotional support, and altered body image, to name a few affective aspects of giving care. Furthermore, if caregivers have the knowledge and the skills ability to perform a skill and they do not, their "affective domain" may be the culprit. Affective aspects of competency cannot be overlooked. To see examples of behavioral objectives related to each level of domain, refer to the appendixes of this book. Decision making, or critical thinking, is also an important element to competence (Caie-Lawrence et al., 1995; Shaffer & Kobs, 1997; Robinson & Barberris, 1995). In a study of 35 nurse managers and 100 staff nurses, there was not a statistically significant correlation between critical thinking and self-concept; however, there was a correlation between higher critical thinking ability among nurses educated at the baccalaureate level (Beeken, 1997). Skills labs should focus on skills that are "essential for job performance and specific to each practitioner" (Joint Commission, 1996). Needs should be selected based on frequency and criticality. Most important are needs that directly impact quality and safety of patient care (Lockhart & Bryce, 1996; del Bueno et al., 1987; Gurvis & Grey, 1995). Competency should be measured if a nurse has not performed a procedure within a certain period of time. When new or updated technology, products, procedures, or services are introduced, there should be education for staff with a follow-up assessment. Furthermore, if there are any changes in clinical practice standards, or if the employee requests a review, skills assessment should take place (Friedman, 1996). Consider teaching and assessing skills that generate frequent questions and those that are relevant to the diagnoses that are most frequently seen in the specific practice (Abruzzese, 1996).

With the growth of home care and resultant increase in the percentage of novice nurses in the specialty, one cannot overlook the skills that are specific to the specialty of home care (Caie-Lawrence et al., 1995). Competence in another specialty, graduation from nursing school, and even previous home care experience do not guarantee competence in home care, for it is a "whole different world" (Caie-Lawrence et al., 1995; Carr, 1991). Examples of skills that are specific to home care nurses involve organizational skills, multiple factor assessment, promotion of patient autonomy, understanding family systems and multiple cultures, extended opportunities for patient communication and patient education (Ark & Nies, 1996), current trends, and other skills (Carr, 1991; Caie-Lawrence et al., 1995; Ward & Rieve, 1995). Time management is completely different in the home care setting. This can possibly be attributable to the volumes of paperwork. One study revealed that only 47% of a nurse's time is spent with direct patient contact, a real concern in a managed care era, which may include capitation (Hedtcke, MacQueen, & Carr, 1992; Remington, 1995). A home care nurse needs to know about current trends in health care such as disease management, case management, customer service, family systems, and home environment factors (Ward & Rieve, 1995; Carr, 1991; Robinson & Barberris, 1995). Due to the early discharge of most patients from the hospital, home care nursing requires competence in "increasingly technical and advanced" skills (Riegel et al., 1996; Alspach, 1996; Paglione, 1991). Some skills related to an ever-increasing number of specialties within home care, such as rehabilitation nursing, cardiac rehabilitation, diabetes management, pulmonary disease management, enterostomal therapy, and behavioral health management, should be included (Nemcek & Egan, 1997; Neal, 1995). With the arrival of many laptop documentation systems and computer-based in-

struction, it is imperative that home care staff are competent in the use of computers (Coffman, 1996; Meyer-Desnoyer & Herrmann, 1996). Nursing competency skills were divided into the following categories at one hospital: basic, generic, advanced, and unit-specific (Gurvis & Grey, 1995). Applying this framework to home care skills yields competencies that are either basic, generic, advanced, or specialty-oriented (Table 9–5). This framework can also be utilized to organize competencies for other disciplines as well. It is also wise to first concentrate on skills that everyone needs, rather than those needed by just a few (Lockhart & Bryce, 1996). The most important skills to a home health organization should be those that are high risk (greater liability)/high frequency (customer demand), and high risk/low frequency (Joint Commission, 1996). However, a competence in a high risk/high frequency skill may possibly be maintained through frequent performance without incident (Abruzzese, 1996). High-risk skills that are not performed on a regular basis should be assessed regularly. If a skill is required on an extremely rare basis, review should be available on an "as needed basis." Because it is difficult to maintain competence in skills that are not routinely performed, many agencies have developed specialty teams so that there are a group of "experts" available at all times.

Frequently overlooked are the competency assessments for managers. There are currently no certification programs available specific to management, although there is home care administrator certification that can be sought through the National Association for Home Care. Depending on the level of education and experience the manager or director has, there may be deficits in knowledge or its application (Finnick et al., 1993). As with other specialties, home care management staff are being faced with altered roles related to streamlining and downsizing (Green, 1994). Unfortunately, uncertainty about the future can lead to apathy and a lack of motivation (Green, 1994). When home care agencies seek to hire managers from within the organization, there are many excellent clini-

Table 9–5 Basic, Generic, Advanced, and Specialty-Related Home Care Nursing Skills

Competency Category	Home Care Related Skills	Ideas for Measurement
Basic	Nursing—physical assessment, vital signs, pulmonary assessment, history taking. Physical therapy—ROM, gait training, resistance training.	Basic skills can be assumed with licensure and education, if performed on a daily basis without incident.
Generic—applicable to all	All discipline—skin integrity. Other skills include nutrition, medications, pain management, referrals to other disciplines as needed.	Simulation of a case: have patient with multiple system failure, socioeconomic challenges, difficulty understanding English, difficulties requiring all disciplines' input. Have nurse enter a 485, then do wound care on mannequin/volunteer. Consider a skills lab where each discipline approaches the mock patient from the perspective of his or her job. Have non-nurses evaluated by those who are experts in that discipline.
Advanced	Nursing—ventilator care, advanced pharmacology, multiple complicated wounds. Physical Therapy—contractures, splinting, decubitus prevention.	Observation of skill in the home, game to review relevant medications, indications, dosages, side effects; Case studies using patients with multiple physical problems and interventions. Have physical therapist demonstrate initial visit, communicate with nurse implementations to be included in the plan of care, and document visit.
Specialty-related	Nursing—infusion, cardiac, psychiatric, maternal-child, rehabilitation. Physical therapy—pediatric, gerontology.	Observation of skill in the home, simulation of case study, content tests for cognitive assessment that are specific to the specialty.

Source: Data from J. Gurvis and M. Grey, The Anatomy of a Competency. *Journal of Nursing Staff Development,* Vol. 11, No. 5, pp. 247–252, © 1995.

cians who lack the knowledge base and skills needed for their management role (Kerns, 1997). On the other hand, experienced hospital managers will find it difficult being the resource for home care nurses until they, too, become competent in home care. As mentioned previously, orienting hospital nurses to home care takes considerable time and effort. Home care and hospice managers are responsible to motivate, which requires that they have self-esteem and competence in other aspects of their role (Green, 1994). Knowledge of leadership and management basics, such as change theory, due process, communication, risk taking, and shared governance, are essential. Interviewing, performance review, supervisory visits, disciplinary ethics, performance improvement, and delegation are all additional skills that can be taught and assessed for competency. Skills related to day-to-day operations include budget planning, strategic planning, and effective communication. It is also significant to note that home care managers are frequently responsible for interdisciplinary teams. Other areas to target for managers or administrators include ethics, labor and other laws, management information systems, marketing and development, organizational management, policy writing, performance improvement, and research (Bryant & Cloonan, 1992). Few managers have a working knowledge of social work, physical therapy, occupational therapy, or other disciplines (Shaffer & Kobs, 1997). Initially, managers may feel threatened being asked to demonstrate competency, until they realize that no value judgments will be made (Vincent, 1996; del Bueno et al., 1987).

Although there are many frameworks that agencies can adapt to meet their needs, it is important that the diverse needs of the population receiving skills lab be considered. Not only are there many ways to categorize and label the skills that are necessary to function in home care, but there are many different levels of performance of each skill. Mastery of one skill may be the prerequisite to becoming competent at another (Benefield, 1996). For example, if a nurse cannot perform basic physical assessment, he or she will not be able to progress to perform the more sophisticated skill of holistic assessment, looking at the patient on many levels.

Attendance Requirements/Promotion

Typically, the skills lab is utilized on an intermittent basis. If space permits, consider setting up the lab permanently to use throughout the year (del Bueno et al., 1987). This eliminates having to relocate equipment, should follow-up be needed or new staff hired. Self-learning modules, games, exercises, videos, and other materials can be stored there for use by nurses throughout the year. How often should a skills lab be scheduled? Although the Joint Commission (1996) states only that it should be evaluated on

a "regular basis," every 6 months to 1 year should suffice (Friedman, 1996). Agencies can implement a skills lab at the same time every year, so the staff can expect them. It is best to avoid scheduling the skills lab during the holiday or vacation seasons. It is also a good idea to avoid the times of year when the weather is most unpredictable.

Home care offers unique time constraints that make it difficult to know what times to schedule labs. Generally, it is best to offer skills labs either early in the morning or late in the afternoon, so that patient care can be accomplished. Some of the variables that can affect ability to attend include patient visits, geographical location, traffic, car maintenance, and poor planning. It is wise to include a question on the needs assessment about the time(s) preferred for skills lab, so that the needs of the majority can be met.

There are variables that influence participation in inservice education programs, including employee resistance (Krisjanson & Scanlan, 1989; Blocker, 1992). The opportunity to grow professionally is key to job satisfaction and retention, according to at least two studies (Stefanik et al., 1994). When marketing any educational programs, this opportunity should be emphasized. There should be a choice of at least two dates and times to attend the skills lab. These times and dates should be based on times of lowest productivity according to organization reports. Policies that indicate the importance of competency assessment within the organization should be in place, and attendance at educational offerings should be in the performance criteria for evaluations of all staff. There should be consequences and an action plan to follow if any staff do not attend. It is up to the organization how to handle documentation of competency that is not measured at the skills lab. For example, issues concerning an overlap in competency measures utilized need to be addressed. In addition, there should be a plan for what to do when employees are out on a family medical leave or vacation or are hired after the skills lab dates. Including evaluation of the skills for the current year in the orientation process is one solution. This is up to the discretion of the organization; however, there is potential danger when a lax attitude is taken. It is an added strain on the staff, patients, and those who assign schedules if a patient requires a skill the staff are not competent to provide.

For agencies unfamiliar with skills labs or other competency measures, it is important for them to see the advantages of participating and to have time to get used to change. Staff should be given the data, such as incident reports, and the needs assessments analysis so that they can see why certain skills have been selected. Promoting the skills lab should not be limited to the staff who will be attending, however. Be sure that administration is invited, perhaps even given a small role. The more buy-in and participation from management, the better. If your organization is part of an alliance or is hospital-based, consider inviting others to attend one or more stations of the lab. Consider "kicking off" the skills lab with some type of activity related to the theme. Occasionally, food items or prizes can be obtained as donations from local businesses, medical supply companies, or pharmaceutical companies. You may even consider informing the local newspaper about the home care skills lab. This can be a wonderful way to market your organization, the home care industry, and the individual professions responsible for care delivery. First it may be best to consult with the appropriate leadership at your organization to have this approved.

Promotional flyers should be posted with all the essential information. Managers should promote the skills lab at team meetings. Voicemails or e-mails should be sent as appropriate. Many agencies utilize an events calendar or an educational calendar that is highly visible to all staff. Employee newsletters, pay stubs, or memos can all be utilized (Bradbury-Golas & Carson, 1994). Skills lab dates can be posted well in advance, then revised only as absolutely necessary. A creative approach goes a long way toward promoting interest in skills labs. The use of music, a "traveling cart" that is decorated with balloons, signs, and provision of snacks, an-

nouncement of a prize drawing, and use of a theme can all lead to increased staff interest and participation. We can all remember with pleasure the creative educational experiences, but so many times the class or conference that utilized a dry lecture seemed endless and like drudgery. There is no limit to implementing creative strategies to encourage someone to want to be the "best home care provider on the planet," only your own imagination.

Educational Planning

After the needs assessment has determined what the staff feel is important, an assessment of previous knowledge, an assessment of learning styles (Gurvis & Grey, 1995), and taking into account the learner's expectations should be considered (Alspach, 1996). The national standards for staff development should be used to assist with educational planning. Staff should mutually set program goals and objectives (Lockhart & Bryce, 1996; Gurvis & Grey, 1995). Skills that are selected for the lab should be the focus of a literature review. Although some use the terms "objectives" and "goals" interchangeably, goals are usually broader than objectives. Typical goals include evaluation and enhancement of competency and specific skills-related objectives (McAnnally & Barnett, 1997). Goals should make a difference in patient care, be measurable, and be written clearly (Gurvis & Grey, 1995). There should be a competency statement, criteria for demonstrating competency, learning options, and evaluation methods (Gurvis & Grey, 1995). The curriculum should be based in the "real world" (Alspach, 1996). A goal might read: "Nurses will increase referrals to appropriate ancillary services from current rate of 2% to 10% by 3 months after completion of skills lab." A corresponding objective might state, "All learners participating in skills lab will score at least 85% on the self-learning module on ancillary services." Regardless of which term you use, whether you write one or both, writing educational objectives may seem like a waste of time. When utilized, they can save time and prevent digressions from the "planned path." Planning is essential to be able to validate outcomes, for without it, there is no point of reference. A clearly defined competency assessment framework is essential (Robinson & Barberris, 1995).

After skills have been selected based on data collection and management consensus has been attained, a search for assistants should be conducted. You may consider posting a list 2 to 6 months before the skills lab, asking staff to sign up. Usually, however, it is more effective to select helpers yourself, because you know which staff would be qualified. Search outside the organization for assistants, particularly if aligned with an acute care facility. The benefits of this are multifaceted. Without incentives to motivate them, most staff are not looking for more work to do. Again, fostering a desire for development among staff must be reinforced with the human resources department and management. Furthermore, you must have the manager's approval to utilize clinical staff. Post the names of those who are "selected" to be on the skills lab committee. Schedule meetings well in advance at the convenience of the committee. Utilize meeting times to outline what your expectations are for those assisting. Take this opportunity to review general guidelines about competency assessment. Evaluators should be trained to use assessment methods, evaluation criteria, and documentation systems (del Bueno et al., 1987). Teach them how to make signs, visuals, and special effects to make their stations more interesting. They will need to know how to assist with writing educational objectives, outlining content, choosing appropriate teaching strategies, and designing audiovisual handouts (Lockhart & Bryce, 1996).

Acquisition of materials can be done by purchasing supplies, borrowing some supplies, seeking donations from area businesses, or a combination. A sample list of supplies needed for a skills lab may include mannequins, infusion equipment, syringes, solution, home infusion pumps, posters, enlarged pictures of procedures being done, theme-related decorations and handouts, certificates of completion, and similar equipment and materials. Some pharmaceutical companies are willing to donate items or assist

with skills labs in some way. Representatives from equipment companies may be willing to demonstrate the use of their equipment for either the educator or a class prior to the skills lab. Home health agencies that are in a partnership or just on good terms with a local hospital or school of nursing should attempt to borrow equipment. Pharmacies also might loan infusion pumps, tubing, and so forth. When home care agencies are a part of an alliance or are hospital-based, it is logical to begin inquiries within that circle initially.

Creative educators can use some everyday items to simulate a home care scenario in some instances. A doll purchased at a garage sale can be equipped with an intravenous access device, colored clay can be used to simulate unusual effects, and old Styrofoam wig forms can be adapted to practice tracheostomy care. To use these objects for teaching, it is important to make sure that they are safe to use, that they closely simulate the actual situation as much as possible, and that they are replaced when they are no longer effective.

Development of written materials for a skills lab can be as simple or as complicated as the educator wishes. A resource manual for each participant was developed by one hospital for its inservices that included objectives, class outlines, schedule for classes, and current articles related to each topic (McGregor, 1990). Although this can be costly, if pages are selected judiciously, there may be greater retention of material, and the staff may use the manual as a future resource.

There are many ways to design skills labs. Regulatory agencies do not specify the number of skills that must be selected, the precise method of evaluation, or the length of time that must be spent on each skill. Sometimes, trial and error will teach you what the best type of schedule is for your organization. Home care agencies have varying amounts of space available, but the skills lab is best when it can remain set up at least 1 to 2 weeks prior to the assessment. Staff should be able to practice, view videotapes, review procedures, and ask questions. Some options include having simulated patient scenarios with case studies, perhaps even getting volunteers to pose as patients. Of course, any invasive procedures will require a mannequin. Another option is to have the staff sign up for dates/times in groups of 6 to 10. Let half of them take a cognitive test reviewing current medications, new procedures, changes in Medicare regulations, and age-appropriate information while the other half demonstrate specific skills in the lab. One hospital evaluated 14 staff members in only 16 hours this way (Taft, 1995). Having them supervise each other after they have been approved is also an option. If you have enlisted help from managers, you should consider letting them supervise the group of staff who are not their own, so that they may gain some perspective.

Teaching strategies used during a skills lab can be limited to self-practice and one-on-one help as needed. Adult learners benefit from knowing what they will be expected to know and having some decision making in the process (Knowles, 1984). Classes should be offered on the topics that will be assessed, literature should be made available, and review and practice should be made possible by setting up skills lab stations well in advance. Using a sample of 150 nurses, the posttest scores of nursing staff after utilizing videos or instructional booklets were as high as the scores of nurses who were taught using a lecture (Flynn et al., 1996). Some creativity is required to meet the unique educational needs of home care staff. Consider audiotaping the information that is needed, so that the staff can listen to it in their cars. If you choose to do this, be sure to make it interesting and concise. Ask for volunteers to be in a video performing the targeted skills correctly and have the video available prior to the lab. Try placing small bits of information in unlikely places to get the staff thinking about the skills lab and the specific skills. Small case studies similar to the scenarios to be used in the skills lab can spark interest.

Finally, when the staff are assessed, it is best to incorporate all three domains of learning (cognitive, skills, and affective) into simulated patient scenarios. First of all, these scenarios can more accurately measure what the staff can do on the job. Secondly, performance requires more than just recitation of a memorized list of facts and tables, which staff usually forget after testing anyway. And lastly, simulations offer opportunities to break the tension by injecting a little humor. Any learning options should be varied, simple, and experiential, allowing the learner to have control and "direct his own learning" (Gurvis & Grey, 1995).

Documentation of competency assessment should be maintained in the human resources file. This documentation should include orientation elements such as the CBO and skills self-assessment. It is important to record scores of posttests or to indicate that a passing grade was obtained after defining what constitutes passing, but filing of posttests is not necessary. It is best to utilize an ongoing listing of educational activities in which the employee has participated. Documentation of ongoing competency can be very time-consuming. It is proposed that the initial list used to self-assess skills competency be designed to support continued competency assessment. This saves space in files and also summarizes competency in one location.

There are many types of software available to maintain educational attendance in an ongoing manner. One of these is Edukeep 2000, an educational database that can be used to print out quarterly summaries of programs, department attendance, or individual educational summaries. Data are entered after a group attendance sheet is given to the secretary, a completed posttest is graded and passing, or an employee attends a continuing education offering and turns in the verification. Some home care agencies may find one of these programs useful.

Evaluation

Evaluation measures must clearly define expectations for the evaluator and the learner, and they should be consistent with the intent of the competency statement (Gurvis & Grey, 1995). One of the most important aspects of evaluation is that it should not be limited to the end of the program. According to adult learning principles developed by Knowles (1984), regular feedback facilitates learning (Strzelecki & Brobst, 1997). There should be a relaxed and mentoring environment for the participants in the skills lab setting. It is best if the participant is corrected immediately if he or she is performing incorrectly and given another chance to demonstrate.

Evaluation of educational activities can be formatted to convert easily into a quality monitoring activity (Jeska et al., 1992). According to Abruzzese (1996), there are four components of evaluation: impact, content, outcome, and process. The RSA Evaluation model illustrates the elements that are contained under each component (Exhibit 9–4). To evaluate the impact of a skills lab or any inservice, measurements need to be taken of cost-effectiveness, quality of patient care, turnover of staff, and risk management. Content evaluation is the measurement of knowledge of skills that have been gained, which again reinforces the need to gather baseline data on every employee upon hire. Outcome measurement occurs when assessment is done for changes in practice that take place as a result of the education. And lastly, evaluation of process requires measurement of overall happiness with the learning experience including comfort, teaching methods, whether objectives were met, content, and faculty and administration opinion. Not every level of evaluation needs to be done with every program (Abruzzese, 1996).

To construct process evaluation questions, one must be sure to avoid bias (Abruzzese, 1996). To determine if the evaluation is biased, it is best to have it reviewed by many. This will also determine if it is clearly understood, "user friendly," and the correct length. Although most agencies have some evaluation form they already use, it is important to consider some factors about evaluations. Abruzzese (1996) wisely admonishes that it is best when using Likert scales to spell out what each number represents on the rating scale to avoid confusion; although the scale is widely used, there are many ways in which it is utilized. It is best not to force learners to decide if an aspect of the skills lab was "all good" or "all bad," but to provide an opportunity

for them to say something was "neutral," "not applicable to my job," or "average."

Once any educational opportunity has been completed, whether it be orientation, an inservice, or skills lab, give every participant enough time to complete an evaluation of the process (Exhibit 9–5). Unfortunately, evaluations are usually completed at the very end of an educational offering, when participants may feel intellectually drained and anxious to go home. It is not unusual for learners to just circle any number to complete an obligation and be done. Signatures should be optional on evaluations (Abruzzese, 1996). Anonymity may result in more honest evaluations, but on the day of the skills lab, it can also be interesting to open up a discussion about what could be better and what was good about the skills lab. To be sure that everyone turns one in, evaluations may be numbered, small number cards given to them upon receipt of their completed evaluation, and a prize drawing conducted using the cards. If participants do not complete the evaluation immediately, they may forget to do so or they may not remember how they felt about the experience. Design the evaluation to be simple, easy to complete, and free from bias. Always write a summary of the evaluations to present to administration and to help plan next year's lab.

Common tools used to measure mastery of content information are self-rating scales, pretests/posttests, group work exercises, return demonstrations, and affective tests and scales (Abruzzese, 1996). Multiple-choice questions are easier to correct, but not as valid a measurement as determining what was learned and the intent of the learner for application of that learning to their clinical practice (Abruzzese, 1996). It is important that evaluation tools do not lose their validity by becoming outdated or so difficult that very few nurses can "pass" (Abruzzese, 1996).

Of utmost importance is the evaluation of learning outcomes (McGregor, 1990). Be sure to ask each learner what his or her level of performance of the skill was prior to the lab. These data were already collected with the needs as-

Exhibit 9–4 RSA Evaluation Model

Process evaluation
General happiness with the learning experience; sample items to evaluate are:
- Faculty
- Objectives
- Content
- Teaching and learning methodologies
- Physical facilities
- Administration

Content evaluation
- Self-rating scales
- Pretests and posttests
- Group work exercises
- Return demonstrations
- Multiple-choice examinations

Outcome evaluation
Changes in practice on clinical units following a learning experience; some changes might be:

- Integration of a new value
- Habitual use of a new skill
- Creation of a new product
- Institution of a new process

Impact evaluation
Organizational results attributable in part to learning experiences; some examples might be:
- Quality of patient care
- Cost-benefit or cost-effectiveness results
- Decreased turnover of nursing personnel
- Few risk-management incidents

Total program evaluation
Congruence of goals and accomplishments; these can be demonstrated by:
- Critique of advisory committee
- Annual reports to administration
- Reappraisal of goals for next year

Source: Copyright © 1996, R.S. Abruzzese.

sessment, but it is easier to evaluate learning outcomes if you correlate "before" and "after" and write it down as each person completes the lab. Tabulate and summarize posttest scores if a cognitive measurement tool is utilized along with the skills performance.

After the educational intervention, it is appropriate to follow up with a behavior-modification approach, giving the participants time with an experienced mentor to apply the new skill in the clinical setting. Positive feedback at this delicate time is crucial for retention of new skills (Ozcan & Shukla, 1993). There may be some learners who do not perform the skill successfully, even after supervised demonstration and practice. Possible causes for difficulties are a knowledge deficit, a resource deficit, inexperience, lack of critical thinking ability, or perhaps a problem with the system in which the staff are asked to perform (Abruzzese, 1996). There should be an action plan in place for embarrassment-free remediation so that they may

become competent, even if it is to be scheduled in the near future. Remediation should consider the cause. If it is a knowledge deficit, then reteaching is necessary. If it is a lack of motivation, consider ways to challenge and motivate that staff member. It might also be helpful to examine if the poor performance is being "rewarded"; in other words, enabling the worker to avoid a responsibility (Benefield, 1996). Regardless, the employee should not be assigned to any patients requiring performance of that skill until competence is demonstrated. If someone doesn't attain the minimal score that is desired as per your organization procedures, he or she should be permitted to review the information and take the test again. This cycle may be repeated as many times as the organization deems appropriate. There are times when a performance issue simply cannot be remediated through education, for example, if poor performance relates to outside stressors or attitudinal problems. Even competent staff can have serious problems with productivity. According to Benefield (1996), today's home care nurse must have the necessary skills, and, after remediation, if there continues to be a problem, transfer or termination may be the solution for the organization to remain viable.

Three to 6 months after the skills lab is a good time to assess how managers and clinical staff are applying the skills that were taught in the lab (Abruzzese, 1996). This evaluation can also provide an overview of what was taught, because review increases knowledge retention (Knowles, 1984). These evaluations must, of course, be specific enough to be measurable and be clearly defined. To successfully measure outcomes, a good baseline assessment is required. Nurses need to demonstrate the outcomes of the

things they do, for behind every project is an opportunity to further the cause of nursing, specifically home care nursing.

With increasing pressure from regulatory bodies, the increase in litigious activity, the pressure from payers to demonstrate a quality product, and the emphasis on performance quality, the home care organization must seriously consider how it can meet the challenges presented to provide its customers with the quality outcomes they deserve. Budgets must be adjusted to include salary for an educator. The educator should be freed of other administrative or managerial duties so that a research-based competency program can be initiated and maintained. When competency issues are compromised, we all ultimately suffer.

Exhibit 9–5 Orientation and Inservice Evaluation Tools

Orientation Evaluation Tool

	Strongly Agree		Agree		Strongly Disagree
	1	2	3	4	5
1. Learning objectives were clearly identified.	1	2	3	4	5
2. Orientation was organized in a logical manner.	1	2	3	4	5
3. I feel ready to practice independently.	1	2	3	4	5
4. Reference material was appropriate and readily available.	1	2	3	4	5
5. There was adequate time:					
For self-study	1	2	3	4	5
Spent in the clinical setting	1	2	3	4	5
6. I have a general understanding of home care.	1	2	3	4	5
7. Preceptor was receptive to my needs.	1	2	3	4	5
8. Preceptor displayed proficient to expert knowledge in his/her role.	1	2	3	4	5
9. Preceptor provided both positive and negative comments.	1	2	3	4	5
10. Orientation has been a positive experience.	1	2	3	4	5

Comments: _____

Source: Orientation Evaluation Tool reprinted from Astarita, T.M., Competency Based Orientation in Home Care: One Agency's Approach, *Home Health Care Management and Practice*, Vol. 8, No. 4, p. 48, © 1996, Aspen Publishers, Inc.

continues

Exhibit 9–5 continued

Inservice Evaluation Tool

Title of Program _____ Date _____

	Strongly Agree		Agree	Strongly Disagree
	1	2	3	4	5
1. Objectives were clearly identified.	1	2	3	4	5
2. Learning objectives were met.	1	2	3	4	5
3. Program content was consistent with objectives.	1	2	3	4	5
4. Speaker demonstrated in-depth knowledge of topic.	1	2	3	4	5
5. Audiovisual equipment was appropriate.	1	2	3	4	5
6. Physical facilities were conducive to learning.	1	2	3	4	5
7. Program will assist me in performing my job.	1	2	3	4	5
8. Handouts were helpful and appropriate.	1	2	3	4	5

Comments: _____

_____

_____

_____

REFERENCES

Abruzzese, R.S. (1996). Evaluation in nursing staff development. In R.S. Abruzzese (Ed.), *Nursing staff development: Strategies for success* (2nd ed.) (pp. 242–258). St. Louis, MO: Mosby-Year Book, Inc.

Alspach, G. (1992). Concern and confusion over competence. *Critical Care Nurse, 12*(4), 9–11.

Alspach, G. (1996). *Designing competency assessment programs: A handbook for nurses and health-related professionals.* Pensacola, FL: National Nursing Staff Development Organization.

Ark, P.D., & Nies, M. (1996). Knowledge and skills of the home healthcare nurse. *Home Healthcare Nurse, 14*(4), 292–297.

Astarita, T.M., Materna, G., & Savage, C. (in press). Perceived knowledge level among home health nurses: A descriptive study. *Home Health Care Management and Practice.*

Bartz, C., & Srsic-Stoehr, K.M.. (1994). Nurses' views on preceptorship programs and preceptor and preceptee experiences. *Journal of Nursing Staff Development, 10*(3), 153–158.

Beacon Health Corporation. (1996). Conditions of participation. *Federal register: Rules and regulations* (Edition 2.51) (pp. 1–14). Washington, DC: Health Care Financing Administration.

Beeken, J. (1997). The relationship between critical thinking and self-concept in staff nurses and the influence of these characteristics on nursing practice. *Journal of Nursing Staff Development, 13*(5), 272–278.

Benedum, E., Kalup, M., & Freed, D. (1990). A competency achievement program for direct caregivers. *Nurse Manager, 21*(5), 32–35.

Benefield, L.B. (1996). Productivity in home healthcare: Maintaining and improving nurse performance. Part II. *Home Healthcare Nurse, 14*(10), 803–812.

Benner, P. (1984). *From novice to expert: Excellence and power in clinical nursing practice.* Menlo Park, CA: Addison-Wesley.

Blocker, V.T. (1992). Organizational models and staff preparation: A survey of staff development departments. *Journal of Continuing Education in Nursing, 23*(6), 259–262.

Bloom, B.S. (1956). *Cognitive domain, taxonomy of educational objectives. Handbook 1.* New York: David McKay.

Bradbury-Golas, K., & Carson, L. (1994). Nursing skills fair: Gaining knowledge with fun and games. *Journal of Continuing Education in Nursing, 25*(1), 32–34.

Brent, N.J. (1994). Orientation to home healthcare nursing is an essential ingredient of risk management and employee satisfaction. *Home Healthcare Nurse, 10*(2), 9–10.

Brent, N.J. (1996). The home healthcare nurse and the state nurse practice act: Gaining familiarity is as easy as 1-2-3. *Home Healthcare Nurse, 14*(10), 788–789.

Bryant, S., & Cloonan, P. (1992). Graduate home health education: A survey of home health educators and agency personnel. *Journal of Nursing Education, 31*(1), 29–32.

Caie-Lawrence, J., Peploski, J., & Russell, J.C. (1995). Training needs of home healthcare nurses. *Home Healthcare Nurse, 13*(2), 53–61.

Carney, K. (1997). Clinical nurse specialists: A market advantage. *Caring, 14*(6), 16.

Carr, P. (1991). A whole different world. *Home Healthcare Nurse, 9*(4), 6–7.

Coffman S. (1996). Applying adult education principles to computer education. *Journal of Nursing Staff Development, 12*(5), 260–263.

Community Health Accreditation Program. (1993). National League for Health Care, Inc. and the Community Health Accreditation Program, Inc. *Standards of Excellence for Home Care Organizations.* New York: Author.

del Bueno, D.J., Weeks, L., & Brown-Stewart, P. (1987). Clinical assessment centers: A cost-effective alternative for competency development. *Nursing Economics, 5*(1), 21–26.

Ellis, C. (1992). Incorporating the affective domain into staff development programs. *Journal of Nursing Staff Development, 8*(3), 127–130.

Finnick, M., Crosby, F., & Ventura, M.R. (1993). Staff development challenge. Assuring nurses' competency in quality assessment and improvement. *Journal of Nursing Staff Development, 9*(3), 136–140.

Flynn, E.R., Wolf, Z.R., McGoldrick, T.B., Jablonski, R.A.S., Dean, L.M., & McKee, E.P. (1996). Effect of three teaching methods on a nursing staff's knowledge of medication error risk reduction strategies. *Journal of Nursing Staff Development, 12*(1), 19–25.

Friedman, M.M. (1996). Competence assessment: How to meet the intent of the Joint Commission on Accreditation of Healthcare Organizations' management of human resource standards. *Home Healthcare Nurse, 14*(10), 771–774.

Friedman, M.M. (1997). Contracted services survey process. *Home Healthcare Nurse, 15*(10), 675–678.

Garland, G.A. (1996). Self report of competence: A tool for the staff development specialist. *Journal of Nursing Staff Development, 12*(4), 191–197.

Gingerich, B.S., & Ondeck, D.A. (1997). *Home care human resources manual.* Gaithersburg, MD: Aspen Publishers.

Green, P.H. (1994). Meeting the learning needs of home health nurses. *Journal of Home Health Care Practice, 6*(4), 25–32.

Gurvis, J., & Grey, M. (1995). The anatomy of a competency. *Journal of Nursing Staff Development, 11*(5), 247–252.

Hedtcke, C.S., MacQueen, L., & Carr, A. (1992). How do home health nurses spend their time? *Journal of Nursing Administration, 22*(1), 18–22.

Hefty, L.V., Kenyon, V., Martaus, T., Bell, M.L., & Snow, L. (1992). A model skills list for orienting nurses to community health agencies. *Public Health Nursing, 9*(4), 228–233.

Jeska, S.B., Fischer, K.J., & McClellan, M.G. (1992). *Quality indicators for nursing staff development.* Pensacola, FL: National Nursing Staff Development Organization.

Joint Commission on Accreditation of Healthcare Organizations. (1996). *Joint Commission accreditation manual for home care.* Oakbrook Terrace, IL: Author.

Kalnins, I. (1989). Home health agency preferences for staff nurse qualifications and practices in hiring and orientation. *Public Health Nursing, 6*(2), 55–61.

Kelly, K.J. (1992). *Nursing staff development: Current competence, future focus.* Philadelphia: J.B. Lippincott.

Kerns, R.D. (1997). Orientation to management. *Home Health Care Management and Practice, 9*(4), 6–10.

Knowles, M.S. (1984). *The adult learner: A neglected species.* Houston, TX: Gulf Publishing Company.

Kobs, A. (1997). Competence: The shot heard around the nursing world. *Nursing Management, 28*(2), 10–13.

Kramer, M., & Schmalenberg, C. (1988). Learning from success: Autonomy and empowerment. *Nursing Management, 24*(5), 58–64.

Krisjanson, L.J., & Scanlan, J.M. (1989). Assessment of continuing nursing education needs: A literature review. *Journal of Continuing Education in Nursing, 20*(3), 118–123.

Leidy, K. (1990). Effective screening and orientation of independent contract nurses. *Journal of Continuing Education in Nursing, 23*(2), 64–69.

Lockhart, J.S., & Bryce, J. (1996). A comprehensive plan to meet the unit-based education needs of nurses from several specialty units. *Journal of Nursing Staff Development, 12*(3), 135–138.

Lohrman, J. (1992). *Competency-based orientation for critical care nursing.* St. Louis, MO: Mosby-Year Book, Inc..

McAnnally, R., & Barnett, J. (1997). Reorganizing competency programs. *Nursing Management, 28*(9), 33.

McGregor, R.J. (1990). A framework for developing staff competencies. *Journal of Nursing Staff Development, 6*(2), 79–84.

McGuire D.B., & Harwood, K.V. (1989). The CNS as researcher. In A.B. Hamric & J.A. Spross (Eds.), *The clinical nurse specialist in theory and practice* (2nd ed.) (pp. 169–204). Philadelphia: W.B. Saunders.

McMillan, J.H. (1997). *Classroom assessment: Principles and practice for effective instruction.* Needham Heights, MA: Allyn & Bacon.

Meyer-Desnoyer, J., & Herrmann, G. (1996). Using computers to manage staff development. In R.S. Abruzzese (Ed.), *Nursing staff development: Strategies for success* (2nd ed.) (pp. 156–185). St. Louis, MO: Mosby-Year Book.

Miller, M.M., & Daly, B.J. (1996). Home health care nursing: There is a difference. *Home Healthcare Management and Practice, 8*(4), 64–70.

Neal, L.J. (1995). The rehabilitation CNS in the home health setting. *Clinical Nurse Specialist, 9*(6), 293–298.

Nemcek, M.A., & Egan, P.B. (1997). Specialty nursing improves home care. *Caring Magazine, 16*(6), 12–18.

O'Hagan, K. (1996). Social work competence: An historical perspective. In K. O'Hagan (Ed.), *Competence in social work practice.* Bristol, PA: J. Kingsley, Publishers.

Ondeck, D. (1997). Competency assessment for maternal-child nursing. *Home Health Care Management and Practice, 9*(3), 78–80.

Ozcan, Y.A., & Shukla, R.K. (1993). The effect of a competency-based targeted staff development program on nursing productivity. *Journal of Nursing Staff Development, 9*(2), 78–84.

Paglione, M.A. (1991). Training home health nurses in IV therapy: A collaborative effort. *Home Healthcare Nurse, 9*(2), 23–27.

Remington, L. (1995). Five trends driving the home care industry. *The Remington Report, 3*(3), 20–23.

Revis, K.S., Thompson, C., Williams, M., Bezanson, J., & Cook, K.L. (1996). Nursing orientation: A continuous quality improvement story. *Clinical Nurse Specialist, 10*(2), 89–93.

Riegel, B., Gates, D.M., Gocka, I., Medina, L., Odell, C., Rich, M., & Finken, J.S. (1996). Effectiveness of a program of early hospital discharge of cardiac surgery patients. *Journal of Cardiovascular Nursing, 11*(1), 63–75.

Robinson, S.M., & Barberris, R.C. (1995). Competency assessment: A systematic approach. *Nursing Management, 26*(2), 40–44.

Salvatori, P. (1996). Clinical competence: A review of the health care literature with a focus on occupational therapy. *Canadian Journal of Occupational Therapy, 63*(4), 260–271.

Schwerin, J., Gaster, K., Krolikowski, J., & Sherman-Justice, D. (1994). Staff nurse leadership and professional growth in the mentor role. *Journal of Nursing Staff Development, 10*(3), 139–144.

Scrima, D. (1987). Assessing staff competency. *Journal of Nursing Administration, 17*(2), 41–45.

Shaffer, F., & Kobs, A. (1997). Measuring competencies of temporary staff. *Nursing Management, 28*(5), 41–45.

Sherman, A.W., Bohlander, G.W., & Snell, S.A. (1996). *Managing human resources.* Cincinnati: Southwestern College Publishing.

Snow, L., Hefty, L.V., Kenyon, B., Bell, M.L., & Martaus, T. (1992). Making the fit: Orienting new employees to community health nursing agencies. *Public Health Nursing, XX*(1), 58–64.

Stark, J. (1995). Critical thinking: Taking the road less traveled. *Nursing 95, 25*(11), 52–56.

Stefanik, R.L., Cassandra K., Edwards-Beckett, J., Copeland, S.G., Hoffman, M., Hulls, P., Freese, L., Opperman, C., & Timmerman, R. (1994). Perceptions of nursing staff development. A replication study. *Journal of Nursing Staff Development, 10*(3), 115–119.

Strzelecki, S., & Brobst, S.A. (1997). The development of an acute care case manager orientation. *Journal of Nursing Staff Development, 13*(5), 266–271.

Taft, C.S. (1995). A cost-effective competency program for a rehabilitation unit. *Rehabilitation Nursing, 20*(3), 164–167.

Van Ort, S., & Woodtli, A. (1989). Home health care. Providing a missing link. *Journal of Gerontological Nursing, 15*(9), 4–9.

Vincent, R. (1996). Assessment in the workplace. In H. Goldstein & T. Lewis (Eds.), *Assessment: Problems, developments and statistical issues* (pp. 231–241). New York: John Wiley.

Ward, M.D., & Rieve, J. (1995). Disease management: Case management's return to patient-centered care. *Journal of Care Management, 1*(4), 7–12.

Wolf, A. (1996). Vocational assessment. In H. Goldstein & T. Lewis (Eds.), *Assessment: Problems, developments and statistical issues* (pp. 209–230). New York: John Wiley.

Yoder Wise, P.S. (1996). Learning needs assessment. In R.S. Abruzzese (Ed.), *Nursing staff development: Strategies for success* (2nd ed.) (pp. 188–207). St. Louis, MO: Mosby-Year Book, Inc.

CHAPTER 10

Performance Improvement

"Whether you think you can, or you think you can't, you're right."
—Author unknown

The home care staff-development department should have its own objectives and strategic plan, which are aligned with and supported by the strategic plan for the organization. This plan should be constructed based on financial goals, current performance-improvement data, future programs to be offered by the organization, specific organizational needs, and sound educational principles. After developing an annual plan, approval should be granted from administration and managers so that the plan will be supported and short-term goals established. As the plan is developed, a systematic evaluation process should also be implemented, as explained in Chapter 7. General items to be included in this evaluation are cost, savings, impact upon care delivery, risk management, customer satisfaction, productivity, and recruitment/retention. Not only will these items demonstrate outcomes for the competency evaluation program, but they will also justify the role of staff development in home care.

PERFORMANCE IMPROVEMENT AND COMPETENCY

There are three primary ways in which competency of staff interrelates with performance improvement. First of all, there are implications for competency program development so that all staff are competent in the rudiments of performance improvement on a personal and organizational level. All staff must recognize the need for

performance improvement within the facility, and those who don't should be educated about its importance. Secondly, the components of performance improvement must be applied directly to the staff development department to ensure that it is well-functioning and justified. With present and future reimbursement issues, the necessity for staff development must be clearly demonstrated if the position is to be supported. Finally, staff competency is an organizational prerequisite for administering quality care. If clinical staff are not competent, it will lower the quality of care being given, as measured by the quality indicators (Table 10–1).

Staff Competencies for Performance Improvement

Performance-improvement activities require a multidisciplinary commitment at the patient care level, especially from nurses (Finnick, Crosby, & Ventura, 1993). If the staff are not competent in skills that specifically impact organizational performance improvement plans, such as assessment, surveillance, and documentation, data collection will be adversely affected. Staff must be taught that their clinical decisions can affect the finances and the overall quality of the organization (Katz, 1996; Bruce, 1992). Monitoring tools for measurement of competency can be derived from Joint Commission standards, which are revised on a regular basis (Western, 1994). In addition, the Community

Table 10–1 Competency Implications from Joint Commission Performance Improvement Standards

Joint Commission Performance Improvement Standard	Implication for Competency Programs
PI.1 Requires written documentation describing organizational approach for design, measurement, assessment, and improvement of performance. Performance improvement activities should be conducted with collaboration.	• Leadership and other staff must be trained regarding the basic principles and methods of performance improvement. • Competency policy for all staff should clearly delineate how staff performance deficits are remediated. • Contract staff competency assessment relevant to performance improvement must be done. • Competency program performance improvement activities should be the primary responsibility of staff development, but saturate the organization to ensure consistency in data collection. • Performance improvement teams should be multidisciplinary and include staff development.
PI.2 Design of processes should be consistent with the mission, vision, and plans of the organization.	• Any processes relevant to competency assessment should be consistent with the organization's mission, vision, and other plans, should meet patient and staff needs, should be based on current information, and should be based on the outcomes and performance elsewhere (benchmarking tools such as OASIS). For example, a needs assessment should be done prior to creating a competency program, and customer satisfaction surveys can help educators review the competency program for adequacy.
PI.3 and PI.4 Data collection is performed systematically and includes assessment of the environment of the organization and the patient; after collection, it must be assessed, using appropriate statistical techniques.	• According to organizational policy, baseline measurement should be done prior to education so that efficacy of programs can be measured by comparing pretests and posttests. • Priorities for performance improvement emphasize high risk, high volume, or problem prone. • There should also be a policy in the organization for how useful and necessary data that are collected from sources, such as customer surveys or infection control reports, translate into educational programs. • Staff must be competent in the areas of safety, security, hazardous material and wastes, emergency preparedness, fire prevention, equipment, and utility systems; and they must be able to collect data appropriately per organizational policy. • What are the implications for future programs? • Education records are maintained. • Those collecting data are competent with statistical techniques such as control charts or histograms.

Source: Data from *1997–98 Home Care Standards, Performance Improvement.* Joint Commission on Accreditation of Healthcare Organizations.

Health Accreditation Program has developed an outcomes-based data system called "Benchmarks for Excellence in Home Care." This software demonstrates standards on quality monitoring and improvement (Zink, 1996).

Home care is an autonomous specialty, requiring each clinician to have strong assessment skills. There is no one with whom to consult for validation of findings. The degree of competence that is required for other specialties certainly should not be less, but there is definitely no place in home care for "weak links." Data collection in the clinical setting requires accuracy in both interpretation and reporting. For example, if the patient develops infections that were not present upon admission to home care (termed nosihusial infections), they must be recognized and recorded accurately. Failure to do so can mask deficits in clinician technique or materials, perpetuating increased occurrences. Documentation is unique in home care in that a clear description of assessment findings, interventions, and the patient's response to them are alone not sufficient. There are specific guidelines that must be followed for the visit to be reimbursed, to ensure that home care will be approved for the ensuing certification period, and to serve as a reference for the interdisciplinary team. There are clinical records unique to home care as well. Nurses must complete a multidisciplinary plan of care when the patient is admitted. The clinician in home care will be the point of service where organizational effectiveness is measured and will be held accountable for achieving outcomes (Medford, 1996). Tools such as Outcome and Assessment Information Set (OASIS) will provide data for benchmarking home care organizations with others, yet will require education prior to their implementation (Gingerich & Ondeck, 1997). In addition, formal multidisciplinary communication is not as readily accessible in home care as it is in other disciplines. Communication must be clear and complete for the patient to receive a high quality of care. The home care staff should not have to rely on the patient for information pertinent to his or her care. All clinicians in an organization must be well-equipped to document at the basic level before they can even begin to understand systems used to measure outcomes (Medford, 1996). Documentation is a key element in a performance-improvement program. It is the role of staff development to include cognitive, affective, and performance evaluations of all clinical staff competencies relevant to understanding and implementing a performance-improvement program. Competency in performance improvement involves core elements such as being able to define performance improvement, understanding one's role in the process, recognizing relevant federal, state, and other guidelines, implementing performance improvement, and managing data (Finnick et al., 1993). The *Manual of Home Care Nursing Orientation* (Humphrey & Milone-Nuzzo, 1996) has an excellent chapter on quality management in home care that can be used as a resource when educating staff about this important topic.

The Value of Performance Improvement in Competency Programs

Not only must the organization have a performance-improvement program, but the staff development educator should have one as well, to demonstrate the effectiveness of the education department. This can be achieved by being visible, being viable, and being valid (Avillion, 1994). Orienting new staff and maintaining competency is no longer an option when regulatory agencies are considered, and it is an important aspect of risk management (Brent, 1994). A well-presented, competency-based orientation may assist with recruitment, and opportunities to increase professional competency on an ongoing basis may lead to increased staff retention (Stefanik et al., 1994). A high rate of turnover is very costly for the agency; recruitment costs alone in 1992 were calculated to be $397.92 per employee (Zahrt, 1992). This figure does not include orientation and the impact a novice to home care has on productivity until he or she increases competency, nor does it include the remuneration to the departing staff member for vacation time, etc. Research indicates that competency-based staff development improves the skills of nurses (Scrima, 1987) and increases the time spent in direct patient care (Ozcan & Shukla, 1993). Further research is needed to support the benefits of competency-based education in the home care setting, but when the cost of educating staff is weighed against the cost of ignorance, education is cost-effective. However, educators must establish quality indicators for their competency-based education program that will continue to support this. The National Nursing Staff Development Organization has published quality indicators for staff development (Jeska, Fischer, & McClellan, 1992). The quality indicators have been taken from the American Nurses Association (ANA) Standards of Nursing Staff Development (Appendix A). The components of a quality management program within staff development are identification of values, a definition of quality, development of standards, measurement and appraisal systems, and evaluation and action systems (Jeska et al., 1992). Identifying the values set forth by the department is essential for marketing within the organization. The purpose and principles that guide the department should be clearly outlined. Quality must be quantified and measurable, so a concise definition is required. Where quality begins and ends must be articulated, using percentages and dates as appropriate. Objective measurements are required to serve as a framework for evaluation of all programs. How the staff-development department is measured is up to the individual organization; however, it is suggested that the ANA standards serve as guidelines. Measurements can be direct, such as participant evaluations, staff surveys, or pretest/posttest scores, or indirect measurements such as productivity measures, chart audit reports, and occupational exposure reports. A department should progressively improve when measured by its measurement framework, for continuous performance improvement is a "customer-oriented, data driven process that facilitates management of change" (Revis, Thompson, Williams, Bezanson, &

Cook, 1996). Once deficits are revealed, an action plan should be implemented with subsequent evaluation and revision as necessary. The nursing process of assessment, diagnosis, planning, implementation, and evaluation can be applied to performance improvement within the staff development department.

Quality Data Synthesis and Application to Educational Programs

The contributions of staff development to the home care organization should originate from established needs for educational interventions within the organization. It is essential that the organization "collects, aggregates, and analyzes data on staff competence to identify and respond to staff learning needs" (Joint Commission, 1996, p. 380). Staff development must learn of any organizational changes related to quality before they are implemented if they are to be a resource to staff (Katz, 1996). In other words, not only should educators receive appropriate referrals when a performance issue is possibly related to an educational need, but educational offerings should take place prior to design of "performance improvement processes, data collection systems, and monitoring" (Joint Commission, 1996, p. 58). Other sources, such as customer complaints, staff requests, incident reports, infection control summaries, and productivity reports, can be used to develop educational programs. Performance quality deficits that may be corrected through the use of educational programs include lack of mastery using equipment that is new to the staff, lack of knowledge about a specific disease process, or affective deficits including poor customer service. Education can serve not only to influence the cognitive, affective, or motor domains of competency, but may also increase motivation and desire for staff to do a better job. The effectiveness of educational interventions on performance improvement should be summarized, measuring performance before and after the educational intervention. Performance improvement should be a cycle for improving organizational performance (Humphrey & Milone-Nuzzo, 1996), but education is not the only part of organizational performance improvement. Organizations that seek accreditation through the Joint Commission must meet the criteria outlined in the current performance improvement standards. There are 1996 Joint Commission performance-improvement standards that directly relate to competency issues (Table 10–1).

Budgetary Performance Improvement Considerations for Home Care Competency

Educators must consistently evaluate the cost of competency programs and seek the best way to be effective yet efficient (Sheridan & Frost-Hartzer, 1996). For example, competency-based orientation can have high initial start-up costs, but can pay for itself if the staff assessment reveals that staff are competent in certain areas that will not require education. In addition, self-directed learning can free the educator, decreasing educational costs (Voorhees, 1996). When projecting costs of competency-based orientation and education, the educator should at least consider the cost of materials, labor, and additional overhead. In addition, planning, implementing, and evaluation costs can be added. This is referred to as "comprehensive cost accounting" (Sheridan & Frost-Hartzer, 1996). Staff development departments can be adversely affected when the organization suffers financially (Sheridan & Frost-Hartzer, 1996).

Financial goals are foremost in the minds of many as health care reform affects how each organization is reimbursed for services. Some smaller organizations may not feel that hiring an educator is necessary. Certainly, all organizations will require some allocation in the budget to meeting educational needs, if they are maintaining certification in the current market. When they must compensate the qualified staff-development educator, some may see little need to provide the educator with a budget to use for programs. It behooves the educator to perpetu-

ally justify not only the effectiveness of his or her programs but the cost-effectiveness as well. If organizations recognize that retention of employees that can result from staff-development programs is saving thousands of dollars, there will be support for staff development.

A basic summary of budget terms is included in this section for those who are not familiar with organizational budgets, for an educator must have this knowledge to know which funds should be requested to support competency programs. An operating budget is the first step in work planning (Bruce, 1992) and includes the day-to-day operating costs of the department (Sheridan & Frost-Hartzer, 1996). This is used to project expenses for one fiscal year, which is frequently July 1 to June 30 of the next year (Sheridan & Frost-Hartzer, 1996). Some categories that should be included in the annual operational education budget include educational books and materials for use by the educator, library resources, computer software for computer-assisted learning or presentations, honoraria for speakers, and education obtained outside the organization. Some organizations prefer to budget any allotted educational conferences or outside seminars under the specific discipline, rather than under staff development. Miscellaneous teaching materials, such as markers, chalk, and poster board, must be budgeted. Purchases of copier paper, postage, and small office supplies must also be anticipated, unless these items are absorbed by the organization as a whole. A category for entertainment/food should be included for refreshments to serve from time to time during educational programs and mileage for supervisory visits as needed. Creativity can help stretch educational dollars only so far, so the organization must be willing to support the educational programs.

A capital budget is used to allocate funds from the capital account for any major expense. Capital funds may be obtained through donations and gifts to the organization, often by satisfied "customers." According to Bruce (1992), this is any expense greater than $500, but this may vary between organizations. Major expenses can be stretched over more than 1 fiscal year to enable them to be purchased. Some purchases that may be made using capital funds include educational tools such as overheads, computers, laser pointers, write-on boards, mannequins, and so forth. The availability of these funds varies from organization to organization and year to year. It is expected that items obtained through capital funds will last for 3 to 7 years (Sheridan & Frost-Hartzer, 1996).

Once the funds have been allocated to the department, the educator must use them wisely. There are times when a budget is approved when the organization is doing very well financially. The educator must realize that, should there be a change in the financial status of the organization, there may be some adjustment to the amount of funds available. It is wise for the educator to approve educational attendance at conferences with discretion, rotating the privilege among the staff. Should there be financial difficulties at the organization, large purchases should be postponed.

Cost containment is just one aspect of performance improvement. With reimbursement issues foremost on the minds of organizations, a balance must be achieved between cost effectiveness and delivery of quality patient care. Performance improvement is inherent to the nursing process, but each employee in the organization must embrace the concepts. Professional preparatory programs may not adequately present the principles of performance improvement to the future health care worker (Finnick, et al., 1993), so it is essential that the educator serve as a resource to all staff. Modeling performance improvement initiatives and maintaining a department that is beyond reproach in its pursuit of quality is important, as well.

The educator and each employee must share a partnership in the organization as a whole. They must capture the mission, vision, and strategic goals of the organization, applying them to their practice and striving to produce a quality product or outcome. Not only should the educator take an active part, but he or she should also be one of the first to know of failures and successes so adjustments can be made to educational programs as needed. If permitted to do so, the educator can serve as an invaluable resource in assisting an organization to improve its performance.

REFERENCES

Avillion, A.E. (1994). Political savvy in staff development: Building an indispensable department. *Journal of Continuing Education in Nursing, 25*(4), 152–154.

Brent, N.J. (1994). Orientation to home healthcare nursing is an essential ingredient of risk management and employee satisfaction. *Home Healthcare Nurse, 10*(2), 9–10.

Bruce, C. (1992). Financial concepts in home healthcare. *Journal of Nursing Administration, 22*(5), 29–34.

Finnick, M., Crosby, F., & Ventura, M.R. (1993). Staff development challenge: Assuring nurses' competency in quality assessment and improvement. *Journal of Nursing Staff Development, 9*(3), 136–140.

Gingerich, B.S., & Ondeck, D.A. (1997). From our vantage point. *Home Health Digest, 3*(4), 4–5.

Humphrey, C.J., & Milone-Nuzzo, P. (1996). *Manual of home care nursing orientation.* Gaithersburg, MD: Aspen Publishers.

Jeska, S.B., Fischer, K.J., & McClellan, M.G. (1992). *Qual-ity indicators for nursing staff development.* Pensacola, FL: National Nursing Staff Development Organization.

Joint Commission on Accreditation of Healthcare Organizations. (1996). *Comprehensive accreditation manual for home care. Vol I: Standards.* Oakbrook Terrace, IL: Author.

Katz, J.M. (1996). Managing the dual dimensions of quality. In R.S. Abruzzese (Ed.), *Nursing staff development: Strategies for success* (2nd ed.) (pp. 302–324). St. Louis, MO: Mosby-Year Book, Inc.

Medford, J. (1996). Order in a new era: Outcome documentation. *Caring, 15*(6), 18–23.

Ozcan, Y.A., & Shukla, R.K. (1993). The effect of a competency-based targeted staff development program on nursing productivity. *Journal of Nursing Staff Development, 9*(2), 78–84.

Revis, K.S., Thompson, C., Williams, M., Bezanson, J., & Cook, K.L. (1996). Nursing orientation: A continuous quality improvement story. *Clinical Nurse Specialist, 10*(2), 89–93.

Scrima, D. (1987). Assessing staff competency. *Journal of Nursing Administration, 17*(2), 41–45.

Sheridan, D.R., & Frost-Hartzer, P. (1996). Documenting effectiveness: Budget and cost considerations. In R.S. Abruzzese (Ed.), *Nursing staff development: Strategies for success* (2nd ed.) (pp. 122–140). St. Louis, MO: Mosby-Year Book, Inc.

Stefanik, R.L., Cassandra, K., Beckett, J.E., Copeland, S.G., Hoffman, M., Hulls, P., Freese, L., Opperman, C., & Timmerman, R. (1994). Perceptions of nursing staff de-velopment: A replication study. *Journal of Nursing Staff Development, 10*(3), 115–119.

Voorhees, M. (1996). Using competency-based education in the perioperative setting. *Nursing Management, 27*(8), 35–38.

Western, P. (1994). QA/QI and nursing competence: A combined model. *Nursing Management, 25*(3), 44–46.

Zahrt, L.M. (1992). The cost of turnover in a home care agency. *Caring, 12*(4), 60–67.

Zink, M.R. (1996). Home care accreditation with the community health accreditation program: Part I: Overview. *Home Healthcare Nurse, 14*(8), 590–594.

CHAPTER 11

Tort Liability of Home Health Care Organizations and Their Employees

Joshua H. Soven and Corrine Parver

The home health care industry is booming. Between 1990 and 1996, the number of people receiving home health care services increased from 1.7 million to 3.9 million, while the number of Medicare dollars spent on the industry rose from $2.6 billion to approximately $18 billion.[1] These increases reflect the growing recognition that certain health care services traditionally provided in hospitals and nursing homes can be provided with equal if not greater efficiency in the patient's home, and that many patients prefer receiving home care.[2]

The expansion of the home health care industry, however, has not been without cost. As the industry has grown, there has been increasing concern that regulators and the industry need to take reasonable measures to ensure the competency of home health care organizations ("HCOs") and their employees ("clinicians").[3] Prompted by these concerns, federal and state governments have issued, and are continuing to issue, regulations governing the qualifications of HCOs and clinicians, and have increased resources for enforcement of those regulations.

This increased focus on competency in the home health care industry highlights the fact that HCOs, clinicians, employees that HCOs hire to evaluate clinicians ("competency evaluators"), and even certification associations that assess HCO and clinician competency face significant risk of legal liability from individuals injured by the industry. Moreover, the risk of such liability is increasing because efforts to control medical costs are causing patients of all ages to spend less time in hospitals and receive more care at home, much of which is provided by the home health care industry.[4] Consequently, HCOs are serving individuals who are often in need of greater monitoring and more complicated care than the individuals treated by the industry in the past.[5] Litigation risks also are growing because HCOs are caring for younger patients, who generally are more likely to bring lawsuits than older persons.

This chapter focuses on the most fundamental liability that confronts the industry related to competency assessment—liability based on the law of "torts." Tort law allows persons to recover damages from those persons who have injured them in violation of a legal duty or obligation.[6] We first discuss the potential tort liability confronting HCOs and then evaluate liability issues facing clinicians and competency evaluators. Lastly, we discuss the potential tort exposure faced by independent organizations that certify the competency of HCOs and clinicians. At the end of each section, we make general recommendations concerning how the home care industry can reduce tort liability risks.

TORT LIABILITY OF HCOs

When a person is injured because he or she received improper home health care, the HCO that provided the care is almost certain to be sued. HCOs are the primary targets in such suits because plaintiffs (and their lawyers) usually conclude that, of the potential defendants, the HCO has the most resources.[7] There are several types of tort actions that are brought against HCOs, each of which we discuss in turn.

Negligence

Most lawsuits filed against HCOs claim that the HCO is liable for damages caused by the negligence of a clinician who failed to provide a patient with proper care.[8] Under a legal principle known as "respondeat superior," an employer is liable for the torts of its employees if these torts are committed when the employee is acting within the scope of his or her employment.[9] However, conduct by employees outside the normal scope of their employment, such as acts engaged in for personal motives intended to harm someone, generally are not covered by the respondeat superior doctrine.[10]

To recover on a negligence claim, a party must prove that:

1. there existed a duty of the defendant to the plaintiff to exercise a standard of care;
2. the defendant failed to conform to the required standard;
3. a reasonably close causal connection existed between the defendant's failure to conform to the standard of care and the plaintiff's damages; and
4. the plaintiff incurred actual loss or damages.[11]

The critical threshold issue in a negligence case against an HCO is determining the appropriate standard of care and whether the HCO conformed to that standard. In such cases, the standard of care is determined by looking to generally accepted industry practices in providing the type of care that is at issue. For example, in a 1995 New York case, a patient with multiple sclerosis (MS) sued an HCO. The court rejected the HCO's position that its clinicians only had a duty to perform household tasks, finding that the clinician had been instructed about the symptoms of MS patients and the emergency circumstances under which an ambulance should be called.[12]

The standard of care in negligence cases against HCOs also may be determined by looking to applicable laws and regulations. Where government requirements provide that a certain procedure must be followed in providing a particular service, a clinician's failure to use that procedure can serve as a basis for finding that the clinician's HCO breached a legal duty to the patient. Thus, in *Roach v. Kelly Health Care, Inc.*, an Oregon court held that a jury should be instructed that an HCO's failure to adhere to state regulations concerning the delegation of supervisory functions required a finding that the HCO was negligent.[13] As noted, there recently has been a flurry of regulations passed at the federal and state levels concerning competency in the home health care industry. These are precisely the types of government mandates that often are used to demonstrate that an HCO (through its clinician) was negligent in providing home health care services.

Negligent Hiring and Supervision

HCOs also face potential liability from claims that they negligently hired a clinician who was incompetent or unfit.[14] The tort of "negligent hiring" is intended to protect the public against the risk created by exposing the public to potentially dangerous individuals. To succeed in a negligent hiring action, the claimant must prove that:

1. the employer knew or should have known that the employee in question had a particular unfitness for the position so as to create a danger of harm to third persons;
2. the unfitness was known or should have been known at the time of hiring; and
3. the particular unfitness proximately caused the claimed injury.[15]

A similar cause of action exists for negligent supervision.

The critical distinction between a negligent hiring and a negligence action is that a negligent hiring claim allows the plaintiff to recover damages from an employer for injuries caused by an employee's conduct that is outside the scope of employment.[16] Examples of such conduct include intentional assault or other acts in which the person intends to harm the home health care recipient. Damages from such conduct are recoverable in negligent hiring cases because the tort of negligent hiring is designed to reduce the risk created by employers' exposing members of the public to potentially dangerous individuals.[17]

As in negligence claims, the critical threshold issue in resolving a negligent hiring action is determining the appropriate standard of care. Again, the standard is determined by looking to generally accepted industry practices and government regulations. Government regulations are potentially particularly significant in negligent hiring cases because many new regulations concern HCO hiring standards, such as requirements that HCOs conduct criminal background checks for certain employees.[18] An HCO's failure to adhere to such requirements in the hiring of a clinician who subsequently injures a patient will expose the HCO to a potential negligent hiring claim.

Lingar v. Live-In Companions, Inc.[19] demonstrates how an HCO can be held liable for negligent hiring. In this action, a husband and wife sued an HCO, alleging that the HCO's clinician, who was hired to care for the husband, had in fact abandoned the husband and stolen several items from the couple's home. The clinician had a substantial criminal record when he was hired by the HCO. In reversing the trial court's dismissal of the plaintiffs' claim, the appeals court found that the couple's negligent hiring claim should go to the jury because the HCO had used a "sketchy and meager application form [that] was wholly insufficient to yield adequate information pertaining to the [clinician's] background, criminal history and experience."[20] As discussed below, development and implementation of a thorough initial competency screening process are vital to avoid the type of negligent hiring liability at issue in *Lingar*.

Fraud and Misrepresentation

A third type of tort action that threatens HCOs is based on claims that an HCO has engaged in fraud or misrepresentation by overstating or misrepresenting the types of services that the HCO can provide competently. As the home health care industry continues to grow and becomes more competitive, there will be a growing temptation for HCOs to attempt to distinguish themselves in the marketplace through promotion, including comparisons with competitors. It is critically important that, in doing so, HCOs make certain that the information they disseminate is accurate. A patient who hires an HCO based on such a misrepresentation, and then discovers that the HCO cannot provide the represented service—or worse, is injured because the HCO cannot provide the represented service—will have a solid fraud claim against the HCO.

Steps HCOs Can Take To Reduce Tort Liability Risks

Certain measures exist that most HCOs can take to lower their risk of the types of tort liability described above. These recommendations are not exhaustive and HCOs should consult counsel and other appropriate advisers in devising a litigation risk plan.

First, to reduce potential liability from negligence claims, HCOs should make certain that all clinicians are well-trained and that there are procedures in place for HCO evaluators to monitor and continually reassess clinicians' performance and qualifications. Clinicians should never be assigned responsibility for services or tasks for which they are not fully qualified. Any complaints about the services provided by a clinician should be promptly investigated and remedial action should be taken when necessary.

Second, HCOs should make certain that they implement and fully utilize a thorough screening procedure in hiring clinicians and competency evaluators. These screening procedures should adhere to relevant industry standards and comply fully with applicable federal, state, and local regulations. As noted, such regulations are potentially critical in determining whether an HCO has violated a legal duty of care in negligence respondeat superior cases and negligent hiring actions. Further, because regulations are continually updated and modified, HCOs should assign personnel to monitor government actions at all times.

Third, HCOs should develop procedures to ensure the accuracy of information that is disseminated about their organizations and clinicians. The review procedure should involve several persons, including individuals who are not directly responsible for distributing the materials. Errors that are discovered should be conveyed promptly to legal counsel.

Fourth, HCOs should assess carefully their legal corporate structure. An HCO's liability in a tort case may depend on the HCO's corporate form. These issues are complicated and are well beyond the scope of this chapter. HCOs should consult appropriate legal counsel to determine which legal corporate structure minimizes tort and other litigation risks.

Finally, HCOs should make certain that they obtain all appropriate insurance coverage, including all insurance coverage required by law.

TORT LIABILITY OF CLINICIANS

Clinicians are also at risk from potential tort liability. When a recipient of home health care services is injured, he or she also typically sues the clinician who provided the care that caused the injury. Such claims against clinicians almost always allege that the clinician was negligent or reckless in providing home care services.

Although there is no guaranteed method for reducing the potential tort liability of home health care clinicians, consistent use of prudence and common sense goes a long way in minimizing liability risks. Plainly, the clinician should make certain that he or she is properly trained for all services that he or she is required to provide, and licensed or certified accordingly. A clinician uncertain about his or her qualifications to perform a particular service should consult with the

HCO's competency evaluators and superiors to determine whether another individual should be assigned to care for the person at issue.

Clinicians, of course, also should make certain that they diligently perform all functions required by the patient that they have been retained to perform. Difficulties or problems should be reported promptly to the clinician's superiors.

Further, at the time they are hired, clinicians should inquire as to what type of insurance coverage they receive from the HCO's liability insurance policies. Typically, clinicians are fully covered for all claims against them resulting from actions taken that are within the scope of their employment. Deliberate actions taken to harm a patient generally are considered outside the scope of employment and, thus, are not covered by most insurance policies.

TORT LIABILITY OF HOME HEALTH CARE EVALUATORS

Many HCOs hire competency evaluators who are specially trained to evaluate the competency of clinicians and other HCO employees. These competency evaluators also face the risk of tort liability, although their risk is less than that faced by the HCOs and clinicians. The primary risk confronting HCO evaluators is that they will be sued as part of a negligent hiring or supervision claim against the HCO. The evaluator's conduct is potentially at issue in such cases because the evaluator typically has certified that an HCO's clinicians have the necessary skills and backgrounds.

As with clinicians, the best precautions that competency evaluators can take against tort liability are to ensure that they are properly qualified for all tasks they perform and that they perform those tasks carefully and diligently. In addition, evaluators need to ensure that the competency assessment program used by their HCO is thorough and complies fully with all applicable regulations. Recordkeeping in implementing a competency assessment program also is critical. For each individual hired, the HCO, through its evaluator, should document precisely how the clinician was evaluated and the results of that evaluation. Problems or doubts uncovered by an evaluator should be noted and brought to the attention of appropriate superiors before any employee is hired.

Moreover, like clinicians, evaluators should make certain that they fully understand the insurance coverage that is provided to them for tort liability. As noted, such insurance issues are complicated and should be reviewed with legal counsel.

TORT LIABILITY OF HOME HEALTH CARE CERTIFYING ASSOCIATIONS

The increased scrutiny of competency in the home health care industry is likely to cause greater use of independent industry associations that certify the competency of HCOs and clinicians (referred to herein as "home health care certification associations" or "certification associations"). Although these certification associations play no role in treating patients, they nonetheless face some risk of tort liability from claims for injuries to recipients of home health care services.

Development of Inadequate Certification Standards

Certification associations face potential liability from suits that allege that the association is responsible for an injury caused to a patient because the association did not utilize adequate standards to assess the treating clinician's competency. A majority of cases analyzing negligence claims against certification associations (primarily in the context of product certification) have held that the associations do not owe a duty of care to the consumers and, thus, cannot be held liable for the consumer's injuries.[21] For example, a federal Appeals Court recently dismissed a student's negligence claim against two agencies that had accredited a school attended by the student, deciding that the agencies did not

"owe a tort law duty to students who attend the schools accredited by th[e] agencies."[22]

A growing minority of courts in product certification cases has decided, however, that certification associations do in fact have a duty to consumers to develop adequate certification standards and has allowed recovery of damages for injuries resulting from the certification bodies' failure to develop such standards.[23] For example, the American Association of Blood Banks ("AABB"), which issues guidelines used by the nation's blood banks, was found to owe a duty of care to patients to issue guidelines sufficient to ensure public safety based on current medical knowledge.[24] The plaintiffs in *Snyder v. American Ass'n of Blood Banks* alleged that, in the early 1980s, the AABB negligently failed to recommend that its members utilize screening measures needed to reduce the risk of the transmission of the AIDS virus through blood transfusions. In finding that the AABB owed a duty of care to patients, the courts used language that illustrates their flexibility to determine whether a duty of care exists and highlights the potential risk to home health care certification associations:

> [T]he question of whether one owes a duty to another is "largely a question of fairness or policy" whose resolution requires the "weighing of the relationship of the parties, the nature of the risk, and the public interest in the proposed solution." The unique and dominant role of AABB in blood-banking and the extent of its control over its institutional members create the requisite relationship between it and the ultimate recipient whose safety is its avowed paramount concern.[25]

Such decisions clearly show that the greater the role assumed by home health care certification organizations in assessing HCO and clinician competency, the more likely a court is to conclude that certification associations owe a duty of care to home health care patients.

Misrepresenting the Qualifications of an Individual Home Health Care Provider to Consumers

Home health care certification associations also risk tort liability if they represent that a clinician is qualified when the clinician in fact is not properly trained to provide home care services. The potential for this type of liability will be particularly significant if the certification organization communicates its certification decisions to consumers.

A patient alleging that an association misrepresented the competency of a home health care worker would likely seek to recover damages by bringing a fraud claim. The critical elements in proving fraud are that the patient demonstrate that the certification association intended the patient to rely on its statements concerning the clinician's abilities and that the patient did in fact rely on the certification association's statements. While such facts are not easy to prove, courts have shown a willingness in recent cases to give plaintiffs the benefit of the doubt when there is reason to believe that a certification group knowingly failed to apply its certification criteria to an applicant.

Recently, a federal court in the District of Columbia allowed a plaintiff to proceed to trial with a fraud claim against an education accreditation agency after the plaintiff presented evidence showing that the agency certified a school even though the agency lacked sufficient information to determine whether the certification was accurate.[26] The court held that the "intent" requirement was satisfied because the agency should reasonably have known that its certification decision would be communicated to the students.[27] With regard to the reliance element, the court accepted the plaintiff's statement that she considered the agency's accreditation when selecting her school.[28]

If home health care certification associations assume a role where their certification decisions are communicated to the public, as seems likely to occur, it is highly probable that consumers will come to rely on their decisions. Such reliance allows consumers who are dissatisfied with their home health care services to bring credible fraud lawsuits against home health care certification associations.

A related potential tort claim against home health care certification associations is that the certification association overstated the abilities of an otherwise qualified HCO or clinician. The risk here is that, even if the certification association properly certifies the individual at issue, the certification association, in an effort to promote the industry, represents that an HCO (or clinician) can provide services that it is not qualified to perform.[29] As with the potential fraud action described above, the outcome of such cases will depend heavily on the ability of the patient bringing the suit to prove that he or she relied on the certification association's alleged misstatements and was harmed by such reliance.

Minimizing the Risk

To reduce the risk of tort liability, home health care certification associations should use all reasonable procedures required to develop and implement certification criteria that are sufficient to evaluate HCO and clinician competency.[30] In developing these standards, certification associations should allow all segments of the industry to participate in developing the certification criteria and also seek the advice of independent experts. Careful written records explaining the reasons for the adoption of certification standards should be maintained. A certification association's ability to demonstrate that its standards are appropriate will serve as a powerful deterrent to tort litigation, and convincing evidence in defeating a claim if one is brought.

Certification associations also should implement appropriate safeguards to ensure that the individuals responsible for administering their competency standards and certification tests are thoroughly screened to determine *their* competence and willingness to apply the certification association's criteria in good faith. The risk of association tort liability soars if a plaintiff can demonstrate that an association knowingly certified an unqualified applicant by failing to apply its own standards. To the extent possible, redundancies should be built into the certification process, such that no individual or small group of individuals has authority to certify a worker or organization.

In addition, certification decisions should be carefully documented through use of a detailed evaluation form. Requiring documentation of certification decisions will reduce the risk that unqualified individuals are certified and ensure that there is a clear written record to defend any charge of wrongdoing by the association.

To further reduce litigation risks, clinicians should be required to be recertified at regular intervals.[31] Requiring periodic recertification will reduce the likelihood that unqualified clinicians are able to practice for a long period of time, and thus reduce liability risks.

Finally, as described above, knowing or careless misrepresentations about an HCO or the profession in general present the greatest risk of tort liability to home health care certification associations. Certification associations have powerful incentives to portray their industry in the best possible light. Consequently, there is the potential for certification associations to imply that an industry or its members can provide services that they may not be qualified to provide. To minimize the risk of claims based on overstatements, home health care certification associations should carefully screen information that they distribute to make certain the information is accurate.[32] In particular, materials that an individual HCO or clinician requests be disseminated should be subject to review by impartial persons to verify the accuracy of the materials.

CONCLUSION

The use of competency assessment and certification standards in the home health care industry has the potential to increase the quality of the industry and facilitate healthy growth. The risks of liability raised here are important and should be carefully considered, but they are not insurmountable obstacles. Through careful planning, HCOs and home health care certification associations can implement certification requirements that improve the industry and substantially reduce the risks of tort litigation and liability.

REFERENCES

1. Robert A. Rosenblatt, "Many Home-Care Firms Unqualified, Study Says," *L.A. Times*, July 28, 1997, sec. A, p. 6.

2. *See, e.g.*, Sue MacDonald, Smart Shopping: What you need to know when looking for home health-care services. *Cincinnati Enquirer*, Oct. 16, 1996, sec. E, p. 1; General Accounting Office, report to the Honorable Ron Wyden, U.S. Senate, *Long-Term Care: Some States Apply Criminal Background Checks to Home Care Workers,* September 1996, 1.

3. *See* General Accounting Office, Medicare Home Health Agencies, Certification Process Ineffective in Excluding Problem Agencies, Report to the Special Committee on Aging, U.S. Senate, December 1997; *Medicare Home Health Agencies: Certification Process Is Ineffective in Excluding Problem Agencies*, statement of Leslie G. Aronovitz before the Special Committee on Aging, U.S. Senate, July 28, 1997.

4. *See* Marshall B. Kapp, *Improving Choices Regarding Home Care Services: Legal Impediments and Empowerments*, 10 St. Louis U. Pub. L. Rev. 441, 455–456 (1991).

5. Kapp, *Improving Choices Regarding Home Care Services*, 455–456.

6. *See Black's Law Dictionary* 1489 (6th ed. 1990).

7. *See* Sandra H. Johnson, *Quality-Control Regulation of Home Health Care*, 26 Hous. L. Rev. 901, 911 (1989).

8. *See, e.g.*, *Obstetrician and Home Health Care Service Found Liable for Failure to Monitor Blood Pressure of Woman During High Risk Pregnancy*, 17 Verdicts, Settlements & Tactics 119 (Mar. 1997) (HCO found partially responsible for death of 28-year-old woman because clinician failed to inform the woman's treating physician about her elevated blood pressure); *Eaton v. Comprehensive Care America, Inc.*, 233 A.D.2d 875 (N.Y. App. Div. 1996) (HCO liable for damages caused by clinician's allowing stroke patient to smoke unattended); *Lauth v. Olstein Home Health Care, Inc.*, 678

So. 2d 447 (Fla. Dist. Ct. App. 1996) (provider of home nursing services liable for damages caused by clinician's failure to provide proper care); Anne Krueger, "$200,000 Awarded for Abusive Care," *San Diego Union-Tribune*, Aug. 20, 1996, sec. B, p. 2 (judgment against HCO for abuse inflicted by HCO's clinician); *Kansas City Star*, Dec. 21, 1991, Johnson County/Metro section, p. 2 (HCO sued because clinician allegedly was negligent in not replacing a tracheotomy tube).

9. *Restatement (Second) of Agency* §§ 219, 228. The states have adopted several different definitions of the term "scope of employment."

10. *Restatement (Second) of Agency* §§ 219, 228.

11. W. Page Keeton, et al., *Prosser and Keeton on the Law of Torts* 164–65 (5th ed. 1984).

12. *Walker v. Ehcci Home Care Services, Inc.*, 211 A.D.2d 402, 403 (N.Y. App. Div. 1995).

13. 742 P.2d 1190, 1196 (Or. Ct. App. 1987).

14. *E.g., Lingar v. Live-In Companions, Inc.*, 692 A.2d 61, 64 (N.J. Super. Ct. App. Div. 1997). *See generally* Marshall B. Kapp, *Malpractice Liability in Long-Term Care: A Changing Environment*, 24 Creighton L. Rev. 1235, 1241-42 (1991) (discussing tort corporate liability).

15. *E.g., Mueller v. Community Consol. Sch. Dist. 54*, 678 N.E.2d 660, 663 (Ill. App. Ct. 1997).

16. *Lingar*, 692 A.2d at 65; Rodolfo A. Camacho, *How to Avoid Negligent Hiring Litigation*, 14 Whittier L. Rev. 787, 791–93 (1993).

17. *Lingar*, 692 A.2d at 65; *see* Bill Torpy, "Ex-nurse's Aide Given Life Plus 40 in Death, Assault," *Atlanta Journal & Constitution*, May 31, 1991, sec. E, p. 2 (American Home Health Care sued for $25 million as a result of murder by company's clinician).

18. *See* Henriette Campagne, *Home Health Care Legislation Filed*, Mass. Law. Wkly., Oct. 13, 1997, at 29 (Massachusetts criminal background check legislation); Mary Zahn, "Care Safeguards Receive Final Legislative Approval: Measure Includes Checks to Prevent Hiring of Serious Criminals as Health Aides," *Milwaukee Journal Sentinel*, Sept. 30, 1997, p. 8 (Wisconsin criminal background check legislation); "Rules check home health providers," *Chicago Sun Times*, June 8, 1997, p. 4.

19. 692 A.2d 61 (N.J. Super. Ct. App. Div. 1997).

20. *Lingar*, 692 A.2d at 66.

21. *See, e.g., Sizemore v. Georgia-Pacific Corp.*, Civ. A. Nos. 6:94-2894 3, 6:94-2895 3, and 6:94-2896 3, 1996 WL 498410, at *8 (D.S.C. Mar. 8, 1996) ("weight of authority has rejected product injury claims such as these [product liability claims] against trade associations based on negligence"), *aff'd without op. sub nom. Sizemore v. Hardwood Plywood & Veneer Ass'n*, 114

F.3d 1177 (4th Cir. 1997); *Evenson v. Osmose Wood Preserving, Inc.*, 760 F. Supp. 1345, 1348-49 (S.D. Ind. 1990) (wood preservers trade association did not owe duty to plaintiff allegedly injured by exposure to wood preserving chemicals); *Beasock v. Dioguardi Enters., Inc.*, 494 N.Y.S.2d 974, 978-79 (N.Y. Sup. Ct. 1985) (automotive trade association which published tire and rim standards could not be held liable for injuries caused by tire explosion); *State v. Joint Comm'n on Accreditation of Hosps., Inc.*, 470 So. 2d 169, 176-77 (La. Ct. App. 1985) (hospital accreditation agency did not owe legal duty to patients of the hospital); *see also Foster v. Greenville County Med. Soc'y*, 367 S.E.2d 468, 470 (S.C. Ct. App. 1988) (medical society had no duty to patient injured by member doctor about whom society had received complaint).

22. *Keams v. Tempe Technical Inst., Inc.*, 110 F.3d 44, 47 (9th Cir. 1997).

23. *Prudential Property & Cas. Ins. Co. v. American Plywood Ass'n*, No. 93-2026, 1994 U.S. Dist. LEXIS 12067, at *6 (S.D. Fla. Aug. 3, 1994) (plywood association owed homeowners a duty of care to promulgate adequate construction standards); *United States Lighting Serv., Inc. v. Llerrad Corp.*, 800 F. Supp. 1513, 1515-17 (N.D. Ohio) (Underwriters Laboratories, Inc. had a duty to consumer purchasers of products with UL label), *vacated on joint motion*, 807 F. Supp. 439 (N.D. Ohio 1992); *King v. National Spa & Pool Inst., Inc.*, 570 So. 2d 612, 616 (Ala. 1990) (trade association that promulgated standards concerning swimming pools was under a legal duty to exercise due care in promulgating the standards); *Winget v. Colfax Creosoting Co.*, 626 So. 2d 370, 371-72 (La. Ct. App. 1993) (company that certified that utility pole complied with federal regulations could potentially be held liable for lineman killed when pole broke), *writ denied*, 633 So. 2d 580 (La. 1994); *Peterson v. Multnomah County Sch. Dist. No. 1*, 668 P.2d 385, 393 (Or. Ct. App. 1983) (upholding jury finding that organization that undertook obligation to make safety regulations to high schools had a duty to students to avoid negligence in making the recommendations).

24. *See Snyder v. American Ass'n of Blood Banks*, 676 A.2d 1036 (N.J. 1996); *Weigand v. University Hosp. of New York Univ. Med. Ctr.*, 659 N.Y.S.2d 395, 400 (N.Y. Sup. Ct. 1997).

25. *Snyder v. American Ass'n of Blood Banks*, 659 A.2d 482, 492 (N.J. Super. Ct. App. Div. 1995) (citations omitted), *aff'd*, 676 A.2d 1036 (N.J. 1996).

26. *Armstrong v. Accrediting Council for Continuing Educ. & Training, Inc.*, 961 F. Supp. 305, 310 (D.D.C. 1997).

27. *Armstrong*, 961 F. Supp. at 311.

28. *Armstrong*, 961 F. Supp. at 311.

29. Thus, in *Collins v. American Optometric Ass'n*, 693 F.2d 636 (7th Cir. 1982), the plaintiff sued an optometrists' professional association, alleging that he was

misled by the association's materials which stated that optometrists were qualified to diagnose glaucoma. The court denied the claim, finding that the plaintiff failed to identify documents issued by the association which influenced his decision to seek treatment. *Id*. at 641.

30. *See* George D. Webster et al., *The Law of Associations* § 12.04[5] (1997).

31. *See* Webster et al., The Law of Associations, § 12.04[5].

32. *See* Webster et al., The Law of Associations, § 12.04[5].

APPENDIX A

Standards of Practice

Exhibit A–1

ANA STANDARDS OF NURSING STAFF DEVELOPMENT

STANDARD 1. ADMINISTRATION

Administration of the provider unit is consistent with the organization's mission, philosophy, purpose, and goals. The organizational structure facilitates the provision of learning activities for nurses.

Criteria

1. The organization's mission, philosophy, and purpose contain statements that support the professional development of nurses.
2. There is an identifiable provider unit responsible for nursing staff development and/or continuing education functions.
3. The provider unit has a written philosophy, purpose, and goals that are congruent with ANA standards.
4. The goals and objectives of the provider unit are written, reviewed annually, and revised as needed.

5. Documentation verifies that educational activities are consistent with the provider unit's stated philosophy, purpose, and goals.
6. An organizational chart demonstrates lines of authority and communication within the organization, including the provider unit.
7. The provider unit administrator and educators are integrally involved in organizational activities through participation on committees, task forces, and projects.
8. Written policies and procedures guide the operation of the provider unit.
9. The provider unit is guided by cost/benefit principles in order to achieve optimal effectiveness and efficiency.
10. The provider unit administrator prepares and manages a financial plan that supports the goals of the provider unit.
11. Overall evaluation of the provider unit includes participant feedback and measurement of outcomes as they relate to the philosophy, purpose, and attainment of goals of the provider unit.
12. The provider unit monitors its performance through the unit's and organization's quality management program.

Source: Reprinted with permission from *Standards for Nursing Professional Development: Continuing Education and Staff Development,* pp. 7–12, © 1994, American Nurses Association.

187

STANDARD 2. HUMAN RESOURCES

Qualified administrative, educational, and support personnel are responsible for achieving the goals of the provider unit.

Criteria

1. The number of educational staff and support personnel is sufficient to meet the goals of the provider unit.
2. The administrator of the provider unit has a baccalaureate or higher degree in nursing, and a graduate degree in nursing or a related field. The administrator demonstrates managerial and educational knowledge and skills.
3. Each member of the educational staff has a baccalaureate or higher degree in nursing and has demonstrated relevant educational, content, and clinical expertise in addition to interest and ability in providing education to adult learners. A graduate degree in nursing or a related field is preferred.
4. Position descriptions delineate the qualifications, responsibilities, authority, and accountability of the educational and support staff and the person administratively responsible for the provider unit.
5. The process and criteria for the selection and evaluation of all staff are clearly delineated.
6. The educational and management expertise of the provider unit administrator is developed, maintained, and enhanced through orientation, self-evaluation, and ongoing professional development.
7. The educational and clinical expertise of the educational staff is developed, maintained, and enhanced through orientation, self-evaluation, and ongoing professional development.

STANDARD 3. MATERIAL RESOURCES AND FACILITIES

Material resources and facilities are adequate to achieve the goals and implement the functions of the provider unit.

Criteria

1. A financial plan sufficient for meeting provider unit goals and objectives is identifiable.
2. Facilities, materials, equipment, and educational technologies appropriate to the educational activities offered by the provider unit are provided.
3. Support services necessary for nursing educational activities are readily available to the provider unit— e.g., library information services, printing, and audiovisual development.
4. Physical facilities are selected to accommodate various teaching methods, provide environmental comfort, and allow accessibility for the target audience.
5. The appropriateness and effectiveness of material resources and facilities are evaluated by learners as part of their evaluation of each educational activity.
6. The adequacy of space, materials, equipment, and budget necessary for implementation of the goals of the provider unit is evaluated and documented annually.

STANDARD 4. EDUCATIONAL DESIGN

Principles of education and adult learning are used to design educational activities.

Criteria

1. The learner participates in assessing, planning, implementing, and evaluating educational activities.
2. Educational activities reflect the identified needs of the target audience and/or organizational priorities and relate to nursing knowledge or nursing practice.
3. Educational activities are designed to support critical thinking and new ideas, professional growth, open communication, and collaborative relationships.
4. The design for each educational activity includes documentation of a needs assessment, description of the target audi-

ence, educational objectives, content outline, teaching methods, evaluation strategies, and designation of appropriate physical facilities and resources.

5. The purpose, objectives, content, teaching methods, materials, and evaluation of educational activities are developed by educators, with input from the presenters and representatives of the intended audience.

6. The presenters are qualified by education and experience in the content area to be taught.

7. Content, teaching methods, and evaluation strategies are consistent with the objectives of the educational activity.

8. Publicity regarding educational activities reaches the intended audience in a timely manner.

9. Educators assume a facilitative role in all aspects of the educational process.

10. Educational activities are evaluated and changes made based on analysis of the results.

11. The evaluation design includes a mechanism for feedback to the learner when appropriate.

12. Presenters receive evaluative feedback for their component of an educational activity.

STANDARD 5. RECORDS AND REPORTS

The provider unit establishes and maintains a recordkeeping and report system.

Criteria

1. All aspects of educational activities are documented and records are maintained in compliance with departmental, organizational, and external agency requirements.

2. Mechanisms are in place for systematic, easy retrieval of data on educational activities and participants.

3. Records are confidential and are available only to authorized individuals.

4. Periodic reports are made to appropriate organizational and/or agency representatives to document and evaluate progress toward attainment of provider unit and organization goals.

STANDARD 6. PROFESSIONAL PRACTICE

The professional development educator role is practiced in a manner that enhances learners' competence to provide quality health care and enhance their contributions to the profession.

Criteria

1. Educators promote lifelong learning as an essential and integral component of professional practice.

2. Educators model behaviors that reflect continued personal and professional growth.

3. Educators facilitate the process for learners to assume responsibility for maintaining competence in practice.

4. Educators apply management principles in the design and delivery of learning activities.

5. Educators promote an understanding of the cultural differences that affect health care consumers and learners.

6. Educators facilitate the initiation and adoption of changes in health care.

7. Educators foster the use of systematic analysis of issues in health care.

8. Through consultation, educators assist individuals, departments, organizations, and other entities in designing and facilitating professional development educational activities.

9. Educators monitor issues and trends in nursing and health care, and develop strategies to facilitate appropriate outcomes.

10. Educators integrate research and current literature into educational activities.

11. Educators provide learning opportunities which enable nurses to utilize research findings in practice.
12. Educators engage in systematic inquiry ranging from problem solving to research on topics such as health care outcomes, issues, concepts and theories, and the learning process.
13. Ethical principles are integrated into the practice of continuing education and staff development.

Exhibit A–2

ANA STANDARDS OF HOME HEALTH NURSING PRACTICE

STANDARD I. ORGANIZATION OF HOME HEALTH SERVICES

All home health services are planned, organized, and directed by a master's-prepared professional nurse with experience in community health and administration.

Rationale

The nurse executive with community health experience builds from the resources of the community, using administrative knowledge to plan and direct services to meet the complex needs of individuals and families within their homes and communities.

Structure Criteria

1. A written organizational plan exists that is current and that delineates lines of authority, accountability, and communication.
2. A written statement of the mission, philosophy, and goals of the organization exists; it reflects the organization's purpose, gives direction to its programs, and sets the parameters of practice.
3. The organization has written policies and procedures that provide all personnel with acceptable methods of meeting their designated responsibilities.
4. An information system facilitates assessment and documentation of client care.
5. An established quality assurance program measures both clinical and administrative aspects of the organization.
6. The organization has a strategic plan that includes an analysis of the marketplace,

existing and projected programs, and financial resources.
7. The chief executive officer should be a nurse with preparation in community health nursing at the master's or doctoral level.
8. In all instances, client services are directed by a master's-prepared registered nurse who is a member of the senior management staff.

Process Criteria

These criteria are divided into criteria for the nurse executive and the director of client services. In the absence of a nurse executive, the director of client services, as a member of the senior management staff, actively participates in activities that are otherwise the prerogative of the nurse executive.

The nurse executive—

1. Establishes the organization's philosophy and goals.
2. Establishes personnel policies.
3. Establishes an information system for assessing and documenting client care.
4. Establishes a budget and a budget-monitoring system.
5. Assures the development of a marketing plan.
6. Develops the long-term strategic plan for the organization.
7. Remains politically active and aware of local, state, and national legislative and regulatory trends.
8. Assumes responsibility for the evaluation and analysis of the organization through a quality assurance program.
9. Maintains compliance with pertinent local, state, and federal laws and regulations.

Source: Reprinted with permission from *Standards of Home Health Nursing Practice*, pp. 5–19, © 1986, American Nurses Association.

10. Actively participates in community organizations.
11. Actively participates in professional organizations.
12. Creates an environment that facilitates the provision of care of high quality and promotes individual professional growth.
13. Initiates a relationship with academic institutions to promote clinical experiences, joint appointments, and research.
14. Promotes the professional image of nursing.
15. Assures the employment of qualified personnel.
16. Provides leadership to the governing body and/or advisory board and implements decisions made.
17. Collaborates with community leaders in assessing, planning, implementing, and evaluating programs for home health services.

The director of client services—

1. Establishes performance standards and measurable criteria.
2. Formulates service policies.
3. Establishes and implements a quality assurance system.
4. Implements the organization's personnel policies.
5. Encourages, supports, and participates in research.
6. Participates in the development and improvement of organization policies.
7. Collaborates with the community in identifying home health needs and developing services.
8. Assumes responsibility for coordinating client services, including case management and appropriate staffing.
9. Manages those who supervise and/or deliver client care.
10. Encourages interdisciplinary collaboration.
11. Participates in management decisions, including budget development and implementation.

12. Implements orientation and staff development programs.

Outcome Criteria

1. The organization is in compliance with all licensing and regulatory requirements.
2. The established quality assurance program is used to revise and improve services.

STANDARD II. THEORY

The nurse applies theoretical concepts as a basis for decisions in practice.

Rationale

The theoretical concepts for home health nursing are derived from nursing and other related disciplines; the resulting insights are integrated into a foundation for practice. The actions of the nurse are based on theoretical concepts.

Structure Criteria

1. Reference materials discussing the conceptual bases for practice are accessible in the practice setting.
2. Relevant continuing education programs are accessible.

Process Criteria

The nurse generalist—

1. Examines personal and professional assumptions about home health practice as a specialized area of community health nursing.
2. Considers alternative theoretical concepts.
3. Uses theoretical concepts and critical thinking in practice to identify patterns and incongruencies, and to generate and test hypotheses.
4. Shares theoretical information with colleagues, individuals, families, and the community.

In addition to the above, the nurse specialist—

1. Formulates new theoretical concepts to be used as a basis for decisions in practice.
2. Serves as a consultant to the nurse generalist regarding theoretical concepts.

Outcome Criteria

1. Nursing actions are consistent with recognized nursing theories and established knowledge.
2. Recognized nursing theories and knowledge are evaluated and tested within the practice setting.

STANDARD III. DATA COLLECTION

The nurse continuously collects and records data that are comprehensive, accurate, and systematic.

Rationale

Data collection is an essential prerequisite to the assessment of the individual, family, and community. The process allows the nurse to reach sound conclusions and plan interventions based in both scientific and social theories. Data collection reflects reality and is the basis upon which the nurse repeatedly evaluates care.

Structure Criteria

1. The organization has a nursing information system that permits the following:
   a. Systematic and thorough data collection
   b. Simple, accessible, and complete retrieval
   c. Confidentiality
   d. Setting of priorities for services to individuals and families
   e. Collection of aggregate demographic data

2. A record-keeping system provides for concise, comprehensive, accurate, and continuous recording.
3. The practice setting permits the nurse access to records of assigned clients in a timely manner.

Process Criteria

The nurse generalist—

1. Collects and records data in a standardized, systematic, and concise form.
2. In conjunction with the family and individual, collects data in the following areas:
   a. Health history
   b. Physical assessment
   c. Growth and development
   d. Mental and emotional status
   e. Family dynamics
   f. Economic, environmental, and community factors affecting health
   g. Cultural and religious factors affecting health
   h. Knowledge, satisfaction, and motivation affecting health
   i. Strengths that promote and maintain health
   j. Risk factors affecting health
   k. Receptivity to health care
   l. Client and family expectations
3. Conducts or participates in an ongoing interdisciplinary process of revising and reviewing the data base on the individual and family.
4. Communicates appropriate data to other persons involved in the individual's or family's care.
5. Participates in the design of the nursing information system.

In addition, the nurse specialist—

1. Performs assessment and records data for a select group of individuals and families who require the advanced assessment skills the specialist is able to provide.

2. Designs and manages the nursing information system.
3. Serves as a consultant to and educator of the nurse generalist in implementation of the nursing information system.

Outcome Criteria

1. Nursing information is synthesized and recorded in a standardized and retrievable format.
2. The data base is kept current and accurately reflects the individual's or family's present clinical status.
3. The data base is complete.

STANDARD IV. DIAGNOSIS

The nurse uses health assessment data to determine nursing diagnoses.

Rationale

Nursing diagnosis is an integral part of the assessment process. Nursing diagnosis is the nurse's identification (by independent judgment) of the individual's or family's actual or potential health problems or needs. Nursing's logical basis for intervention rests on the identification of those diagnoses that flow from nursing theories and scientific knowledge.

Structure Criteria

The practice setting provides opportunities for—

1. Use of nursing diagnosis by the professional nurse.
2. Exchange of information and research findings among peers regarding the scientific premises underlying nursing diagnoses.
3. Validation of diagnoses by colleagues, individuals, and families.

Process Criteria

The nurse generalist—

1. Formulates and revises nursing diagnoses through comprehensive and continuing assessment.
2. Collaborates with other health personnel to assure that diagnoses are congruent with the individual's or family's clinical status.
3. Communicates the nursing diagnoses obtained during health assessment to appropriate members of the health care team.
4. Documents the nursing diagnosis in a standardized, systematic, and concise form.

In addition, the nurse specialist—

1. Participates in or conducts research involving the formulation, validation, or revision of nursing diagnoses.
2. Serves as a consultant to the nurse generalist in the formulation of nursing diagnoses.

Outcome Criteria

1. Nursing diagnoses are recorded in a manner that facilitates planning, evaluation, and research.
2. Evidence exists that nursing diagnoses are used by other health care team members in planning care.
3. Nursing diagnoses are validated with colleagues, individuals, and families, as appropriate.

STANDARD V. PLANNING

The nurse develops care plans that establish goals. The care plan is based on nursing diagnoses and incorporates therapeutic, preventive, and rehabilitative nursing actions.

Rationale

Planning guides nursing interventions and facilitates desired outcomes. Care plans, specifying goals and interventions, are based on nursing diagnoses and the medical treatment plan. The client and family participate in the planning process.

Structure Criteria

The practice setting provides—

1. The necessary resources to initiate planning for clients prior to discharge from hospitals, nursing homes, and other health facilities.
2. The necessary resources for the development of plans derived from the nursing diagnoses and medical treatment plan.
3. Mechanisms for plans to be recorded, retrieved, updated, and communicated in a timely manner.
4. Criteria for the acceptance of the client for home health services, to be used as guidelines in determining whether the services the client needs may be safely and appropriately delivered in the home.

Process Criteria

The nurse generalist—

1. Initiates development of the client care plan in partnership with the client, family, physician, and other health care professionals as indicated. This care plan—
   a. Reflects relevant theoretical concepts and research findings.
   b. Includes measurable goals and/or behavioral objectives, including an expected date of accomplishment.
   c. Identifies a sequence of actions for achieving the goals, including assignment of support staff.
   d. Proposes contingency actions.
   e. Proposes alternatives for continuity of care for long-term needs.
   f. Lists resources necessary to accomplish the plan.
   g. Estimates costs and benefits.
2. Revises the plan as goals and objectives are achieved or changed.
3. Records the plan in a standardized, systematic, and concise form.

In addition, the nurse specialist provides consultation to the nurse generalist in planning care for clients.

Outcome Criteria

1. The client, family, physician, and other health care providers participate in the planning process as appropriate.
2. The plan is initiated prior to the client's admission to home health services.
3. The plan exists in a concise, standardized, and retrievable form.
4. The plan evidences revision and deletion of actions as goals and objectives are achieved or changed.

STANDARD VI. INTERVENTION

The nurse, guided by the care plan, intervenes to provide comfort, to restore, improve, and promote health, to prevent complications and sequelae of illness, and to effect rehabilitation.

Rationale

The nurse implements the care plan to achieve the desired goals and objectives. The nurse provides direct care, incorporates preventive measures in the client's care, teaches the family and nonprofessional caregivers methods to promote the client's recovery, and provides comfort and support during a terminal illness.

Structure Criteria

1. The nurse is the case manager.
2. A mechanism exists to provide the initial and periodic assessment of client needs by a registered nurse to assure safe, adequate, and appropriate care.
3. Independent nursing functions are employed to enhance the medical treatment plan and enrich the services provided to the client.

4. A mechanism exists for reviewing staffing patterns and revising them in accord with client care needs.
5. Intervention skills are maintained and increased through professional development.

Process Criteria

The nurse generalist—

1. Implements interventions that are based on applicable scientific theories.
2. Intervenes with the concurrence and/or participation of the client and family.
3. Administers medically prescribed medications and treatments.
4. Treats physical and psychological responses to changes in health status, level of independence, and treatments.
5. Teaches prevention or control of disease progression or disability.
6. Coordinates client services provided by other health professionals while serving as an advocate for the client and family.
7. Supervises and evaluates ancillary personnel who provide care to clients and families.
8. Informs the client and family about the client's health status, health care resources, and treatments.
9. Teaches the client and family self-care concepts and skills.
10. Reviews interventions and revises them in accord with responses of the client and family.
11. Ensures continuity of care.
12. Documents interventions and responses of the client and family.

In addition, the nurse specialist functions as a consultant to the nurse generalist in nursing interventions.

Outcome Criteria

1. The client and family demonstrate self-care to the extent of their ability.

2. There is measurable evidence of progress toward goal achievement.
3. The client and family use community resources appropriately.
4. Problems, interventions, and responses of the client and family are recorded in a systematic, retrievable, and timely manner.
5. There is documented evidence that interdisciplinary services are in accord with client needs and capability.

STANDARD VII. EVALUATION

The nurse continually evaluates the client's and family's responses to interventions in order to determine progress toward goal attainment and to revise the data base, nursing diagnoses, and plan of care.

Rationale

Nursing practice is a dynamic process that responds to alterations in data, diagnoses, or plans previously made. Evaluation of the quality of care is an essential part of all health services. The effectiveness of nursing care depends on the continuing reassessment of the client's and family's health needs and appropriate revision of the plan.

Structure Criteria

1. There is an ongoing, organized quality assurance program to evaluate care; the nurse is an active participant in this program.
2. Supervision and consultation is available within the practice setting to allow the nurse to evaluate the results of nursing interventions and to develop alternate plans when appropriate.
3. The nurse has access to current information regarding changes in the client situation that might warrant revision of the plan of care.

4. Resources are sufficient to allow the nurse to coordinate care and evaluate the care delivered.
5. There is a mechanism by which the client or family is able to participate in the evaluation process and revision of the plan of care.

Process Criteria

The nurse generalist—

1. Clearly documents the evaluation results and revisions of the plan of care, as well as the results of care.
2. Uses baseline and current data to measure progress toward goal achievement.
3. Plans for continuing evaluation of nursing care to assure that evaluation is timely and complete.
4. In conjunction with the client and family, revises priorities, goals, and interventions as indicated in the evaluation process.
5. Evaluates client progress on a continuing basis, using structure, process, and outcome criteria.

In addition, the nurse specialist—

1. Pursues validations, suggestions, and new information related to the provision of nursing care.
2. Conducts a program-and-service evaluation, using structure, process, and outcome criteria of health care. This evaluation may include the following:
   a. A cost-benefit analysis
   b. A study of recording systems
   c. A review of the quality of interventions
   d. An examination of immediate and long-term client care outcomes intended and unintended, expected and actual
3. Conducts evaluation research with appropriate consultation.
4. Serves as a consultant to the nurse generalist in evaluating results of the plan of care.

5. Initiates and develops quality assurance programs.

Outcome Criteria

1. There is evidence that the data base, diagnosis, and plan of care are revised in accord with continuing evaluations.
2. There is evidence that the client and family participate in the evaluation and revision of the plan of care.
3. There is evidence that program evaluation is used to make program decisions.
4. Evaluation of interventions is documented in a manner that contributes to the effectiveness of nursing actions and to research.

STANDARD VIII. CONTINUITY OF CARE

The nurse is responsible for the client's appropriate and uninterrupted care along the health care continuum, and therefore uses discharge planning, case management, and coordination of community resources.

Rationale

Without specific nursing interventions, gaps and fragmentation occur in the delivery of health care services, causing the client's condition to be compromised.

Structure Criteria

1. The home health organization makes available to institutions experienced community health nurses to provide consultation to facilitate discharge planning.
2. A formal referral system is in place. The referral system includes a timely, reciprocal exchange of pertinent information between referral services.
3. The home health organization has available current listings and descriptions of community resources.

4. A formal orientation to case management is provided to nursing staff.
5. The home health organization encourages and supports case management as a tool for effective client care.
6. The home health organization assists staff in developing and using community resources.

Process Criteria

Discharge Planning

The nurse generalist—

1. Identifies and plans for services to meet health care needs during transition from one system to another.
2. Initiates the discharge process for the institution at the time of referral to the home health care agency.
3. Initiates appropriate referral and seeks feedback.

In addition, the nurse specialist provides consultation to the nurse generalist regarding discharge planning.

Case Management

The nurse generalist—

1. Assesses the total health care needs of the client and family, including physiological, psychological, intellectual, social, emotional, spiritual, environmental, and educational needs.
2. Assesses and coordinates all appropriate resources of the client, family, and community to meet the needs of the client and family.
3. Coordinates the delivery of all services to the client according to prioritized needs, with the safety of the client as the primary consideration.

In addition, the nurse specialist—

1. Provides consultation to the nurse generalist regarding case management.

2. May provide direct care to high-risk clients with complex needs.

Coordination of Community Resources

The nurse generalist—

1. Uses or helps the client use formal and informal services available in the community, such as meals on wheels, Medicaid, day care, neighbors, and religious and social organizations.
2. Networks with professional resources in the community to expand and improve client care services.

In addition, the nurse specialist—

1. Provides consultation to the nurse generalist in identifying resources within the community.
2. Develops professional networks and resources within the community.

Outcome Criteria

1. There is evidence that coordinated and appropriate home health services are provided.
2. There is evidence of appropriate interdisciplinary coordination, including case conferences and ongoing communication.
3. There is documented exchange of information between referral sources.
4. The client has a written plan for discharge from the home health agency.
5. There is documented evidence in the client record of appropriate and coordinated use of community resources.

STANDARD IX. INTERDISCIPLINARY COLLABORATION

The nurse initiates and maintains a liaison relationship with all appropriate health care providers to assure that all efforts effectively complement one another.

Rationale

The complexity of home health care delivery systems requires a multidisciplinary approach to delivery of services, necessitating the strong support and active participation of all the health professions. Nurses must actively promote the collaborative planning and interventions required to ensure high-quality home health services.

Structure Criteria

1. Opportunities for interdisciplinary collaboration are encouraged and provided within the practice setting.
2. Opportunities for participation with other colleagues in policy making and overall planning for the agency and the community are provided within the practice setting.

Process Criteria

The nurse generalist—

1. Participates in the formulation of goals, plans, and decisions.
2. Recognizes and respects colleagues and their contributions.
3. Consults and plans with colleagues.
4. Articulates nursing knowledge and skills so colleagues may appropriately integrate them in the care of the client.
5. Assures the integration and coordination of the contributions of colleagues into an overall plan of care.
6. Collaborates with other disciplines in education, supervision, and research.

In addition, the nurse specialist provides consultation to the nurse generalist regarding appropriate and effective interdisciplinary collaboration.

Outcome Criteria

1. There is evidence that the nurse is an integral member of the interdisciplinary team.

2. There is documented evidence that interdisciplinary collaboration exists.

STANDARD X. PROFESSIONAL DEVELOPMENT

The nurse assumes responsibility for professional development and contributes to the professional growth of others.

Rationale

Scientific, cultural, social, and political changes in society require a commitment from the nurse to the continuing pursuit of knowledge to enhance professional growth and to facilitate client care.

Structure Criteria

1. Policies exist that provide for a continuing education needs assessment.
2. A mechanism is in place to provide continuing education opportunities.
3. There are opportunities for participation in professional organizational activities.
4. Current professional texts and periodicals are available in the practice setting.

Process Criteria

The nurse generalist—

1. Participates in continuing education programs, such as in-service sessions, conventions, institutes, and workshops, to increase knowledge and skills.
2. Assists others in identifying areas of educational needs and communicates new knowledge to others.
3. Initiates and participates in peer review and other means of evaluation to assure the quality of nursing practice.
4. Incorporates changes in the nurse's practice suggested by peer review and continuing education.

5. Demonstrates professional responsibility by active participation in appropriate professional organizations.

In addition, the nurse specialist—

1. Plans, develops, and conducts quality assurance activities, including continuing education programs.
2. Serves as a role model for the nurse generalist.

Outcome Criteria

Evidence exists that the nurse—

1. Participates in the peer review process and continuing education programs.
2. Incorporates new information and methods into practice.
3. Meets continuing education requirements for relicensure and recertification as appropriate.

STANDARD XI. RESEARCH

The nurse participates in research activities that contribute to the profession's continuing development of knowledge of home health care.

Rationale

Improvement of the practice of home health nursing depends upon a commitment of the nurse to participate in research activities, to disseminate research findings, and to use research findings in practice.

Structure Criteria

1. Reference material regarding research in home health nursing and related disciplines is accessible in the practice setting.
2. The incorporation of validated research findings in the provision of care to clients, families, and communities is recognized within the practice setting.

3. Agency policy is supportive of research in home health nursing.
   a. The agency serves as a site for research related to home health nursing by its personnel and/or external researchers.
   b. The agency recognizes and supports research initiatives of staff nurses.
   c. A formal mechanism exists within the agency for review of proposed research studies, including a review of their ethical implications.

Process Criteria

The nurse generalist—

1. Critically reads reported research and applies valid findings to practice.
2. Identifies researchable problems related to practice.
3. Participates in agency-based research projects under the supervision of qualified nurse researchers.

In addition, the nurse specialist, with appropriate consultation and/or collaboration of doctorally prepared nurse researchers—

1. Defines researchable problems relevant to home health nursing theory and practice.
2. Participates in the design of research studies appropriate to the agency setting.
3. Prepares proposals for support of research projects from internal and external sources.
4. Participates in all phases of project implementation, including data collection, analysis, and interpretation.
5. Ensures that research findings are accurately reported and disseminated.
6. Serves as a resource to the nurse generalist in the identification and evaluation of research findings for application to home health nursing practice.

Outcome Criteria

1. Research activities occur within the practice setting.
2. Evidence exists that the practice of home health nursing reflects the incorporation of currently validated findings from research.
3. Evidence exists that the knowledge base of home health nursing is continuously augmented and updated by the findings of relevant research studies.

STANDARD XII. ETHICS

The nurse uses the code for nurses established by the American Nurses Association as a guide for ethical decision making in practice.

Rationale

The nurse is responsible for providing health care to individuals in a setting where the client must trust the nurse to make significant judgments about health care. The nurse must assure that the home is the appropriate setting for the care provided and that the nurse and other providers are prepared by education and experience to provide the care needed by the client. The Code for Nurses provides the parameters within which the nurse makes ethical judgments.

Structure Criteria

1. The home health organization's administration provides a formal mechanism for resolving ethical dilemmas.
2. Continuing education programs are provided that identify and support discussions of moral, ethical, and legal issues.

Process Criteria

The nurse generalist—

1. Participates with other colleagues in identifying and discussing ethical conflicts.
2. Advocates for the client, particularly in the areas of confidentiality and informed consent.

In addition, the nurse specialist provides consultation to the nurse generalist regarding ethical issues.

Outcome Criterion

Evidence exists that nurses adhere to the Code for Nurses established by the American Nurses Association.

Exhibit A–3

STANDARDS FOR SOCIAL WORK IN HOME HEALTH CARE

HISTORICAL OVERVIEW

Medical Social Services have been an integral part of the provision of health services since 1905. The U.S. Public Health Service, in 1955, endorsed the physician-oriented organized home care program, designed to provide medical and social services to patients at home through a professional group minimally composed of a physician, nurse and social worker. The Social Security Amendments of 1965 under Title XVIII (Medicare) allowed federal reimbursement of health care and social services. Medicare legislation has not only provided for reimbursement for social work services on a level equal to nursing and other skilled care, but has recognized that home health care must include services which strive to improve the patient's total functioning.

DEFINITION OF HOME HEALTH CARE

Home health care provides a broad range of comprehensive services to help people of all ages who are in need of short-term acute rehabilitative care or long-term maintenance in order to remain in their own homes. Home care serves people who are generally frail and/or disabled, who do not have an adequate family or informal support system, or whose social, mental health, financial or environmental needs are not met. Thus, home care cannot be viewed as only medical service. Home health care includes an array of services—nursing, rehabilitative therapies, social work, personal care, homemaking—to aid the individual in achieving and sustaining the highest level of health, activity, and independence. Such services are typically provided through community-based or hospital affiliated

specialized home health programs both on a for-profit and not-for-profit basis.

ROLE OF THE SOCIAL WORKER IN HOME HEALTH CARE

With changes in the structuring, financing and, to some extent, philosophy of health care delivery, patients are being discharged from hospitals to home care earlier, often more debilitated and at greater risk than in the past. Advances in technology allow certain medical procedures which had been limited to in-hospital care to be completed in the home. An additional stress has been placed on family caregivers who must learn the technical aspects of caring for their relative while trying to cope with increased dependency needs and the role shifts that may result from illness. As the patient moves from health to illness and struggles to return to health, the family is often required to provide 24-hour care which may turn part of the household into a patient care facility. Stress is generated and disturbs the equilibrium of family life. Roles change, relationships become strained, space shrinks, money dwindles, and efforts are focused on technical medical procedures and caregiving issues.

An interdisciplinary approach is needed to treat the patient-family system in the context of their social milieu. The social worker assists patients and their families to adapt and plan in the home environment. Relief of stress, crisis intervention, assistance with financial problems, advocacy with community agencies, information and referral, assistance with planning, emotional support, appropriate counseling, and interpretation of and education about family and patient's needs to other health care staff and service providers, are the components of the social work role in helping patients adjust to their situations and in helping families sustain the patient at home rather than resort to premature or unnecessary institutionalization.

Social and emotional rehabilitation and advocacy must be recognized as critical components in achieving and sustaining optimum states of health independence in individuals of all ages. The goal of social work's participation in home health care is the improvement and maintenance of the social, emotional, environmental, functional, physical and mental health status of patient and family.

In addition to the National Association of Social Workers core standards for social work in health care settings, the following standards for social work in home health are presented.

STANDARD 1

Social workers in home health settings shall have knowledge of chronic, acute and terminal illnesses, physical disabilities and the resultant age-specific impact on individual and family systems.

Interpretation

Social workers in home health agencies must have knowledge of acute, chronic and terminal illnesses as well as permanent and temporary disabling conditions. They must be familiar with the usual course of the illness or condition, therapeutic interventions, and adaptations which will be necessary by clients and their families. Social workers must also be familiar with the general concerns of special populations. They must be aware that these illnesses are often long-term and permanent, resulting in functional losses, social isolation and economic pressures which can impact on the individual's and family's ability to cope.

STANDARD 2

Social workers in home health settings should support and advocate for appropriate home health care for people with chronic, acute and/or terminal illnesses.

Interpretation

Medical advances have provided technologies which can be used to maintain at home people with multiple medical problems. At the same time, an increase in federally funded community support programs provides home-based services for people with disabilities, chronic and/or acute illnesses. Home health care social workers must be advocates for the maintenance of these individuals, families, agencies and the community resources and programs to support them. Advocacy must also be pursued on a state and federal level in support of legislation promoting home care.

STANDARD 3

When provided independently, social work services in home health settings shall be provided by a social worker with a graduate degree from a school of social work accredited by the council on social work education; and two years of post-masters experience, one of which is in a health/clinical setting; and licensure and/or certification at the applicable level. When provided within the context of an organization where there is a social work department and/or social work supervision, services may be provided by a social worker with a graduate degree or baccalaureate degree from a Council on Social Work education accredited program.

Interpretation

Independent provision of services applies to 1) solo or autonomous practice, consultation or contracted services; 2) practice within an organization where there is only one social worker responsible for providing social work services; and 3) to directors of social work departments or those responsible for supervision and training of other social work staff.

STANDARD 4

The home health social worker shall integrate social work intervention with that of other members of the interdisciplinary team.

Interpretation

The complex problems experienced at home by special populations should be assessed and addressed from a variety of perspectives. A collaborative team approach has the potential for being more comprehensive, more efficient and more responsive to clients' needs. The home health social worker must integrate the psychosocial plan and interventions with the other services being offered and educate the entire team to the psychosocial needs of the client and client's family.

STANDARD 5

The home health social worker shall work to achieve an appropriate continuum of care, assuring the clients of ongoing services to meet their needs.

Interpretation

The home health social worker must consider all social work services as part of a continuum of care including the family, referring agencies and institutions and other community social workers. When possible, he/she must work closely with initial referral sources to insure the patient an appropriate discharge plan and safe transition into the home. Likewise, prior to the discharge of the patient from home care, when indicated, the social worker must establish the necessary linkages to community resources or other facilities to assure that needs are met.

STANDARD 6

The functions of the social worker in home health settings shall include specific services to the client population, the staff of the agency, and the community.

Source: Copyright © 1989, National Association of Social Workers, Inc.

Interpretation

The social work functions include the services listed in core Standard 4 of the NASW Standards for Social Workers in Health Care Settings.

---

*Standard 1. Clinical social workers shall function in accordance with the ethics and the stated standards of the profession, including its accountability procedures.

Standard 2. Clinical social workers shall have and continue to develop specialized knowledge and understanding of individuals, families, and groups and of therapeutic and preventive interventions.

Standard 3. Clinical social workers shall respond in a professional manner to all persons who seek their assistance.

Standard 4. Clinical social workers shall be knowledgeable about the services available in the community and make appropriate referrals for their clients.

Standard 5. Clinical social workers shall maintain their accessibility to clients.

Standard 6. Clinical social workers shall safeguard the confidential nature of the treatment relationship and of the information obtained within that relationship.

Standard 7. Clinical social workers shall maintain access to professional case consultation.

Standard 8. Clinical social workers shall establish and maintain professional offices and procedures.

Standard 9. Clinical social workers shall represent themselves to the public with accuracy.

Standard 10. Social workers shall engage in the independent private practice of clinical social work only when qualified to do so.

Standard 11. Clinical social workers shall have the right to establish an independent private practice.

Exhibit A–4

STANDARDS OF PRACTICE FOR PHYSICAL THERAPY AND THE ACCOMPANYING CRITERIA

PREAMBLE

The physical therapy profession is committed to providing an optimum level of service delivery and to striving for excellence in practice. The House of Delegates of the American Physical Therapy Association, as the formal body that represents the profession, attests to this commitment by adopting and promoting the following *Standards of Practice for Physical Therapy.* These *Standards of Practice for Physical Therapy* are the profession's statement of conditions and performances that are essential for provision of high-quality physical therapy. The *Standards* provide a foundation for assessment of physical therapy practice.

I. LEGAL/ETHICAL CONSIDERATIONS

A. Legal Considerations

The physical therapist complies with all the legal requirements of jurisdictions regulating the practice of physical therapy.

The physical therapist assistant complies with all the legal requirements of jurisdictions regulating the work of the assistant.

Note: The *Standards of Practice for Physical Therapy* are promulgated by APTA's House of Delegates; the *Criteria* for the *Standards* are promulgated by APTA's Board of Directors. The *Criteria* are listed with bullets beneath the *Standards* to which they apply.

Source: Reprinted from *Standards of Practice for Physical Therapy and the Accompanying Criteria,* with permission of the American Physical Therapy Association.

B. Ethical Considerations

The physical therapist practices according to the *Code of Ethics* of the American Physical Therapy Association.

The physical therapist assistant complies with the *Standards of Ethical Conduct for the Physical Therapist Assistant* of the American Physical Therapy Association.

II. ADMINISTRATION OF THE PHYSICAL THERAPY SERVICE

A. Statement of Mission, Purpose, and Goals

The physical therapy service has a statement of mission, purposes, and goals that reflects the needs and interests of the individuals served, the physical therapy personnel affiliated with the service, and the community.

The statement:

- Defines the scope and limitations of the service.
- Lists the goals and objectives of the service.
- Is reviewed annually.

B. Organizational Plan

The physical therapy service has a written organizational plan.

The plan:

- Describes relationships within the service and, where the physical therapy service is part of a larger organization, between the physical therapy service and other components of the organization.
- Ensures that the service is directed by a physical therapist.

- Defines supervisory structures within the service.
- Reflects current personnel functions.

C. Policies and Procedures

The physical therapy service has written policies and procedures that reflect the operation of the service and that are consistent with the mission, purposes, and goals of the service.

The policies and procedures, which are reviewed regularly and revised as necessary, address pertinent information including (but not limited to) the following:

- Clinical education.
- Clinical research.
- Interdisciplinary collaboration.
- Criteria for access to, initiation of, continuation of, referral of, and termination of care.
- Equipment maintenance.
- Environmental safety.
- Fiscal management.
- Infection control.
- Job/position descriptions.
- Competency assessment.
- Medical emergencies.
- Patient/client care policies and protocols.
- Patient/client rights.
- Personnel-related policies.
- Quality/performance improvement.
- Documentation.
- Staff orientation.

The policies and procedures meet the requirements of state law and external agencies.

D. Administration

A physical therapist is responsible for the direction of the physical therapy service.

The director:

- Ensures compliance with local, state, and federal requirements.
- Ensures compliance with current APTA documents, including *Standards of Practice for Physical Therapy, Guide for Pro-*

fessional Conduct, and *Guide for Conduct of the Affiliate Member.*
- Ensures that services provided are consistent with the mission, purposes, and goals of the service.
- Ensures that services are provided in accordance with established policies and procedures.
- Reviews and updates policies and procedures.
- Provides training that assures continued competence of physical therapy support personnel.
- Provides for continuous in-service training on safety issues and for periodic safety inspection of equipment by qualified individuals.

E. Fiscal Management

The director of the physical therapy service, in consultation with staff and appropriate administrative personnel, is responsible for planning for, and allocation of, resources. Fiscal planning and management of the service is based on sound accounting principles.

The fiscal management plan includes:

- Preparation and monitoring of a budget that provides for optimum use of resources.
- Accurate recording and reporting of financial information.
- Conformance with legal requirements.
- Cost-effective utilization of resources.
- A fee schedule that is consistent with cost of services and that is within customary norms of fairness and reasonableness.

F. Quality/Performance Improvement

The physical therapy service has a written plan for continuous improvement of the performance of services provided.

The plan:

- Provides evidence of ongoing review and evaluation of the service.

- Provides a mechanism for documentation of performance improvement.
- Is consistent with requirements of external agencies, if applicable.

G. Staffing

The physical therapy personnel affiliated with the physical therapy service have demonstrated competence and are sufficient to achieve the mission, purposes, and goals of the service.
The service:

- Meets all legal requirements regarding licensure and/or certification of appropriate personnel.
- Provides staff expertise that is appropriate to the patients/clients served.
- Provides for appropriate staff-to-patient/client ratios.
- Provides for appropriate ratios of support staff to professional staff.

H. Staff Development

The physical therapy service has a written plan that provides for appropriate and ongoing staff development.
The plan:

- Provides for consideration of self-assessments, individual goal setting, and organization needs in directing continuing education and learning activities.
- Includes strategies for long-term learning and professional development.

I. Physical Setting

The physical setting is designed to provide a safe and accessible environment that facilitates fulfillment of the mission and achievement of the purposes and goals of the physical therapy service. The equipment is safe and sufficient to achieve the purposes and goals of physical therapy.

The physical setting:

- Meets all applicable legal requirements for health and safety.
- Meets space needs appropriate for the number and type of patients/clients served.

The equipment:

- Meets all applicable legal requirements for health and safety.
- Is inspected routinely.

J. Interdisciplinary Collaboration

The physical therapy service collaborates with all appropriate disciplines.
The collaboration includes:

- An interdisciplinary team approach to patient/client care.
- Interdisciplinary patient/client and family education.
- Interdisciplinary staff development and continuing education.

III. PROVISION OF SERVICES

A. Informed Consent

The physical therapist has sole responsibility for providing information to the patient/client and for obtaining the patient's/client's informed consent in accordance with jurisdictional law before initiating physical therapy.
The information provided to the patient/client should include the following:

- A clear description of the proposed intervention/treatment.
- A statement of material (decisional) risks associated with the proposed intervention/treatment.
- A statement of expected benefits of the proposed intervention/treatment.
- A comparison of the benefits and risks possible both with and without intervention/treatment.

- An explanation of reasonable alternatives to the recommended intervention/treatment.

Informed consent requires:

- Consent by a competent adult.
- Consent by a parent/legal guardian as the surrogate decision maker when the adult patient/client is not competent or when the patient/client is a minor.
- The patient's/client's acknowledgment of understanding and consent before the intervention/treatment proceeds.

B. Initial Examination and Evaluation

The physical therapist performs and documents an initial examination and evaluates the results to identify problems and determine the diagnosis prior to intervention/treatment.

The examination:

- Is documented, dated, and signed by the physical therapist who performed the examination.
- Identifies the physical therapy needs of the patient/client.
- Incorporates appropriate objective tests and measures to facilitate outcome measurement.
- Documents sufficient data to establish a plan of care.
- May result in recommendations for additional services to meet the needs of the patient/client.

C. Plan of Care

The physical therapist establishes and provides a plan of care for the individual based on the results of the examination and evaluation and on patient/client needs.

The physical therapist involves the patient/client and appropriate others in the planning, implementation, and assessment of the intervention/treatment program.

The physical therapist, in consultation with appropriate disciplines, plans for discharge of

the patient/client taking into consideration goal achievement, and provides for appropriate follow-up or referral.

The plan of care includes:

- Realistic goals and expected functional outcomes.
- Intervention/treatment, including its frequency and duration.
- Documentation that is dated and signed by the physical therapist who established the plan of care.

D. Intervention/Treatment

The physical therapist provides, or delegates and supervises, the physical therapy intervention/treatment consistent with the results of the examination and evaluation and plan of care.

The physical therapist documents, on an ongoing basis, services provided, responses to services, and changes in status relative to the plan of care.

The intervention/treatment is:

- Provided under the ongoing personal care or supervision of the physical therapist.
- Provided in such a way that delegated responsibilities are commensurate with the qualifications and legal limitations of the physical therapy personnel involved in the intervention/treatment.
- Altered in accordance with changes in individual response or status.
- Provided at a level that is consistent with current physical therapy practice.
- Interdisciplinary when necessary to meet the needs of the patient/client.

Documentation of the services provided includes:

- Date and signature of the physical therapist and/or of the physical therapist assistant when permissible by law.

E. Reexamination and Reevaluation

The physical therapist reexamines and reevaluates the individual continually and modifies or discontinues the plan of care accordingly. The physical therapist:

- Periodically documents, dates, and signs the patient/client reexamination and modifications of the plan of care.

F. Discharge/Discontinuation of Treatment or Intervention

The physical therapist discharges the patient/client from physical therapy intervention/treatment when the goals or projected outcomes for the patient/client have been met.

Physical therapy intervention/treatment shall be discontinued when the goals are achieved, the patient/client declines to continue care, the patient/client is unable to continue, or the physical therapist determines that intervention/treatment is no longer warranted.

Discharge documentation shall include:

- The patient's/client's status at discharge and functional outcomes/goals achieved.
- Dating and signing of the discharge summary by the physical therapist.
- When a patient/client is discharged prior to goal achievement, the patient's/client's status and the rationale for discontinuation.

IV. EDUCATION

The physical therapist is responsible for individual professional development. The physical therapist assistant is responsible for individual career development.

The physical therapist participates in the education of physical therapist students, physical therapist assistant students, and students in other health professions. The physical therapist assistant participates in the education of physical therapist assistant students and other student health professionals.

The physical therapist educates and provides consultation to consumers and the general public regarding the purposes and benefits of physical therapy.

The physical therapist educates and provides consultation to consumers and the general public regarding the roles of the physical therapist and the physical therapist assistant.

The physical therapist educates and provides consultation to consumers and the general public regarding the roles of the physical therapist, the physical therapist assistant, and other support personnel.

V. RESEARCH

The physical therapist applies research findings to practice and encourages, participates in, and promotes activities that establish the outcomes of physical therapist patient/client management.

The physical therapist supports collaborative and interdisciplinary research.

VI. COMMUNITY RESPONSIBILITY

The physical therapist demonstrates community responsibility by participating in community and community agency activities, educating the public, formulating public policy, or providing pro bono physical therapy services.

The physical therapist demonstrates community responsibility by participating in community and community agency activities; educating the public, including prevention and health promotion activities; formulating public policy; or providing pro bono physical therapy services.

Standards:
Adopted by the House of Delegates
June 1980
Amended June 1985, June 1991, June 1996

Criteria:
Adopted by the Board of Directors
November 1985
Amended March 1989, March 1991, March 1993, November 1994, March 1995

Exhibit A–5

STANDARDS OF PRACTICE FOR OCCUPATIONAL THERAPY

PREFACE

These standards are intended as recommended guidelines to assist occupational therapy practitioners in the provision of occupational therapy services. These standards serve as a minimum standard for occupational therapy practice and are applicable to all individual populations and the programs in which these individuals are served.

These standards apply to those registered occupational therapists and certified occupational therapy assistants who are in compliance with regulation where it exists. The term *occupational therapy practitioner* refers to the registered occupational therapist and to the certified occupational therapy assistant, both of whom are in compliance with regulation where it exists.

The minimum educational requirements for the registered occupational therapist are described in the current *Essentials and Guidelines of an Accredited Educational Program for the Occupational Therapist* (American Occupational Therapy Association [AOTA], 1991a). The minimum educational requirements for the certified occupational therapy assistant are described in the current *Essentials and Guidelines of an Accredited Educational Program for the Occupational Therapy Assistant* (AOTA, 1991b).

STANDARD I: PROFESSIONAL STANDING

1. An occupational therapy practitioner shall maintain a current license, registration, or certification as required by law.

Source: Reprinted with permission from *Reference Manual of the Official Documents of the American Occupational Therapy Association, Inc.,* pp. 129–136, American Occupational Therapy Association, Inc., Bethesda, Maryland.

2. An occupational therapy practitioner shall practice and manage occupational therapy programs in accordance with applicable federal and state laws and regulations.
3. An occupational therapy practitioner shall be familiar with and abide by AOTA's (1994) *Occupational Therapy Code of Ethics (American Journal of Occupational Therapy,* 48, 1037–1038).
4. An occupational therapy practitioner shall maintain and update professional knowledge, skills, and abilities through appropriate continuing education or in-service training or higher education. The nature and minimum amount of continuing education must be consistent with state law and regulation.
5. A certified occupational therapy assistant must receive supervision from a registered occupational therapist as defined by official AOTA documents. The nature and amount of supervision must be provided in accordance with state law and regulation.
6. An occupational therapy practitioner shall provide direct and indirect services in accordance with AOTA's standards and policies. The nature and scope of occupational therapy services provided must be in accordance with state law and regulation.
7. An occupational therapy practitioner shall maintain current knowledge of the legislative, political, social, and cultural issues that affect the profession.

STANDARD II: REFERRAL

1. A registered occupational therapist shall accept referrals in accordance with

AOTA's *Statement of Occupational Therapy Referral* (AOTA, 1994) and in compliance with appropriate laws.

2. A registered occupational therapist may accept referrals for assessment or assessment with intervention in performance areas, performance components, or performance contexts when individuals have or appear to have dysfunctions or potential for dysfunctions.

3. A registered occupational therapist, responding to requests for service, may accept cases within the parameters of the law.

4. A registered occupational therapist shall assume responsibility for determining the appropriateness of the scope, frequency, and duration of services within the parameters of the law.

5. A registered occupational therapist shall refer individuals to other appropriate resources when the therapist determines that the knowledge and expertise of other professionals is indicated.

6. An occupational therapy practitioner shall educate current and potential referral sources about the process of initiating occupational therapy referrals.

STANDARD III: SCREENING

1. A registered occupational therapist, in accordance with state and federal guidelines, shall conduct screening to determine whether intervention or further assessment is necessary and to identify dysfunctions in performance areas.

2. A registered occupational therapist shall screen independently or as a member of an interdisciplinary team. A certified occupational therapy assistant may contribute to the screening process under the supervision of a registered occupational therapist.

3. A registered occupational therapist shall select screening methods that are appro-

priate to the individual's age and developmental level; gender; education; cultural background; and socioeconomic, medical, and functional status. Screening methods may include, but are not limited to, interviews, structured observations, informal testing, and record reviews.

4. A registered occupational therapist shall communicate screening results and recommendations to appropriate individuals.

STANDARD IV: ASSESSMENT

1. A registered occupational therapist shall assess an individual's performance areas, performance components, and performance contexts. A registered occupational therapist conducts assessments individually or as part of a team of professionals, as appropriate to the practice settings and the purposes of the assessments. A certified occupational therapy assistant may contribute to the assessment process under the supervision of a registered occupational therapist.

2. An occupational therapy practitioner shall educate the individual, or the individual's family or legal guardian, as appropriate, about the purposes and procedures of the occupational therapy assessment.

3. A registered occupational therapist shall select assessments to determine the individual's functional abilities and problems as related to performance areas, performance components, and performance contexts.

4. Occupational therapy assessment methods shall be appropriate to the individual's age and developmental level; gender; education; socioeconomic, cultural, and ethnic background; medical status; and functional abilities. The assessment methods may include some combination of skilled observation, interview, record review, or the use of stan-

dardized or criterion-referenced tests. A certified occupational therapy assistant may contribute to the assessment process under the supervision of a registered occupational therapist.

5. An occupational therapy practitioner shall follow accepted protocols when standardized tests are used. Standardized tests are tests whose scores are based on accompanying normative data that may reflect age ranges, gender, ethnic groups, geographic regions, and socioeconomic status. If standardized tests are not available or appropriate, the results shall be expressed in descriptive reports, and standardized scales shall not be used.

6. A registered occupational therapist shall analyze and summarize collected evaluation data to indicate the individual's current functional status.

7. A registered occupational therapist shall document assessment results in the individual's records, noting the specific evaluation methods and tools used.

8. A registered occupational therapist shall complete and document results of occupational therapy assessments within the time frames established by practice settings, government agencies, accreditation programs, and third-party payers.

9. An occupational therapy practitioner shall communicate assessment results, within the boundaries of client confidentiality, to the appropriate persons.

10. A registered occupational therapist shall refer the individual to the appropriate services or request additional consultations if the results of the assessments indicate areas that require intervention by other professionals.

STANDARD V: INTERVENTION PLAN

1. A registered occupational therapist shall develop and document an intervention plan based on analysis of the occupa-

tional therapy assessment data and the individual's expected outcome after the intervention. A certified occupational therapy assistant may contribute to the intervention plan under the supervision of a registered occupational therapist.

2. The occupational therapy intervention plan shall be stated in goals that are clear, measurable, behavioral, functional, and appropriate to the individual's needs, personal goals, and expected outcome after intervention.

3. The occupational therapy intervention plan shall reflect the philosophical base of occupational therapy (AOTA, 1979) and be consistent with its established principles and concepts of theory and practice. The intervention planning processes shall include
   a. Formulating a list of strengths and weaknesses.
   b. Estimating rehabilitation potential.
   c. Identifying measurable short-term and long-term goals.
   d. Collaborating with the individual, family members, other caregivers, professionals, and community resources.
   e. Selecting the media, methods, environment, and personnel needed to accomplish the intervention goals.
   f. Determining the frequency and duration of occupational therapy services.
   g. Identifying a plan for reevaluation.
   h. Discharge planning.

4. A registered occupational therapist shall prepare and document the intervention plan within the time frames and according to the standards established by the employing practice settings, government agencies, accreditation programs, and third-party payers. The certified occupational therapy assistant may contribute to the formation of the intervention plan under the supervision of the registered occupational therapist.

STANDARD VI: INTERVENTION

1. An occupational therapy practitioner shall implement a program according to the developed intervention plan. The plan shall be appropriate to the individual's age and developmental level, gender, education, cultural and ethnic background, health status, functional ability, interests and personal goals, and service provision setting. The certified occupational therapy assistant shall implement the intervention under the supervision of a registered occupational therapist.

2. An occupational therapy practitioner shall implement the intervention plan through the use of specified purposeful activities or therapeutic methods to enhance occupational performance and achieve stated goals.

3. An occupational therapy practitioner shall be knowledgeable about relevant research in the practitioner's areas of practice. A registered occupational therapist shall interpret research findings as appropriate for application to the intervention process.

4. An occupational therapy practitioner shall educate the individual, the individual's family or legal guardian, non-certified occupational therapy personnel, and nonoccupational therapy staff, as appropriate, in activities that support the established intervention plan. An occupational therapy practitioner shall communicate the risk and benefit of the intervention.

5. An occupational therapy practitioner shall maintain current information on community resources relevant to the practice area of the practitioner.

6. A registered occupational therapist shall periodically reassess and document the individual's levels of functioning and changes in levels of functioning in the performance areas, performance compo-

nents, and performance contexts. A certified occupational therapy assistant may contribute to the reassessment process under the supervision of a registered occupational therapist.

7. A registered occupational therapist shall formulate and implement program modifications consistent with changes in the individual's response to the intervention. A certified occupational therapy assistant may contribute to program modifications under the supervision of a registered occupational therapist.

8. An occupational therapy practitioner shall document the occupational therapy services provided, including the frequency and duration of the services within the time frames and according to the standards established by the employing facility, government agencies, accreditation programs, and third-party payers.

STANDARD VII: TRANSITION SERVICES

1. The occupational therapy practitioner shall provide community-referenced services, as necessary, to identify occupational performance needs related to transition. Transition involves outcome-oriented actions which are coordinated to prepare or facilitate an individual for change, such as from one functional level to another, from one life stage to another, from one program to another, or from one environment to another.

2. The occupational therapy practitioner shall participate, when appropriate, in preparing a formal individualized transition plan based on the individual's needs and shall assist in the fulfillment of life roles (e.g., independent or community living, self-care, care for others, work, play, and leisure) through activities in such a plan.

3. The occupational therapy practitioner shall facilitate the transition process in cooperation with the individual and the multidisciplinary team or other community support systems (including family members), when appropriate. The registered occupational therapist shall initiate referrals to appropriate community agencies to provide needed services (e.g., direct service, consultation, monitoring).

4. The occupational therapy practitioner shall determine the effectiveness of transition programs and the extent to which individuals have achieved desired transition outcomes (e.g., degree to which the individual is integrated and successful in community living and work environments). This is done in conjunction with the individual and other team members, where appropriate.

STANDARD VIII: DISCONTINUATION

1. A registered occupational therapist shall discontinue service when the individual has achieved predetermined goals or has achieved maximum benefit from occupational therapy services.

2. A registered occupational therapist, with input from a certified occupational therapy assistant where applicable, shall prepare and implement a discharge plan that is consistent with occupational therapy goals, individual goals, interdisciplinary team goals, family goals, and expected outcomes. The discharge plan shall address appropriate community resources for referral for psychosocial, cultural, and socioeconomic barriers and limitations that may need modification.

3. A registered occupational therapist shall document the changes between the initial and current states of functional ability and deficit in performance areas, performance components, and performance contexts. A certified occupational therapy assistant may contribute to the process

under the supervision of a registered occupational therapist.

4. An occupational therapy practitioner shall allow sufficient time for the coordination and effective implementation of the discharge plan.

5. A registered occupational therapist shall document recommendations for follow-up or reevaluation when applicable.

STANDARD IX: CONTINUOUS QUALITY IMPROVEMENT

1. An occupational therapy practitioner shall monitor and document the continuous quality improvement of practice, which may include outcomes of services, using predetermined practice criteria reflecting professional consensus, recent developments in research, and specific employing facility standards.

2. An occupational therapy practitioner shall monitor all aspects of individual occupational therapy services for effectiveness and timeliness. If actual care does not meet the prescribed standard, it must be justified by peer review or other appropriate means within the practice setting. Occupational therapy services shall be discontinued when no longer necessary.

3. A registered occupational therapist shall systematically assess the review process of patient care to determine the success or appropriateness of interventions. Certified occupational therapy assistants may contribute to the process in collaboration with the registered occupational therapist.

STANDARD X: MANAGEMENT

1. A registered occupational therapist shall provide the management necessary for efficient organization and provision of occupational therapy services.

2. A certified occupational therapy assistant, under the supervision of a registered

occupational therapist, may perform the following management functions:

a. Education of members of other related professions and physicians about occupational therapy.
b. Participation in (1) orientation, supervision, training, and evaluation of the performance of volunteers and other noncertified occupational therapy personnel, and (2) developing plans to remediate areas of skill deficit in the performance of job duties by volunteers and other noncertified occupational therapy personnel.
c. Design and periodic review of all aspects of the occupational therapy program to determine its effectiveness, efficiency, and future directions.
d. Systematic review of the quality of service provided, using criteria established by professional consensus and current research, as well as established standards for state regulation; accreditation; American Occupational Therapy Certification Board (AOTCB) certification; and related laws, policies, guidelines, and regulations.
e. Incorporation of a fair and equitable system of admission, discharge, and charges for occupational therapy services.
f. Participation in cross-disciplinary activities to ensure that the total needs of the individual are met.
g. Provision of support (i.e., space, time, money as feasible) for clinical research or collaborative research when such projects have the approval of the appropriate governing bodies (e.g., institutional review board), and the results of which are deemed poten-

tially beneficial to individuals of occupational therapy services now or in the future.

REFERENCES

American Occupational Therapy Association. (1979). The philosophical base of occupational therapy. *American Journal of Occupational Therapy, 33*, 785.

American Occupational Therapy Association. (1991a). Essentials and guidelines of an accredited educational program for the occupational therapist. *American Journal of Occupational Therapy, 45*, 1077–1084.

American Occupational Therapy Association. (1991b). Essentials and guidelines of an accredited educational program for the occupational therapy assistant. *American Journal of Occupational Therapy, 45*, 1085–1092.

American Occupational Therapy Association (1994). Occupational therapy code of ethics. *American Journal of Occupational Therapy, 48*, 1037–1038.

American Occupational Therapy Association (1994). Statement of occupational therapy referral. *American Journal of Occupational Therapy, 48*, 1034.

PREPARED BY

Commission on Practice

Jim Hinojosa, PhD, OTR, FAOTA, Chairperson

Adopted by the Representative Assembly July 1994

Note: This document replaces the *1992 Standards of Practice for Occupational Therapy* (*American Journal of Occupational Therapy, 46*, 1082–1085) and the *1987 Standards of Practice for Occupational Therapy in Schools* (*American Journal of Occupational Therapy, 41*, 804–808), which were rescinded by the 1994 Representative Assembly.

Exhibit A–6

DELIVERY OF SPEECH-LANGUAGE PATHOLOGY AND AUDIOLOGY SERVICES IN HOME CARE

This position paper represents the cumulative effort of the members of the Task Force on Home Care, which included Martha Ackerman, Joanne M. Gray, Dennis C. Hampton, Mary Marshall, Gloria B. Nelson, Ellen Enright-Stacy, Jacqueline Taubman, and Patricia G. Larkins, chair, under the guidance of Nancy G. Becker, then vice president for professional and governmental affairs.

INTRODUCTION

Home care[1] is a rapidly growing field within the health care industry and is expected to be one of the most dynamic segments within health care in the future. Factors contributing to the growth in home care services include (1) a rapidly expanding older population, (2) an increased number of children identified as needing home care, (3) pressure on hospitals to decrease costs by reducing lengths of stay, early discharge, and limiting the number of beds, (4) government and private business stress on cost containment, (5) technology, and (6) consumer need or preference for receiving services within the home.

Initially, home care services were limited to nursing services. However, since 1966 and the establishment of Medicare and Medicaid programs, home care services have grown to include but are not restricted to speech-language-hearing services, home health aide services, homemaker services, nutritional services, occupational therapy, physical therapy, respiratory therapy, and social services. These services are provided to patients of all ages with funding provided by Medicare, Medicaid, county agencies, federal and state grants, foundation grants and contracts, education departments/agencies, court systems, charitable organizations such as United Way, private health insurance, and private payment.

Speech-language pathologists and audiologists are becoming more active in the delivery of services in home care. An example is that the number of speech-language pathologists providing services in home care grew from 858 in 1976 to 2,793 in 1984. Speech-language pathology and/or audiology services may be provided in the home setting and do not need a physician's order, unless required by a specific third-party payer.

The home setting has characteristics different from the traditional settings and presents speech-language pathologists and audiologists with a number of challenges. This position statement, which addresses the delivery of services in the home regardless of payment source, considers the following: (1) components of the home care service delivery system, (2) the roles and professional responsibilities of speech-language pathologists and audiologists in the provision of home care services, and (3) the impact of service needs on personnel preparation.

---

[1]Home care is the provision of professional and personal care services within the patient's home. The individual, family members, and a team of professional and personal care providers work together to deliver these services in a multidisciplinary approach.

Source: Reprinted with permission from Task Force on Home Care. (1995). Delivery of Speech-Language Pathology and Audiology Services in Home Care. *ASHA Desk Reference* (Vol. 4), pp. 13–16. Rockville, MD: American Speech–Language–Hearing Association. © 1995. Reprinted by permission

SERVICE DELIVERY COMPONENTS

Delivery of speech-language pathology and audiology services in home care encompasses components which are unique to this setting as well as components that are generic to the delivery of speech-language pathology and audiology services regardless of work setting. The following list describes selected generic and specialized components considered important to the home setting.

GENERIC COMPONENTS

- **Referrals**—The speech-language pathologist and audiologist receive referrals on patients who are suspected of having a speech-language-hearing disorder or who are in need of speech-language pathology and/or audiology services. In addition, they also recommend appropriate interagency and intra-agency referrals.
- **Assessment**—Norm and criterion-referenced evaluations are used by speech-language pathologists and audiologists to determine if a speech-language-hearing disorder exists. Data are collected and used to determine the patient's diagnosis and rehabilitation potential. In addition, the data are used to develop the patient's treatment plan, expected frequency and duration of treatment, discharge goals, and other recommendations when indicated.
- **Treatment**—The speech-language pathologist and audiologist intervene based upon their established treatment plans. These treatment plans are reassessed and revised as indicated until discharge goals are achieved or the patient has reached maximum potential for benefit from treatment.
- **Family Involvement**—When appropriate, the speech-language pathologist and audiologist involve the people present in the home so as to maximize treatment effectiveness.
- **Recordkeeping**—The speech-language pathologist and audiologist provide appropriate documentation which clearly and succinctly reports services.
- **Utilization of Supportive Personnel**— The speech-language pathologist and au-

diologist may utilize supportive personnel (for example, home care aides, speech-language pathology aides) to provide services under their supervision. Refer to "Guidelines for the Employment and Utilization of Supportive Personnel" (*Asha*, 1981).
- **Supervision**—Speech-language pathologists and audiologists are involved in supervision which primarily involves the tasks and skills of "clinical teaching" related to the interaction between a clinician and client (*Asha*, 1985). This "clinical supervision" may involve supervising peers, clinical fellows, and/or students completing professional education requirements. Tasks involved in supervision, competencies for effective clinical supervision, and preparation for clinical supervisors are found in ASHA's position statement, "Clinical Supervision in Speech-Language Pathology and Audiology" (*Asha*, 1985). On-site supervision is provided to students whenever delivering clinical services.
- **Cultural/Linguistic Factors**—Cultural/linguistic factors may necessitate modification of materials, the format of the evaluation, and diagnostic and treatment approaches as well as the use of a bilingual evaluator and/or translator.
- **Interdisciplinary Management**—The speech-language pathologist and audiologist work with other appropriate professionals to (1) coordinate services, goals, and plans, and (2) ensure appropriate services are provided and continuity of care is maintained.
- **Quality Assurance**—The speech-language pathologist and audiologist evaluate and monitor on an ongoing basis the quality and appropriateness of speech-language-hearing services provided. When problems are identified through peer review, action plans are developed by the speech-language pathologist and audiologist to resolve these problems. Follow-up evaluations are then conducted in order to demonstrate problem resolution.

Specialized Components of Home Care

- **Travel**—The speech-language pathologist and audiologist may travel extensively when providing services in the home. Documentation of time and distance is maintained.
- **Safety/Infection Control**—The speech-language pathologist and audiologist may experience unique environmental and/or health concerns when going into the home. Special precautions related to patient care and personal safety need to be made.
- **Reimbursement**—Third-party payers have varied and specific regulations that allow billing reimbursement for speech-language pathology and audiology services. Speech-language pathologists and audiologists need to familiarize themselves with these requirements.

ROLE OF THE SPEECH-LANGUAGE PATHOLOGIST AND AUDIOLOGIST

Services in the home are generally provided by a team of professionals. The home care team may include the speech-language pathologist, audiologist, home care aide, homemaker, family member or caregiver, nurse, nutritionist, occupational therapist, physical therapist, physician, psychologist, respiratory therapist, social worker, and special education teacher. The home care team is coordinated by a patient care manager. While the registered nurse frequently coordinates the services of the home care team, the speech-language pathologist and audiologist also are qualified to serve as patient care managers.

The professional role of the speech-language pathologist includes but is not limited to:

1. conducting speech, language, and/or oral pharyngeal evaluations;
2. developing and recommending appropriate individual treatment/education programs;
3. providing treatment;
4. referring to other health professionals;
5. instructing and counseling family members, nurses, and other members of the home care team;
6. providing referral and follow-up with other community resources;
7. recommending prosthetic and augmentative communication devices;
8. conducting hearing screenings;
9. providing aural rehabilitation in consultation with an audiologist;
10. participating in admission/discharge planning;
11. providing appropriate documentation;
12. supervising peers, clinical fellows, supportive personnel, and students in training;
13. providing inservice training to agency staff
14. providing public education;
15. conducting research;
16. developing and participating in prevention activities;
17. directing and administering home care services; and
18. maintaining quality control.

The professional role of the audiologist includes but is not limited to:

1. providing hearing evaluations;
2. providing aural rehabilitation or habilitation;
3. evaluating the need for assistive listening devices, alerting systems, and hearing aids;
4. selecting, dispensing, and adjusting hearing aids, assistive listening, and alerting devices;
5. instructing and counseling family member, nurses, and other members of the home care team;
6. providing referrals and follow-up with other community resources;
7. conducting speech-language screenings;
8. participating in admission/discharge planning;
9. providing appropriate documentation;

10. supervising peers, clinical fellows, supportive personnel, and students in training;
11. providing inservice training to agency staff;
12. providing public education;
13. referring to other health professionals;
14. conducting research;
15. developing and participating in prevention activities;
16. directing and administering home care services; and
17. maintaining quality control.

PERSONNEL PREPARATION

The Certificates of Clinical Competence (CCC) in Speech-Language Pathology and Audiology indicate that speech-language pathologists and audiologists have basic knowledge and clinical training related to the provision of services to various patient populations. In order to assure the most efficient and effective delivery of speech-language-audiology services in home care, it is important for speech-language pathologists and audiologists to acquire additional special knowledge and practical experiences in a number of areas unique to home care. This knowledge and experience may be obtained from a variety of sources including graduate education programs, clinical fellowship year, professional practice, and continuing education. Areas of professional knowledge with which speech-language pathologists and audiologists need to be familiar but to which they are not restricted include the following:

1. treatment of neurologically impaired children and adults in the home;
2. provision of services to persons with communication problems and oral pharyngeal disorders resulting from trauma, severe illness, and/or surgery;
3. provision of services to infants and children including knowledge of pre-speech and language development;
4. family intervention techniques;
5. observation of patients within the home environment;
6. drugs/medications/illnesses and disabilities and their effects on communication;
7. infection control;
8. roles and responsibilities of other health care professionals;
9. participation on an interdisciplinary team;
10. medical terminology;
11. documentation required in home care; and
12. reimbursement and legislative issues impacting service delivery in home care.

Exhibit A–7

MEDICARE CONDITIONS OF PARTICIPATION

PART 484—CONDITIONS OF PARTICIPATION: HOME HEALTH AGENCIES

Subpart A—General Provisions

SEC.
484.1 Basis and scope.
484.2 Definitions.
484.4 Personnel qualifications.

Subpart B—Administration

SEC.
484.10 Condition of participation: Patient rights.
484.12 Condition of participation: Compliance with Federal, State, and local laws, disclosure and ownership information, and accepted professional standards and principles.
484.14 Condition of participation: Organization, services, administration.
484.16 Condition of participation: Group of professional personnel.
484.18 Condition of participation: Acceptance of patients, plan of care, medical supervision.

Subpart C—Furnishing of Services

SEC.
484.30 Condition of participation: Skilled nursing services.

Note: At the time of this writing, the Health Care Financing Administration has proposed changes to the Conditions of Participation. Proposed changes can be found at the end of this exhibit.

Source: Reprinted from *Federal Register*, pp. 1–14, January 1996; pp. 11029–11035, March 1997.

484.32 Condition of participation: Therapy services.
484.34 Condition of Participation: Medical social services.
484.36 Condition of participation: Home health aide services.
484.38 Condition of participation: Qualifying to furnish outpatient physical therapy or speech pathology services.
484.48 Condition of participation: Clinical records.
484.52 Condition of participation: Evaluation of the agency's program.

Subpart A—General Provisions

§484.1 Basis and scope.

This part implements the requirements of sections 1861(o) and 1891(a) of the Act for HHA services and also sets forth the additional requirements considered necessary to ensure the health and safety of patients.

§484.2 Definitions.

As used in this part, unless the context indicates otherwise—"Bylaws or equivalent" means a set of rules adopted by an HHA for governing the agency's operation.

"Branch office" means a location or site from which a home health agency provides services within a portion of the total geographic area served by the parent agency. The branch office is part of the home health agency and is located sufficiently close to share administration, supervision, and services in a manner that renders it unnecessary for the branch independently to meet the conditions of participation as a home health agency.

"Clinical note" means a notation of a contact with a patient that is written and dated by a member of the health team, and that describes signs and symptoms, treatment and drugs administered and the patient's reaction, and any changes in physical or emotional condition.

"HHA" stands for home health agency.

"Nonprofit agency" means an agency exempt from Federal income taxation under section 501 of the Internal Revenue Code of 1954.

"Parent home health agency" means the agency that develops and maintains administrative controls of subunits and/or branch offices.

"Primary home health agency" means the agency that is responsible for the services furnished to patients and for implementation of the plan of care.

"Progress note" means a written notation, dated and signed by a member of the health team that summarizes facts about care furnished and the patient's response during a given period of time.

"Proprietary agency" means a private profit-making agency licensed by the State.

"Public agency" means an agency operated by a State or local government.

"Subdivision" means a component of a multi-function health agency, such as the home care department of a hospital or the nursing division of a health department, which independently meets the conditions of participation for HHAs. A subdivision that has subunits or branch offices is considered a parent agency.

"Subunit" means a semi-autonomous organization that—

(1) Serves patients in a geographic area different from that of the parent agency; and

(2) Must independently meet the conditions of participation for HHAs because it is too far from the parent agency to share administration, supervision, and services on a daily basis.

"Summary report" means the compilation of the pertinent factors of a patient's clinical notes and progress notes that is submitted to the patient's physician.

"Supervision" means authoritative procedural guidance by a qualified person for the accomplishment of a function or activity. Unless otherwise specified in this part, the supervisor must be on the premises to supervise an individual who does not meet the qualifications specified in §484.4.

§484.4 Personnel qualifications

Staff required to meet the conditions set forth in this part are staff who meet the qualifications specified in this section.

"Administrator, home health agency". A person who:

(a) Is a licensed physician, or

(b) Is a registered nurse, or

(c) Has training and experience in health service administration and at least 1 year of supervisory or administrative experience in home health care or related health programs.

"Audiologist". A person who:

(a) Meets the education and experience requirements for a Certificate of Clinical Competence in audiology granted by the American Speech-Language-Hearing Association; or

(b) Meets the educational requirements for certification and is in the process of accumulating the supervised experience required for certification.

"Home health aide". Effective for services furnished after August 14, 1990, a person who has successfully completed a State-established or other training program that meets the requirements of §484.36(a) and a competency evaluation program or State licensure program that meets the requirements of §484.36(b) or (e), or a competency evaluation program or State licensure program that meets the requirements of §484.36(b) or (e). An individual is not considered to have completed a training and competency evaluation program, or a competency evaluation program if, since the individual's most recent completion of this program(s), there has been a continuous period of 24 consecutive months during none of which the individual furnished services described in §409.40 of this chapter for compensation.

"Occupational therapist". A person who:

(a) Is a graduate of an occupational therapy curriculum accredited jointly by the Committee on Allied Health Education and Accreditation of the American Medical Association and the American Occupational Therapy Association; or

(b) Is eligible for the National Registration Examination of the American Occupational Therapy Association; or

(c) Has 2 years of appropriate experience as an occupational therapist, and has achieved a satisfactory grade on a proficiency examination conducted, approved, or sponsored by the U.S. Public Health Service, except that such determinations of proficiency do not apply with respect to persons initially licensed by a State or seeking initial qualification as an occupational therapist after December 31, 1977.

"Occupational therapy assistant." A person who:

(a) Meets the requirements for certification as an occupational therapy assistant established by the American Occupational Therapy Association; or

(b) Has 2 years of appropriate experience as an occupational therapy assistant, and has achieved a satisfactory grade on a proficiency examination conducted, approved, or sponsored by the U.S. Public Health Service, except that such determinations of proficiency do not apply with respect to persons initially licensed by a State or seeking initial qualification as an occupational therapy assistant after December 31, 1977.

"Physical therapist". A person who is licensed as a physical therapist by the State in which practicing and

(a) Has graduated from a physical therapy curriculum approved by:

(1) The American Physical Therapy Association, or

(2) The Committee on Allied Health Education and Accreditation, of the American Medical Association, or

(3) The Council on Medical Education of the American Medical Association and the American Physical Therapy Association, or

(b) Prior to January 1, 1966:

(1) Was admitted to membership by the American Physical Therapy Association, or

(2) Was admitted to registration by the American Registry of Physical Therapists, or

(3) Has graduated from a physical therapy curriculum in a 4 year college or university approved by a State department of education; or

(c) Has 2 years of appropriate experience as a physical therapist, and has achieved a satisfactory grade on a proficiency examination conducted, approved, or sponsored by the U.S. Public Health Service except that such determinations of proficiency do not apply with respect to persons initially licensed by a State or seeking qualification as a physical therapist after December 31, 1977; or

(d) Was licensed or registered prior to January 1, 1966, and prior to January 1, 1970, had 15 years of full-time experience in the treatment of illness or injury through the practice of physical therapy in which services were rendered under the order and direction of attending and referring doctors of medicine or osteopathy; or

(e) If trained outside the United States,

(1) Was graduated since 1928 from a physical therapy curriculum approved in the country in which the curriculum was located and in which there is a member of the World Confederation for Physical Therapy.

(2) Meets the requirements for membership in a member organization of the World Confederation for Physical Therapy.

"Physical therapy assistant". A person who is licensed as a physical therapy assistant, if applicable, by the state in which practicing, and

(1) Has graduated from a 2-year college-level program approved by the American Physical Therapy Association; or

(2) Has 2 years of appropriate experience as a physical therapy assistant, and has achieved a satisfactory grade on a proficiency examination conducted, approved, or sponsored by the U.S. Public Health Service, except that these determinations of proficiency do not apply with respect to persons initially licensed by a State or seeking initial qualification as a physical therapy assistant after December 31, 1977.

"Physician". A doctor of medicine, osteopathy, or podiatry legally authorized to practice medicine and surgery by the State in which such function or action is performed.

"Practical (vocational) nurse". A person who is licensed as a practical (vocational) nurse by the State in which practicing.

"Public health nurse". A registered nurse who has completed a baccalaureate degree program approved by the National League for Nursing for public health nursing preparation or post registered nurse study that includes content approved by the National League for Nursing for public health nursing preparation.

"Registered nurse (RN)". A graduate of an approved school of professional nursing, who is licensed as a registered nurse by the State in which practicing.

"Social work assistant". A person who:

(1) Has a baccalaureate degree in social work, psychology, sociology, or other field related to social work and has had at least 1 year of social work experience in a health care setting, or

(2) Has 2 years of appropriate experience as a social work assistant and has achieved a satisfactory grade on a proficiency examination conducted, approved, or sponsored by the U.S. Public Health Service, except that these determinations of proficiency do not apply with respect to persons initially licensed by a State or seeking initial qualification as a social work assistant after December 31, 1977.

"Social worker". A person who has a master's degree from a school of social work accredited by the Council on Social Work Education, and has 1 year of social work experience in a health care setting.

"Speech pathologist". A person who:

(1) Meets the education and experience requirements for a Certificate of Clinical Competence in (speech pathology or audiology) granted by the American Speech-Language-Hearing Association; or

(2) Meets the educational requirements for certification and is in the process of accumulating the supervised experience required for certification.

Subpart B—Administration

§484.10 Condition of participation: Patient rights.

The patient has the right to be informed of his or her rights. The HHA must protect and promote the exercise of these rights.

(a) Standard. Notice of rights. (1) The HHA must provide the patient with a written notice of the patient's rights in advance of furnishing care to the patient or during the initial evaluation visit before the initiation of treatment.

(2) The HHA must maintain documentation showing that it has complied with the requirements of this section.

(b) Standard: Exercise of rights and respect of property and person. (1) The patient has the right to exercise his or her rights as a patient of the HHA.

(2) The patient's family or guardian may exercise the patient's rights when the patient has been judged incompetent.

(3) The patient has the right to have his or her property treated with respect.

(4) The patient has the right to voice grievances regarding treatment or care that is (or fails to be) furnished, or regarding the lack of respect for property to anyone who is furnishing services on behalf of the HHA and must not be subjected to discrimination or reprisal for doing so.

(5) The HHA must investigate complaints made by a patient or the patient's family or guardian regarding treatment or care that is (or fails to be) furnished, or regarding the lack of respect for the patient's property by anyone furnishing services on behalf of the HHA, and must document both the existence of the complaint and the resolution of the complaint.

(c) Standard: Right to be informed and to participate in planning care and treatment. (1) The patient has the right to be informed in advance about the care to be furnished, and of any changes in the care to be furnished.

(i) The HHA must advise the patient in advance of the disciplines that will furnish care, and the frequency of visits proposed to be furnished.

(ii) The HHA must advise the patient in advance of any change in the plan of care before the change is made.

(2) The patient has the right to participate in the planning of the care.

(i) The HHA must advise the patient in advance of the right to participate in planning the care or treatment and in planning changes in the care or treatment.

(ii) The HHA complies with the requirements of Subpart I of Part 489 of this chapter relating to maintaining written policies and procedures regarding advance directives. The HHA must inform and distribute written information to the patient, in advance, concerning its policies on advance directives, including a description of applicable State law. The HHA may furnish advance directives information to a patient at the time of the first home visit, as long as the information is furnished before care is provided.

(d) Standard: Confidentiality of medical records. The patient has the right to confidentiality of the clinical records maintained by the HHA. The HHA must advise the patient of the agency's policies and procedures regarding disclosure of clinical records.

(e) Standard. Patient liability for payment. (1) The patient has the right to be advised, before care is initiated, of the extent to which payment for the HHA services may be expected from Medicare or other sources, and the extent to which payment may be required from the patient. Before the care is initiated, the HHA must inform the patient, orally and in writing, of—

(i) The extent to which payment may be expected from Medicare, Medicaid, or any other Federally funded or aided program known to the HHA;

(ii) The charges for services that will not be covered by Medicare; and

(iii) The charges that the individual may have to pay.

(2) The patient has the right to be advised orally and in writing of any changes in the information provided in accordance with paragraph (e)(1) of this section when they occur. The HHA must advise the patient of these changes orally and in writing as soon as possible, but no later than 30 calendar days from the date that the HHA becomes aware of a change.

(f) Standard: Home health hotline. The patient has the right to be advised of the availability of the toll-free HHA hotline in the State. When the agency accepts the patient for treatment or care, the HHA must advise the patient in writing of the telephone number of the home health hotline established by the State, the hours of its operation, and that the purpose of the hotline is to receive complaints or questions about local HHAs. The patient also has the right to use this hotline to lodge complaints concerning the implementation of the advance directive requirements.

§484.12 Condition of participation: Compliance with Federal, State, and local laws, disclosure and ownership information, and accepted professional standards and principles.

(a) Standard: Compliance with Federal, State, and local laws and regulations. The HHA and its staff must operate and furnish services in compliance with all applicable Federal, State, and local laws and regulations. If state or applicable local law provides for the licensure of HHAs, an agency not subject to licensure is approved by the licensing authority as meeting the standards established for licensure.

(b) Standard: Disclosure of ownership and management information. The HHA must comply with the requirements of Part 420, Subpart C of this chapter. The HHA also must disclose the following information to the State survey agency at the time of the HHA's initial request for certification, for each survey, and at the time of any change in ownership or management:

(1) The name and address of all persons with an ownership or control interest in the HHA as defined in §§420.201, 420.202, and 420.206 of this chapter.

(2) The name and address of each person who is an officer, a director, an agent or a managing employee of the HHA as defined in §§420.201, 420.202, and 420.206 of this chapter.

(3) The name and address of the corporation, association, or other company that is responsible for the management of the HHA, and the name and address of the chief executive officer and the chairman of the board of directors of that corporation, association, or other company responsible for the management of the HHA.

(c) <u>Standard</u>: Compliance with accepted professional standards and principles. The HHA and its staff must comply with accepted professional standards and principles that apply to professionals furnishing services in an HHA.

§484.14 Condition of participation: Organization, services, and administration.

Organization, services furnished, administrative control, and lines of authority for the delegation of responsibility down to the patient care level are clearly set forth in writing and are readily identifiable. Administrative and supervisory functions are not delegated to another agency or organization and all services not furnished directly, including services provided through subunits are monitored and controlled by the parent agency. If an agency has subunits, appropriate administrative records are maintained for each subunit.

(a) <u>Standard</u>: Services furnished. Part-time or intermittent skilled nursing services and at least one other therapeutic service (physical, speech, or occupational therapy; medical social services; or home health aide services) are made available on a visiting basis in a place of residence used as a patient's home. An HHA must provide at least one of the qualifying services directly through agency employees, but may provide the second qualifying service and additional services under arrangements with another agency or organization.

(b) <u>Standard</u>: Governing body. A governing body (or designated persons so functioning) assumes full legal authority and responsibility for the operation of the agency. The governing body appoints a qualified administrator, arranges for professional advice as required under §484.16, adopts and periodically reviews written bylaws or an acceptable equivalent, and oversees the management and fiscal affairs of the agency.

(c) <u>Standard</u>: Administrator. The administrator, who may also be the supervising physician or registered nurse required under a paragraph (d) of this section, organizes and directs the agency's ongoing functions; maintains ongoing liaison among the governing body, the group of professional personnel, and the staff; employs qualified personnel and ensures adequate staff education and evaluations; ensures the accuracy of public information materials and activities; and implements an effective budgeting and accounting system. A qualified person is authorized in writing to act in the absence of the administrator.

(d) <u>Standard</u>: Supervising physician or registered nurse. The skilled nursing and other therapeutic services furnished are under the supervision and direction of a physician or a registered nurse (who preferably has at least 1 year of nursing experience and is a public health nurse). This person, or similarly qualified alternate, is available at all times during operating hours and participates in all activities relevant to the professional services furnished, including the development of qualifications and the assignment of personnel.

(e) <u>Standard</u>: Personnel policies. Personnel practices and patient care are supported by appropriate, written, personnel policies. Personnel records include qualifications and licensure that are kept current.

(f) <u>Standard</u>: Personnel under hourly or per visit contracts. If personnel under hourly or per visit contracts are used by the HHA, there is a written contract between those personnel and the agency that specifies the following:

(1) Patients are accepted for care only by the primary HHA.

(2) The services to be furnished.

(3) The necessity to conform to all applicable agency policies including personnel qualifications.

(4) The responsibility for participating in developing plans of care.

(5) The manner in which services will be controlled, coordinated, and evaluated by the primary HHA.

(6) The procedures for submitting clinical and progress notes, scheduling of visits, periodic patient evaluation.

(7) The procedures for payment for services furnished under the contract.

(g) Standard: Coordination of patient services. All personnel furnishing services maintain liaison to ensure that their efforts are coordinated effectively and support the objectives outlined in the plan of care. The clinical record or minutes of case conferences establish that effective interchange, reporting, and coordination of patient care does occur. A written summary report for each patient is sent to the attending physician at least every 62 days.

(h) Standard: Services under arrangements. Services furnished under arrangements are subject to a written contract conforming with the requirements specified in paragraph (f) of this section and with the requirements of section 1861(w) of the Act [42 U.S.C.1495x(w)].

(i) Standard: Institutional planning. The HHA, under the direction of the governing body, prepares an overall plan and a budget that includes an annual operating budget and capital expenditure plan.

(1) Annual operating budget. There is an annual operating budget that includes all anticipated income and expenses related to items that would, under generally accepted accounting principles, be considered income and expense items. However, it is not required that there be prepared, in connection with any budget, an item by item identification of the components of each type of anticipated income or expense.

(2) Capital expenditure plan. (i) There is a capital expenditure plan for at least a 3-year period, including the operating budget year. The plan includes and identifies in detail the anticipated sources of financing for, and the objectives of, each anticipated expenditure of more than $600,000 for items that would under generally accepted accounting principles, be considered capital items. In determining if a single capital expenditure exceeds $600,000, the cost of studies, surveys, designs, plans, working drawings, specifications, and other activities essential to the acquisition, improvement, modernization, expansion, or replacement of land, plant, building, and equipment are included.

Expenditures directly or indirectly related to capital expenditures, such as grading, paving, broker commissions, taxes assessed during the construction period, and costs involved in demolishing or razing structures on land are also included. Transactions that are separated in time, but are components of an overall plan or patient care objective, are viewed in their entirety without regard to their timing. Other costs related to capital expenditures include title fees, permit and license fees, broker commissions, architect, legal, accounting, and appraisal fees; interest, finance, or carrying charges on bonds, notes and other costs incurred for borrowing funds.

(ii) If the anticipated source of financing is, in any part, the anticipated payment from title V (Maternal and Child Health and Crippled Children's Services) or title XVIII (Medicare) or title XIX (Medicaid) of the Social Security Act, the plan specifies the following:

(A) Whether the proposed capital expenditure is required to conform or is likely to be required to conform to current standards, criteria, or plans developed in accordance with the Public Health Service Act or the Mental Retardation Facilities and Community Mental Health Centers Construction Act of 1963.

(B) Whether a capital expenditure proposal has been submitted to the designated planning agency for approval in accordance with section

1122 of the Act (42 U.S.C. 1320a–1) and implementing regulations.

(C) Whether the designated planning agency has approved or disapproved the proposed capital expenditure if it was presented to that agency.

(3) Preparation of plan and budget. The overall plan and budget is prepared under the direction of the governing body of the HHA by a committee consisting of representatives of the governing body, the administrative staff and the medical staff (if any) of the HHA.

(4) Annual review of plan and budget. The overall plan and budget is reviewed and updated at least annually by the committee referred to in paragraph (ii)(3) of this section under the direction of the governing body of the HHA.

(j) Standard: Laboratory services. (1) If the HHA engages in laboratory testing outside of the context of assisting an individual in self-administering a test with an appliance that has been cleared for that purpose by the FDA, such testing must be in compliance with all applicable requirements of Part 493 of this chapter.

(2) If the HHA chooses to refer specimens for laboratory testing to another laboratory, the referral laboratory must be certified in the appropriate specialties and subspecialties of services in accordance with the applicable requirements of Part 493 of this chapter.

§484.16 Condition of participation: Group of professional personnel.

A group of professional personnel which includes at least one physician and one registered nurse (preferably a public health nurse), and with appropriate representation from other professional disciplines, establishes and annually reviews the agency's policies governing scope of services offered, admission and discharge policies, medical supervision and plans of care, emergency care, clinical records, personnel qualifications, and program evaluation. At least one member of the group is neither an owner nor an employee of the agency.

(a) Standard: Advisory and evaluation function. The group of professional personnel meets frequently to advise the agency on professional issues, to participate in the evaluation of the agency's program, and to assist the agency in maintaining liaison with other health care providers in the community and in the agency's community information program. The meetings are documented by dated minutes.

§484.18 Condition of participation: Acceptance of patients, plan of care, and medical supervision.

Patients are accepted for treatment on the basis of a reasonable expectation that the patient's medical, nursing, and social needs can be met adequately by the agency in the patient's place of residence. Care follows a written plan of care established and periodically reviewed by a doctor of medicine, osteopathy, or podiatric medicine.

(a) Standard: Plan of care. The plan of care developed in consultation with the agency staff covers all pertinent diagnoses, including mental status, types of services and equipment required, frequency of visits, prognosis, rehabilitation potential, functional limitations, activities permitted, nutritional requirements, medications and treatments, any safety measures to protect against injury, instructions for timely discharge or referral, and any other appropriate items. If a physician refers a patient under a plan of care that cannot be completed until after an evaluation visit, the physician is consulted to approve additions or modifications to the original plan. Orders for therapy services include the specific procedures and modalities to be used and the amount, frequency, and duration. The therapist and other agency personnel participate in developing the plan of care.

(b) Standard: Periodic review of plan of care. The total plan of care is reviewed by the attending physician and HHA personnel as often as the severity of the patient's condition requires, but at least once every 62 days. Agency professional staff promptly alert the physician to any changes that suggest a need to alter the plan of care.

(c) Standard: Conformance with physician's orders. Drugs and treatments are administered by agency staff only as ordered by the physician. Oral orders are put into writing and signed and dated with the date of receipt by the registered nurse or qualified therapist (as defined in §484.4 of this chapter) responsible for furnishing or supervising the ordered services. Oral orders are only accepted by personnel authorized to do so by applicable State and Federal laws and regulations as well as by the HHA's internal policies. Agency staff check all medicines a patient may be taking to identify possible ineffective drug therapy or adverse reactions, significant side effects, drug allergies, and contraindicated medication, and promptly report any problem to the physician.

Subpart C—Furnishing of Services

§484.30 Condition of participation: Skilled nursing services.

The HHA furnishes skilled nursing services by or under the supervision of a registered nurse and in accordance with the plan of care.

(a) Standard: Duties of the registered nurse. The registered nurse makes the initial evaluation visit, regularly reevaluates the patient's nursing needs, initiates the plan of care and necessary revisions, furnishes those services requiring substantial and specialized nursing skill, initiates appropriate preventive and rehabilitative nursing procedures, prepares clinical and progress notes, coordinates services, informs the physician and other personnel of changes in the patient's condition and needs, counsels the patient and family in meeting nursing and related needs, participates in inservice programs, and supervises and teaches other nursing personnel.

(b) Standard: Duties of the licensed practical nurse. The licensed practical nurse furnishes services in accordance with agency policies, prepares clinical and progress notes, assists the physician and registered nurse in performing specialized procedures, prepares equipment and materials for treatments observing aseptic technique as required, and assists the patient in learning appropriate self-care techniques.

§484.32 Condition of participation: Therapy services.

Any therapy services offered by the HHA directly or under arrangement are given by a qualified therapist or by a qualified therapy assistant under the supervision of a qualified therapist and in accordance with the plan of care. The qualified therapist assists the physician in evaluating level of function, helps develop the plan of care (revising it as necessary), prepares clinical and progress notes, advises and consults with the family and other agency personnel, and participates in in-service programs.

(a) Standard: Supervision of physical therapy assistant and occupational therapy assistant. Services furnished by a qualified physical therapy assistant or qualified occupational therapy assistant may be furnished under the supervision of a qualified physical or occupational therapist. A physical therapy assistant or occupational therapy assistant performs services planned, delegated, and supervised by the therapist, assists in preparing clinical notes and progress reports, and participates in educating the patient and family, and in in-service programs.

(b) Standard: Supervision of speech therapy services. Speech therapy services are furnished only by or under supervision of a qualified speech pathologist or audiologist.

§484.34 Condition of participation: Medical social services.

If the agency furnishes medical social services, those services are given by a qualified social worker or by a qualified social work assistant under the supervision of a qualified social worker and in accordance with the plan of care. The social worker assists the physician and other team members in understanding the significant social and emotional factors related to the health problems, participates in the development of the plan of care, prepares clinical and progress notes, works with the family, uses appropriate community resources, participates in discharge planning and in-service programs, and acts as a consultant to other agency personnel.

§484.36 Condition of participation: Home health aide services.

Home health aides are selected on the basis of such factors as a sympathetic attitude toward the care of the sick, ability to read, write, and carry out directions, and maturity and ability to deal effectively with the demands of the job. They are closely supervised to ensure their competence in providing care. For home health services furnished (either directly or through arrangements with other organizations) after August 14, 1990, the HHA must use individuals who meet the personnel qualifications specified in §484.4 for "home health aide".

(a) Standard: Home health aide training—
(1) Content and duration of training. The aide training program must address each of the following subject areas through classroom and supervised practical training totaling at least 75 hours, with at least 16 hours devoted to supervised training. The individual being trained must complete at least 16 hours of classroom training before beginning the supervised practical training.

(i) Communications skills.

(ii) Observation, reporting and documentation of patient status and the care or service furnished.

(iii) Reading and recording temperature, pulse, and respiration.

(iv) Basic infection control procedures.

(v) Basic elements of body functioning and changes in body function that must be reported to an aide's supervisor.

(vi) Maintenance of a clean, safe, and healthy environment.

(vii) Recognizing emergencies and knowledge of emergency procedures.

(viii) The physical, emotional, and developmental needs of and ways to work with the populations served by the HHA, including the need for respect for the patient, his or her privacy and his or her property.

(ix) Appropriate and safe techniques in personal hygiene and grooming that include—
(A) Bed bath.
(B) Sponge, tub, or shower bath.
(C) Shampoo (sink, tub, or bed).
(D) Nail and skin care.
(E) Oral hygiene.
(F) Toileting and elimination.

(x) Safe transfer techniques and ambulation.

(xi) Normal range of motion and positioning.

(xii) Adequate nutrition and fluid intake.

(xiii) Any other task that the HHA may choose to have the home health aide perform.

"Supervised practical training" means training in a laboratory or other setting in which the trainee demonstrates knowledge while performing tasks on an individual under the direct supervision of a registered nurse or licensed practical nurse.

(2) Conduct of training—
(i) Organizations. A home health aide training program may be offered by any organization except an HHA that, within the previous 2 years has been found—

(A) Out of compliance with requirements of this paragraph (a) or paragraph (b) of this section;

(B) To permit an individual that does not meet the definition of "home health aide" as specified in §484.4 to furnish home health aide services (with the exception of licensed health professionals and volunteers);

(C) Has been subject to an extended (or partial extended survey as a result of having been found to have furnished substandard care (or for other reasons at the discretion of the HCFA or the State);

(D) Has been assessed a civil monetary penalty of not less than $5,000 as an intermediate sanction;

(E) Has been found to have compliance deficiencies that endanger the health and safety of the HHA's patients and has had a temporary management appointed to oversee the management of the HHA;

(F) Has had all or part of its Medicare payments suspended; or

(G) Under any Federal or State laws within the 2-year period beginning on October 1, 1988—

(1) Has had its participation in the Medicare program terminated;

(2) Has been assessed a penalty of not less than $5,000 for deficiencies in Federal or State standards for HHAs;

(3) Was subject to a suspension of Medicare payments to which it otherwise would have been entitled;

(4) Had operated under a temporary management that was appointed to oversee the operation of the HHA and to ensure the health and safety of the HHA's patients; or

(5) Was closed or had its residents transferred by the State.

(ii) Qualifications for instructors. The training of home health aides and the supervision of home health aides during the supervised practical portion of the training must be performed by or under the general supervision of a registered nurse who possesses a minimum of 2 years of nursing experience, at least 1 year of which must be in the provision of home health care. Other individuals may be used to provide instruction under the supervision of a qualified registered nurse.

(3) Documentation of training. The HHA must maintain sufficient documentation to demonstrate that the requirements of this standard are met.

(b) Standard: Competency evaluation and in-service training—(1) Applicability. An individual may furnish home health aide services on behalf of an HHA only after that individual has successfully completed a competency evaluation program as described in this paragraph. The HHA is responsible for ensuring that the individuals who furnish home health aide services on its behalf meet the competency evaluation requirements of this section.

(2) Content and frequency of evaluation and amount of in-service training. (i) The competency evaluation must address each of the subjects listed in paragraph (a)(1)(ii) through (xiii) of this section.

(ii) The HHA must complete a performance review of each home health aide no less frequently than every 12 months.

(iii) The home health aide must receive at least 12 hours of in-service during each 12 month period. The in-service training may be furnished while the aide is furnishing care to patients.

(3) Conduct of evaluation and training—(i) Organizations. A home health aide competency evaluation program may be offered by any organization except as specified in paragraph (a)(2)(i) of this section. The in-service training may be offered by any organization.

(ii) Evaluators and instructors. The competency evaluation must be performed by a registered nurse. The in-service training generally must be supervised by a registered nurse who possesses a minimum of 2 years of nursing experience, at least 1 year of which must be in the provision of home health care.

(iii) Subject areas. The subject areas listed at paragraphs (a)(1)(iii), (ix), (x), and (xi) of this section must be evaluated after observation of the aide's performance of the tasks with a patient. The other subject areas in paragraph (a)(1) of this section may be evaluated through written examination, oral examination, or after observation of a home health aide with a patient.

(4) Competency determination. (i) A home health aide is not considered competent in any task for which he or she is evaluated as "unsatisfactory". The aide must not perform that task without direct supervision by a licensed nurse until after he or she receives training in the task for which he or she was evaluated as "unsatisfactory" and passes a subsequent evaluation with "satisfactory".

(ii) A home health aide is not considered to have successfully passed a competency evaluation if the aide has an "unsatisfactory" rating in more than one of the required areas.

(5) Documentation of competency evaluation. The HHA must maintain documentation which demonstrates that the requirements of this standard are met.

(6) Effective date. The HHA must implement a competency evaluation program that meets the requirements of this paragraph before February 14, 1990. The HHA must provide the preparation necessary for the individual to successfully complete the competency evaluation program. After August 14, 1990, the HHA may use only those aides that have been found to be competent in accordance with §484.36(b).

(c) Standard: Assignment and duties of the home health aide.

(1) Assignment. The home health aide is assigned to a specific patient by the registered nurse. Written patient care instructions for the home health aide must be prepared by the registered nurse or other appropriate professional who is responsible for the supervision of the home health aide under paragraph (d) of this section.

(2) Duties. The home health aide provides services that are ordered by the physician in the plan of care and that the aide is permitted to perform under State law. The duties of a home health aide include the provision of hands-on personal care, performance of simple procedures as an extension of therapy or nursing services, assistance in ambulation or exercises, and assistance in administering medications that are ordinarily self-administered. Any home health aide services offered by an HHA must be provided by a qualified home health aide.

(d) Standard: Supervision.

(1) If the patient receives skilled nursing care, the registered nurse must perform the supervisory visits required by paragraph (d)(2) of this section. If the patient is not receiving skilled nursing care, but is receiving another skilled service (that is, physical therapy, occupational therapy, or speech-language pathology services), supervision may be provided by the appropriate therapist.

(2) The registered nurse (or another professional described in paragraph (d)(1) of this section) must make an on-site visit to the patient's home no less frequently than every 2 weeks.

(3) If home health aide services are provided to a patient who is not receiving skilled nursing care, physical or occupational therapy or speech-language pathology services, the registered nurse must make a supervisory visit to the patient's home no less frequently than every 62 days. In these cases, to ensure that the aide is properly caring for the patient, each supervisory visit must occur while the home health aide is providing patient care.

(4) If home health aide services are provided by an individual who is not employed directly by the HHA (or hospice), the services of the home health aide must be provided under arrangements, as defined in Section 1861(w)(1) of the Act. If the HHA (or hospice) chooses to provide home health aide services under arrangements with another organization, the HHA's (or hospice's) responsibilities include, but are not limited to—(i) Ensuring the overall quality of the care provided by the aide;

(ii) Supervision of the aide's services as described in paragraphs (d)(1) and (d)(2) of this section; and

(iii) Ensuring that home health aides are providing services under arrangements that have met the training requirements of paragraphs (a) and (b) of this section.

(e) Standard: Personal care attendant. Evaluation requirements.

(1) Applicability. This paragraph applies to individuals who are employed by HHAs exclusively to furnish personal care attendant services under a Medicaid personal care benefit.

(2) Rule. An individual may furnish personal care services, as defined in §440.170 of this chapter, on behalf of an HHA after the individual has been found competent by the State to furnish those services for which a competency evaluation is required by paragraph (b) of this section and which the individual is required to perform. The individual need not be determined competent in those services listed in paragraph (a) of this section that the individual is not required to furnish.

§484.38 Condition of participation: Qualifying to furnish outpatient physical therapy or speech pathology services.

An HHA that wishes to furnish outpatient physical therapy or speech pathology services must meet all the pertinent conditions of this part and also meet the additional health and safety requirements set forth in §§405.1717 through 405.1719, 405.1721, 405.1723, and 405.1725 of this chapter to implement section 1861(p) of the Act.

§484.48 Condition of participation: Clinical records.

A clinical record containing pertinent past and current findings in accordance with accepted professional standards is maintained for every patient receiving home health services. In addition to the plan of care, the record contains appropriate identifying information; name of physician; drug, dietary, treatment, and activity orders; signed and dated clinical and progress notes; copies of summary reports sent to the attending physician; and a discharge summary. The HHA must inform the attending physician of the availability of a discharge summary. The discharge summary must be sent to the attending physician upon request and must include the patient's medical and health status at discharge.

(a) Standard: Retention of records. Clinical records are retained for 5 years after the month the cost report to which the records apply is filed with the intermediary, unless State law stipulates a longer period of time. Policies provide for retention even if the HHA discontinues operations. If a patient is transferred to another health facility, a copy of the record or abstract is sent with the patient.

(b) Standard: Protection of records. Clinical record information is safeguarded against loss or unauthorized use. Written procedures govern use and removal of records and the conditions for release of information. Patient's written consent is required for release of information not authorized by law.

§484.52 Condition of participation: Evaluation of the agency's program.

The HHA has written policies requiring an overall evaluation of the agency's total program at least once a year by the group of professional personnel (or a committee of this group), HHA staff, and consumers, or by professional people outside the agency working in conjunction with consumers. The evaluation consists of an overall policy and administrative review and a clinical record review. The evaluation assesses the extent to which the agency's program is appropriate, adequate, effective, and efficient. Results of the evaluation are reported to and acted upon by those responsible for the operation of the agency and are maintained separately as administrative records.

(a) Standard: Policy and administrative review. As a part of the evaluation process the policies and administrative practices of the agency are reviewed to determine the extent to which they promote patient care that is appropriate, adequate, effective, and efficient. Mechanisms are established in writing for the collection of pertinent data to assist in evaluation.

(b) Standard: Clinical record review. At least quarterly, appropriate health professionals representing at least the scope of the program, review a sample of both active and closed clinical records to determine whether established policies are followed in furnishing services directly or under arrangement. There is a continuing review of clinical records for each 62-day period that a patient receives home health services to determine adequacy of the plan of care and appropriateness of continuation of care.

HCFA proposed to amend 42 CFR chapter IV as follows:

PART 484—CONDITIONS OF PARTICIPATION: HOME HEALTH AGENCIES

1. The authority citation for part 484 continues to read as follows:

Authority: Secs. 1102 and 1871 of the Social Security Act (42 U.S.C. 1302 and 1395 (hh)).

2. Part 484 is revised to read as follows:

PART 484—CONDITIONS OF PARTICIPATION: HOME HEALTH AGENCIES

Subpart A—General Provisions
Sec.
484.1 Basis and scope
484.2 Definitions
Subpart B—Patient Care
484.50 Condition of participation: Patient rights.
484.55 Condition of participation: Comprehensive assessment of patients.
484.60 Condition of participation: Care planning and coordination of services.
484.65 Condition of participation: Quality assessment and performance improvement.
484.70 Condition of participation: Skilled professional services.
484.75 Condition of participation: Home health aide services.
Subpart C—Organizational Environment
484.100 Condition of participation: Compliance with Federal, State, and local laws.
484.105 Condition of participation: Organization and administration of services.
484.110 Condition of participation: Clinical records.
484.115 Condition of participation: Personnel qualifications for skilled professionals.

Subpart A—General Provisions

§484.1 Basis and Scope.

(a) *Basis.* This part is based on sections 1861(o) and 1891 of the Act, which establish the conditions that an HHA must meet in order to participate in Medicare, and specify that the Secretary may impose additional requirements that are considered necessary to ensure the health and safety of patients.

(b) *Scope.* The provisions of this part serve as the basis for survey activities for the purpose of determining whether an agency meets the requirements for participation in Medicare.

§484.2 Definitions.

As used in this part—

Branch office means a location or site from which a home health agency provides services within a portion of the total geographic area served by the parent agency. The branch office is part of the home health agency and is located sufficiently close to share administration, supervision, and services in a manner that renders it unnecessary for the branch independently to meet the conditions of participation as a home health agency.

Parent home health agency means the agency that develops and maintains administrative control of branches.

Quality indicator means a specific, valid, and reliable measure of access, care outcomes, or satisfaction, or a measure of a process of care that has been empirically shown to be predictive of access, care outcomes, or satisfaction.

Subpart B—Patient Care

§484.50 Condition of participation: Patient rights.

The patient has the right to be informed of his or her rights. The HHA must protect and promote the exercise of these rights.

(a) *Standard: Notice of rights.*

(1) The HHA must provide the patient with a written notice of the patient's rights in advance of furnishing care to the patient or during the ini-

tial evaluation visit before the initiation of treatment.

(2) The HHA must maintain documentation showing that it has complied with the requirements of this section.

(b) *Standard: Exercise of rights and respect for property and person.*

(1) The patient has the right to exercise his or her rights as a patient of the HHA.

(2) The patient's family or guardian may exercise the patient's rights when the patient has been judged incompetent.

(3) The patient has the right to have his or her property treated with respect.

(4) The patient has the right to voice grievances regarding treatment or care that is (or fails to be) furnished, or regarding the lack of respect for property by anyone who is furnishing services on behalf of the HHA and must not be subjected to discrimination or reprisal for doing so.

(5) The HHA must investigate complaints made by a patient or the patient's family or guardian regarding treatment or care that is (or fails to be) furnished, or regarding the lack of respect for the patient or the patient's property by anyone furnishing services on behalf of the HHA, and must document both the existence of the complaint and the resolution of the complaint.

(c) *Standard: Right to be informed and to participate in planning care and treatment.*

(1) The patient has the right to be informed, in advance, about the care to be furnished, the plan of care, expected outcomes, barriers to treatment, and of any changes in the care to be furnished.

(i) The HHA must advise the patient in advance of the disciplines that will furnish care, and the frequency of visits proposed to be furnished.

(ii) The HHA must advise the patient in advance of any change in the plan of care before the change is made.

(2) The patient has the right to participate in the planning of the care.

(i) The HHA must advise the patient in ad-

vance of the right to participate in planning the care or treatment and in planning changes in the care or treatment.

(ii) The HHA must comply with the requirements of subpart 1 of part 489 of this chapter relating to maintaining written policies and procedures regarding advance directives. The HHA must inform and distribute written information to the patient, in advance, concerning its policies on advance directives, including a description of applicable State law.

(d) *Standard: Confidentiality of medical clinical records.* The patient has the right to confidentiality of the clinical records maintained by the HHA. The HHA must advise the patient of the agency's policies and procedures regarding disclosure of clinical records.

(e) *Standard: Patient liability for payment.*

(1) The patient has the right to be advised, before care is initiated, of the extent to which payment for the HHA services may be expected from Medicare or other sources, and the extent to which payment may be required from the patient. Before the plan of care is initiated, the HHA must inform the patient orally and in writing of:

(i) The extent to which payment may be expected from Medicare, Medicaid, or any other Federally funded or aided program known to the HHA;

(ii) The charges for services that will not be covered by Medicare; and

(iii) The charges that the individual may have to pay.

(2) The patient has the right to be advised orally and in writing of any changes in the information provided in accordance with paragraph (e)(1) of this section when they occur. The HHA must advise the patient of these changes orally and in writing as soon as possible, but no later than 30 calendar days from the date that the HHA becomes aware of a change.

(f) *Standard: Home health hotline.* The patient has the right to be advised of the availability of the toll-free home health hotline in the

State. When the agency accepts the patient for treatment of care, the HHA must advise the patient in writing of the telephone number of the home health hotline established by the State, the hours of its operation, and that the purpose of the hotline is to receive complaints or questions about local HHAs.

§484.55 Condition of participation: Comprehensive assessment of patients.

Each patient must receive, and an HHA must provide, a patient-specific, comprehensive assessment that identifies the patient's need for home care and that meets the patient's medical, nursing, rehabilitative, social, and discharge planning needs.

(a) *Standard: Drug regimen review.* The comprehensive assessment must include a review of the patient's drug regimen in order to identify any potential adverse effects and drug reactions, including ineffective drug therapy, significant side effects, significant drug interactions, duplicate drug therapy, and noncompliance with drug therapy.

(b) *Standard: Initial assessment visit.*

(1) Based on physician's orders, a registered nurse must perform an initial assessment visit to determine the immediate care and support needs of the patient. The initial assessment visit must be held either within 48 hours of referral, or within 48 hours of the patient's return home, or within 48 hours of the physician-ordered start of care date, if that is later.

(2) When rehabilitation therapy service (speech language pathology services, physical therapy, or occupational therapy) is the only service ordered by the physician, the initial assessment visit may be made by the appropriate rehabilitation skilled professional.

(c) *Standard: Timeframe for completion of the comprehensive assessment.* The HHA must complete the comprehensive assessment in a timely manner consistent with the patient's immediate needs, but no later than 5 working days after the start of care.

(d) *Standard: Update of comprehensive assessment.* The comprehensive assessment must include information on the patient's progress toward clinical outcomes, and must be updated and revised—

(1) As frequently as the condition of the patient requires, but not less frequently than every 62 days beginning with the start of care date;

(2) When the plan of care is revised for physician review and

(3) At discharge.

§484.60 Condition of participation: Care planning and coordination of services.

Each patient must have a written plan of care that must specify the care and services necessary to meet the patient-specific needs identified by the physician or in the comprehensive assessment, or both, and the measurable outcomes that the HHA anticipates will occur as a result of implementing and coordinating the plan of care. Patients are accepted for treatment on the basis of a reasonable expectation that the patient's medical, nursing, and social needs can be met adequately by the agency in the patient's place of residence.

(a) *Standard: Plan of care.* All home health services furnished to patients must follow a written plan of care established and periodically reviewed by a doctor of medicine, osteopathy, or podiatric in accordance with §409.42 of this chapter. All patient care orders must be included in the plan of care.

(b) *Standard: Review and revision of the plan of care.*

(1) The plan of care must be reviewed and revised by the physician and the HHA as frequently as the patient's condition requires, but no less frequently than once every 62 days, beginning with the date of start of care. The HHA must promptly alert the physician to any changes in the patient's condition that suggest a need to alter the plan of care or that suggest that measurable outcomes are not being achieved.

(2) A revised plan of care must include current information from the patient's comprehen-

sive assessment and information concerning the patient's progress toward outcomes specified in the plan of care.

(c) *Standard: Conformance with physician orders.*

(1) Services and treatments must be administered by agency staff only as ordered by the physician.

(2) Oral orders must be accepted only by personnel authorized to do so by applicable State and Federal laws and regulations as well as by the HHA's internal policies.

(3) When services are provided on the basis of a physician's oral orders, a registered nurse or qualified therapist responsible for furnishing or supervising the ordered services must put the orders in writing and sign and date the orders with the date of receipt. Oral orders must also be countersigned and dated by the physician.

(d) *Standard: Coordination of care.*

(1) The HHA must maintain a system of communication and integration of services, whether provided directly or under arrangement, that ensures the identification of patient needs and barriers to care, the ongoing liaison of all disciplines providing care, and the contact of the physician for relevant medical issues.

(2) The HHA identifies the level of coordination necessary to deliver care to the patient and involves the patient and care giver in coordination of care efforts.

§484.55 Condition of participation: Quality assessment and performance improvement.

The HHA must develop, implement, maintain, and evaluate an effective, data-driven quality assessment and performance improvement program. The program must reflect the complexity of the HHA's organization and services (including those services provided directly or under arrangement). The HHA must take actions that result in improvements in the HHA's performance across the spectrum of care.

(a) *Standard: Components of quality assessment and performance improvement program.* The HHA's quality assessment and performance improvement program must include, but not be limited to, the use of objective measures to demonstrate improved performance with regard to:

(1) Quality indicator data (derived from patient assessments) to determine if individual and aggregate measurable outcomes are achieved compared to a specified previous time period.

(2) Current clinical practice guidelines and professional practice standards applicable to home care.

(3) Utilization data, as appropriate (for example, numbers of staff, types of visits, hours of services, etc.).

(4) Patient satisfaction measures.

(5) Effectiveness and safety of services (including complex high technology services, if provided), including competency of clinical staff, promptness of service delivery, and whether patients are achieving treatment goals and measurable outcomes.

(b) *Standard: Monitoring performance improvement.* The HHA must take actions that result in performance improvements and must track performance to assure that improvements are sustained over time.

(c) *Standard: Prioritizing improvement activities.* The HHA must set priorities for performance improvement, considering prevalence and severity of identified problems and giving priority to improvement activities that affect clinical outcomes. The HHA must immediately correct any identified problems that directly or potentially threaten the health and safety of patients.

(d) *Standard: External quality assessment and performance improvement program.* The HHA must meet periodic external quality assessment and performance improvement reporting requirements as specified by HCFA.

(e) *Standard: Infection control.* The HHA must maintain an effective infection control program in accordance with the policies and procedures of the HHA and Federal and State requirements.

§484.70 Condition of participation: Skilled professional services.

Skilled professionals who provide services to HHA patients directly or under arrangement must participate in all aspects of care, including an ongoing multidisciplinary evaluation and development of the plan of care, and be actively involved in the HHA's quality assessment and performance improvement program. For purposes of this section, skilled professional services include skilled nursing services, physical therapy, speech language pathology services, and occupational therapy as specified in §409.44, and medical social worker and home health aide services as specified in §409.45.

(a) *Standard: Services of skilled professionals.* Skilled professional services are authorized, delivered, and supervised (that is, given authoritative procedural guidance) only by health care professionals who meet the appropriate qualifications specified under §484.115 and who practice under the HHA's policies and procedures.

(b) *Standard: Provision of services.* The HHA must ensure that a majority, at least 50 percent, of total skilled professional services are routinely provided directly by the HHA. An HHA may provide other skilled professional visits under arrangement as needed.

§484.75 Condition of participation: Home health aide services.

All home health aide services must be provided by individuals who meet the personnel requirements specified in paragraph (a) of this section.

(a) *Standard: Home health aide qualifications.* A qualified home health aide is a person who—

(1) Has successfully completed a State-established or other training program that meets the requirements of paragraph (b) of this section and a competency evaluation program or State licensure program that meets the requirements of paragraph (c) of this section, or a competency evaluation program or State licensure program that meets the requirements of paragraph (c) of this section; or has completed a nurse aide training or competency evaluation program approved by the State as meeting the requirements of §§483.151 through 483.154 of this chapter and is currently listed in good standing on the State nurse aide registry;

(2) Under paragraph (a)(1) of this section, an individual is not considered to have completed a training and competency evaluation program, or a competency evaluation program if, since the individual's most recent completion of this program(s), there has been a continuous period of 24 consecutive months during none of which the individual furnished services described in §409.40 of this chapter for compensation. If a 24-month lapse in furnishing services has occurred, the individual must complete another training and competency evaluation program or a competency evaluation program, as specified in paragraph (a)(1) of this section, before providing services.

(b) *Standard: Home health aide training.—* (1) *Content and duration of training.* The home health aide training must include classroom and supervised practical training that totals at least 75 hours. A minimum of 16 hours of classroom training must precede a minimum of 16 hours of supervised practical training. "Supervised practical training" means training in a practicum laboratory or other setting in which the trainee demonstrates knowledge while performing tasks on an individual under the direct supervision of a registered nurse or licensed practical nurse. The home health aide training program must address each of the following subject areas:

(i) Communication skills, including the ability to read, write, and make brief and accurate oral and written presentations to patients, care givers, and other HHA staff.

(ii) Observation, reporting, and documentation of patient status and the care or service furnished.

(iii) Reading and recording temperature, pulse, and respiration.

(iv) Basic infection control procedures.

(v) Basic elements of body functioning and changes in body function that must be reported to an aide's supervisor.

(vi) Maintenance of a clean, safe, and healthy environment.

(vii) Recognizing emergencies and knowledge of emergency procedures.

(viii) The physical, emotional, and developmental needs of and ways to work with the populations served by the HHA, including the need for respect for the patient, his or her privacy, and his or her property.

(ix) Appropriate and safe techniques in personal hygiene and grooming that include—

(A) Bed bath.

(B) Sponge, tub, or shower bath.

(C) Hair shampoo (sink, tub, or bed).

(D) Nail and skin care.

(E) Oral hygiene.

(F) Toileting and elimination.

(x) Safe transfer techniques and ambulation.

(xi) Normal range of motion and positioning.

(xii) Adequate nutrition and fluid intake.

(xiii) Any other task that the HHA may choose to have the home health aide perform. The HHA is responsible for training the home health aide, as needed, for skills not covered in this basic checklist.

(2) *Conduct of training: Eligible training organizations.* A home health aide training program may be offered by any organization except an HHA that, within the previous 2 years, has been found—

(i) Out of compliance with the requirements of paragraphs (b) or (c) of this section;

(ii) To permit an individual that does not meet the definition of "home health aide" as specified in paragraph (a) of this section to furnish home health aide services (with the exception of licensed health professionals and volunteers);

(iii) Has been subject to an extended (or partial extended) survey as a result of having been found to have furnished substandard care (or for other reasons at the discretion of HCFA or the State);

(iv) Has been assessed a civil monetary penalty of not less than $5,000 as an intermediate sanction;

(v) Has been found to have compliance deficiencies that endanger the health and safety of the HHA's patients and has had a temporary management appointed to oversee the management of the HHA;

(vi) Has had all or part of its Medicare payments suspended, or

(vii) Under any Federal or State law

(A) Has had its participation in the Medicare program terminated;

(B) Has been assessed a penalty of not less than $5,000 for deficiencies in Federal or State standards for HHAs;

(C) Was subject to a suspension of Medicare payments to which it otherwise would have been entitled;

(D) Had operated under a temporary management that was appointed to oversee the operation of the HHA and to ensure the health and safety of the HHA's patients; or

(E) Was closed or had its residents transferred by the State.

(3) *Conduct of training: Qualifications for instructors.* The training of home health aides must be performed by or under the supervision of a registered nurse. Other individuals may be used to provide instruction under the general supervision of the registered nurse.

(4) *Documentation of training.* The HHA must maintain documentation of the aide's successful completion of a home health aide training and competency evaluation program or competency evaluation program or State approved nurse aide training and competency evaluation to demonstrate that the requirements of this standard are met.

(c) *Standard: Competency evaluation.* An individual may furnish home health services on behalf of an HHA only after that individual has successfully completed a competency evaluation program as described in this section.

(1) The HHA must ensure that all individuals who furnish home health aide services to patients meet the competency evaluation requirements of this section. Personal care aides who exclusively provide personal care services to Medicaid patients under a State Medicaid per-

sonal care benefit must meet the requirements specified in paragraph (g) of this section.

(2) The competency evaluation must address each of the subjects listed in paragraphs (b)(l)(ii) through (xiii) of this section. Subject areas specified under paragraphs (b)(l)(iii), (ix), (x), and (xi) of this section must be evaluated by observing the aide's performance of the task with a patient. The remaining subject areas may be evaluated through written examination, oral examination, or after observation of the home health aide with a patient.

(3) A home health aide competency evaluation program may be offered by any organization, except as specified in paragraph (b)(2) of this section.

(4) The competency evaluation must be performed by a registered nurse in consultation with other skilled professionals, as appropriate.

(5) A home health aide is not considered competent in any task for which he or she is evaluated as "unsatisfactory." The aide must not perform that task without direct supervision by a licensed nurse until after he or she received training in the task for which he or she was evaluated as "unsatisfactory" and passes a subsequent evaluation with "satisfactory."

(6) The HHA must maintain documentation that demonstrates the requirements of this standard are met.

(d) *Standard: Inservice training.*

(1) The home health aide must receive at least 12 hours of inservice training in a 12-month period. During the first 12 months of employment, hours may be prorated based on the date of hire. The in-service training may occur while the aide is furnishing care to a patient.

(2) Inservice training may be offered by any organization except one that is excluded under paragraph (b)(2) of this section.

(3) The inservice training must be supervised by a registered nurse.

(e) *Standard: Home health aide assignments.*

(1) The home health aide is assigned to a specific patient by the registered nurse. Written patient care instructions for the home health aide must be prepared by the registered nurse or other appropriate skilled professional (that is, physical therapist, speech language pathologist, or occupational therapist) who is responsible for the supervision of the home health aide as specified under paragraph (f) of this section.

(2) The home health aide provides services that are ordered by the physician in the plan of care and that the aide is permitted to perform under State law. The duties of a home health aide include the provision of hands-on personal care, performance of simple procedures as an extension of therapy or nursing services, assistance in ambulation or exercises, and assistance in administering medications that are ordinarily self-administered.

(3) Home health aides must report changes in the patient's medical, nursing, rehabilitative, and social needs to the registered nurse or other appropriate skilled professional, and complete appropriate records in compliance with the HHA policies and procedures.

(f) *Standard: Supervision.*

(1) If the patient receives skilled nursing care, the registered nurse must perform the supervisory visit required under paragraph (f)(2) of this section. If the patient is not receiving skilled nursing care, but is receiving another skilled service (that is, physical therapy, occupational therapy, or speech-language pathology services), supervision may be provided by the appropriate skilled professional. Documentation of the supervisory visit must be made in the patient's record.

(2) The registered nurse (or another professional described in paragraph (f)(1) of this section) must make an onsite visit to the patient's home no less frequently than every 2 weeks.

(3) If home health aide services are provided to a patient who is not receiving skilled nursing care, physical or occupational therapy, or speech-language pathology services, the registered nurse must make a supervisory visit to the patient's home no less frequently than every 62 days. In these cases, each supervisory visit must occur while the home health aide is providing patient care to ensure that the aide is properly caring for the patient.

(4) If home health aide services are provided by an individual who is not employed directly by the HHA, the services of the home health aide must be provided under arrangement as defined in section 1861(w)(1) of the Act (42 U.S.C. 1395 x(w)). If the HHA chooses to provide home health aide services under arrangement with another organization, the HHA's responsibilities include, but are not limited to—

(i) Ensuring the overall quality of care provided by the aide;

(ii) Supervision of the aide's services as described in paragraphs (f)(1) and (2) of this section; and

(iii) Ensuring that home health aides providing services under arrangement have met the training or competency evaluation requirements, or both, of this condition.

(g) *Standard: Medicaid personal care aide services—Medicaid personal care benefit.*

(1) *Applicability.* This paragraph applies to individuals who are employed by HHAs exclusively to furnish personal care attendant services under a Medicaid personal care benefit.

(2) *Rule.* An individual may furnish personal care services, as defined in §440.170 of this chapter, on behalf of an HHA after the individual has been found competent by the State to furnish those services for which a competency evaluation is required by this section and which the individual is required to perform. The individual need not be determined competent in those services listed in this section that the individual is not required to furnish.

Subpart C—Organizational Environment

§484.100 Condition of participation: Compliance with Federal, State, and local laws.

(a) *Standard: Compliance with Federal, State, and local laws and regulations.* The HHA and its staff must operate and furnish services in compliance with all Federal, State, and local laws and regulations applicable to HHAs. If a state has established licensing requirements for HHAs, all HHAs must be approved by the State licensing authority as meeting those requirements whether or not they are required to be licensed by the State.

(b) *Standard: Disclosure of ownership and management information.* The HHA must comply with the requirements of part 420, subpart C of this chapter. The HHA also must disclose the following information to the State survey agency at the time of the HHA's initial request for certification, for each survey, and at the time of any change in ownership or management.

(1) The name and address of all persons with an ownership or control interest in the HHA as defined in §§420.201, 420.202, and 420.206 of this chapter.

(2) The name and address of each person who is an officer, a director, an agent, or a managing employee of the HHA as defined in §§420.201, 420.202, and 420.206 of this chapter.

(3) The name and address of the corporation, association, or other company that is responsible for the management of the HHA, and the name and address of the chief executive officer and the chairperson of the board of directors of that corporation, association, or other company responsible for the management of the HHA.

(c) *Standard: Licensing.* The HHA and its branches must be licensed in accordance with State licensure laws, if applicable, prior to providing Medicare reimbursed services.

(d) *Standard: Laboratory services.*

(1) If the HHA engaged in laboratory testing outside of the context of assisting an individual in self-administering a test with an appliance that has been cleared for the purpose by the Food and Drug Administration, such testing must be in compliance with all applicable requirements of part 493 of this chapter.

(2) If the HHA chooses to refer specimens for laboratory testing to another laboratory, the referral laboratory must be certified in the appropriate specialties and subspecialties of services

in accordance with the applicable requirements of part 493 of this chapter.

§484.105 Condition of participation: Organization and administration of services.

The HHA must organize, manage, and administer its resources to attain and maintain the highest practicable functional capacity for each patient regarding medical, nursing, and rehabilitative needs as indicated by the plan of care.

(a) *Standard: Governing body.* A governing body (or designated persons so functioning) must assume full legal authority and responsibility for the management and provision of all home health services, fiscal operations, quality assessment and performance improvement, and appoints a qualified administrator who is responsible for the day-to-day operation designated persons to carry out these functions.

(b) *Standard: Primary HHA.* The HHA that accepts the patient becomes the primary HHA and assumes responsibility for the interdisciplinary coordination and provision of services ordered on the patient's plan of care, and continuity of care, whether the services are provided directly or under arrangement.

(c) *Standard: Parent-branch relationship.*
(1) The parent home health agency provides direct support and administrative control of its branches.
(2) The branch office is located sufficiently close to the parent home health agency to effectively share administration, supervision, and services in a manner that renders it unnecessary for the branch separately to meet the conditions of participation as an HHA.

(d) *Standard: Services under arrangement.*
(1) The HHA must ensure that all arranged services provided by other entities or individuals meet the requirements of this part and the requirements of section 1861(w) of the Act (42 U.S.C. 1395x(w)).

(2) An HHA that has a written agreement with another agency or organization to furnish services to the HHA's patients maintains overall responsibility for those services.

(e) *Standard: Services furnished.* Part-time or intermittent skilled nursing services and at least one other therapeutic service (physical, speech, or occupational therapy; medical social services; or home health aide services) are made available on a visiting basis, in a place of residence used as a patient's home. An HHA must provide at least one of the qualifying services directly, but may provide the second qualifying service and additional services under arrangement with another agency or organization.

(f) *Standard: Physical therapy or speech-language pathology services.* An HHA that furnishes outpatient physical therapy or speech language pathology services must meet all of the applicable conditions of this part and the additional health and safety requirements set forth in §§485.711, 485.713, 485.715, 485.719, 485.723, and 485.727 of this chapter.

§484.110 Condition of participation: Clinical records.

A clinical record containing past and current findings is maintained for every patient who is accepted by the HHA for home health service. Information contained in the clinical record must be accurate, available to the patient's physician and appropriate HHA staff, and may be maintained electronically.

(a) *Standard: Contents of clinical record.* The record must include:
(1) The patient's current comprehensive assessment, clinical progress notes, and plan of care;
(2) Responses to medications, treatments, and services;
(3) A description of measurable outcomes relative to goals in the patient's plan of care that have been achieved; and

(4) A discharge summary that is available to physicians upon request.

(b) *Standard: Authentication.* All entries must be legible, clear, complete, and appropriately authenticated and dated. Authentication must include signatures or a secured computer entry by a unique identifier of a primary author who has reviewed and approved the entry.

(c) *Standard: Retention of records.* Clinical records must be retained for 5 years after the month the cost report to which the records apply is filed with the intermediary, unless State law stipulates a longer period of time. The HHA's internal policies must provide for retention of the clinical records even if the HHA discontinues operations. If a patient is transferred to another health facility, a copy of the records or discharge summary must be sent with the patient.

(d) *Standard: Protection of records.* Patient information and the record must be safeguarded against loss or unauthorized use.

§484.115 Personnel qualifications for skilled professionals.

(a) *General qualification requirements.* Except as specified in paragraphs (b) and (c) of this section, all skilled professionals who provide services directly by or under arrangements with an HHA must be legally authorized (licensed or, if applicable, certified or registered) to practice by the State in which he or she performs the functions or actions, and must act only within the scope of his or her State license or State certification or registration.

(b) *Exception for Federally defined qualifications.* The following Federally defined qualifications must be met:

(1) For physicians, the qualifications and conditions as defined in section 1861(r) of the Act and implemented at §410.20 of this chapter.

(2) For speech language pathologists, the qualifications specified in section 1861(ll)(1) of the Act.

(3) For home health aides, the qualifications required by section 1891(a)(3) of the Act and implemented at §484.75.

(c) *Exceptions when no State licensing laws or State certification or registration requirements exist.* If no State licensing laws or State certification or registration requirements exist for the profession, the following requirements must be met:

(1) The administrator of a home health agency must—

(i) Be a licensed physician; or

(ii) Hold an undergraduate degree and—

(A) Be a registered nurse, or

(B) Have education and experience in health service administration, with at least one year of supervisory or administrative experience in home health care or a related health care program, and in financial management.

(2) *An occupational therapist must—*

(i) Be a graduate of an occupational therapy curriculum accredited jointly by the Committee on Allied Health Education and Accreditation of the American Medical Association and the American Occupational Therapy Association; or

(ii) Be eligible for the National Registration Examination of the American Occupational Therapy Association; or

(iii) Have 2 years of appropriate experience as an occupational therapist, and have achieved a satisfactory grade on a proficiency examination conducted, approved, or sponsored by the U.S. Public Health Service, except that such determinations of proficiency do not apply with respect to persons initially licensed by a State or seeking initial qualification as an occupational therapist after December 31, 1977.

(3) *An occupational therapy assistant must—*

(i) Meet the requirements for certification as an occupational therapy assistant established by the American Occupational Therapy Association; or

(ii) Have 2 years of a appropriate experience as an occupational therapy assistant, and have achieved a satisfactory grade on a proficiency examination conducted, approved, or sponsored by the U.S. Public Health Service, except that such determinations of proficiency do not apply with respect to persons initially licensed by a State or seeking initial qualification as an occupational therapy assistant after December 31, 1977.

(4) *Physical therapist.* A person who—

(1) Has graduated from a physical therapy curriculum approved by—

(A) The American Physical Therapy Association;

(B) The Committee on Allied Health Education and Accreditation of the American Medical Association, or;

(C) The Council on Medical Education of the American Medical Association and the American Physical Therapy Association, or;

(ii) Prior to January 1, 1966—

(A) Was admitted to membership by the American Physical Therapy Association;

(B) Was admitted to registration by the American Registry of Physical Therapists or

(C) Has graduated from a physical therapy curriculum in a 4-year college or university approved by a State department of education; or

(iii) Has 2 years of appropriate experience as a physical therapist, and has achieved a satisfactory grade on a proficiency examination conducted, approved, or sponsored by the U.S. Public Health Service except that such determinations of proficiency do not apply with respect to persons initially licensed by a State or seeking qualification as a physical therapist after December 31, 1977; or

(iv) Was licensed or registered prior to January 1, 1966, and prior to January 1, 1970, had 15 years of full-time experience in the treatment of illness or injury through the practice of physical therapy in which services were rendered under the order and direction of attending and referring doctors of medicine or osteopathy; or

(v) If trained outside the United States—

(A) Was graduated since 1928 from a physical therapy curriculum approved in the country in which the curriculum was located and in which there is a member organization of the World Confederation for Physical Therapy;

(B) Meets the requirements for membership in a member organization of the World Confederation for Physical Therapy.

(5) *Physical therapist assistant.* A person who—

(i) Has graduated from a 2-year college-level program approved by the American Physical Therapy Association; or

(ii) Has 2 years of appropriate experience as a physical therapy assistant, and has achieved a satisfactory grade on a proficiency examination conducted, approved, or sponsored by the U.S. Public Health Service, except that these determinations of proficiency do not apply with respect to persons initially licensed by a State or seeking initial qualification as a physical therapy assistant after December 31, 1977.

(6) *Public health nurse.* A registered nurse who has completed a baccalaureate degree program approved by the National League for Nursing for public health nursing preparation or post-registered nurse study that includes content approved by the National League for Nursing for public health nursing preparation.

(7) *Registered nurse.* A graduate of a school of professional nursing.

(8) *Social work assistant.* A person who—

(i) Has a baccalaureate degree in social work, psychology, sociology, or other field related to social work, and has had at least 1 year of social work experience in a health care setting; or

(ii) Has 2 years of appropriate experience as a social work assistant, and has achieved a satisfactory grade on a proficiency examination conducted, approved, or sponsored by the U.S. Public Health Service, except that these determinations of proficiency do not apply with respect to persons initially licensed by a State or seeking initial qualification as a social work assistant after December 31, 1977.

(9) *Social worker.* A person who has a master's degree from a school of social work accredited by the Council on Social Work Education, and has 1 year of social work experience in a health care setting.

(Catalog of Federal Domestic Assistance Program No. 93.773, Medicare—Hospital Insurance; and Program No. 93.774, Medicare—Supplementary Medical Insurance Program)

Dated: July 15, 1996.

Bruce C. Vladeck,

Administrator, Health Care Financing Administration.

Dated: August 16, 1996.

Donna E. Shalala

Secretary

[FR Doc. 97–5316 Filed 3–5–97; 9:45 am]

BILLING CODE 4120–01–P

Competency Templates

Exhibit B–1 Aide Competency Template

Name _____   Date of Hire _____   Employee ID # _____

I. Pre-Hire Professional Competency Verification:

Copy of Diploma(s) in HR File ❏	Comments:
Verification of attendance of 75-hour CNA course & requirements ❏	
Copy of CNA in HR File ❏	
Copy of Current CPR card in HR File ❏	
Competent Performance verified by previous employer or school ❏	

II. Core Clinical Skills Competency—Initial and Ongoing

SKILL	*Initial* Competency Demonstrated (Enter Date)	Evaluation Method DO–Direct Observation SIM–Simulation CA–Chart Audit CT–Cognitive Testing (indicate score)	*Ongoing* Competency Assessment Dates/ Evaluation Method
1. Demonstrate strategies to minimize safety risks in the community.			
2. Demonstrate correct bag technique.			
3. Demonstrate standard precautions against blood and body fluid pathogens. (Use of PPE)			
4. Demonstrate handwashing.			
5. Demonstrate timely and accurate communication with colleagues.			
6. Demonstrate an effective working plan for time management and organization.			
7. Demonstrate at least minimal documentation proficiency.			
8. Demonstrate, organize, and effectively complete at least one home visit.			
9. Incorporate cultural, age-appropriate, family and environmental data into care, teaching, and assessment.			
10. Successfully complete and/or report data appropriately.			
11. Successfully demonstrate map reading and navigational skills.			
12. Monitor and/or report patient response to therapeutic interventions.			
13. Complete mandatory inservice requirements as outlined by organization.			

continues

Exhibit B–1 continued

Name _____   Date of Hire _____

III. HCA Competency Assessment—Initial and Ongoing

SKILL	*Initial* Competency Demonstrated (Enter Date)	Evaluation Method DO–Direct Observation SIM–Simulation CA–Chart Audit CT–Cognitive Testing (indicate score)	*Ongoing* Competency Assessment Dates/Evaluation Method
Reading and recording temperature, pulse, and respirations			
Giving a bed bath			
Giving a sponge bath, tub bath, and shower			
Shampooing (bed, sink, or tub)			
Skin care and back rubs			
Nail care (fingers and toes)			
Toileting and elimination: bedpan, urinal			
Oral hygiene (mouth and denture care)			
Transfer techniques (one or two people assisting, Hoyer lift)			
Ambulation assistance (cane, walker)			
Positioning in bed or chair			
Range of motion exercises			
Maintains a clean, safe environment			
Obtains 12 hours of inservice education annually			
Other:			

(Place pre/post test scores, class dates on line)

RN Evaluator's Signatures, Titles, and Initials: _____

_____

_____

Exhibit B–2 RN Competency Template

Name _____   Date of Hire _____   Employee ID # _____

I. Pre-Hire Professional Competency Verification:

Copy of Diploma(s) in HR File ❏	Comments:
Copy of License in HR File ❏	
Copy of Current CPR card in HR File ❏	
Competent Performance verified by previous employer ❏	
Verification of Certification(s) ❏	

II. Core Clinical Skills Competency—Initial and Ongoing

SKILL	*Initial* Competency Demonstrated (Enter Date)	Evaluation Method DO–Direct Observation SIM–Simulation CA–Chart Audit CT–Cognitive Testing (indicate score)	*Ongoing* Competency Assessment Dates/ Evaluation Methods
1. Demonstrate strategies to minimize safety risks in the community.			
2. Demonstrate correct bag technique.			
3. Demonstrate standard precautions against blood and body fluid pathogens. (Use of PPE)			
4. Demonstrate handwashing.			
5. Demonstrate timely and accurate communication with colleagues.			
6. Demonstrate an effective working plan for time management and organization.			
7. Demonstrate at least minimal documentation proficiency.			
8. Demonstrate, organize, and effectively complete at least one home visit.			
9. Incorporate cultural, age-appropriate, family and environmental data into care, teaching, and assessment.			
10. Successfully complete and/or report data appropriately.			
11. Successfully demonstrate map reading and navigational skills.			
12. Monitor and/or report patient response to therapeutic interventions.			
13. Complete mandatory inservice requirements as outlined by organization.			

continues

Exhibit B–2 continued

Name _____ Date of Hire _____

III. RN Competency Assessment—Initial and Ongoing

SKILL	*Initial* Competency Demonstrated (Enter Date)	Evaluation Method DO–Direct Observation SIM–Simulation CA–Chart Audit CT–Cognitive Testing (indicate score)	*Ongoing* Competency Assessment Dates/Evaluation Method
RESPIRATORY			
Oxygen Therapy:			
Face Mask			
Tracheal Collar			
Transtracheal			
Metered Dose Inhalers			
Suctioning:			
Nasal			
Tracheal			
Tracheostomy:			
Site Care			
Inner Cannula Change			
GASTROINTESTINAL			
Gastric:			
Insertion			
Maintenance			
Colostomy:			
Maintenance			
Irrigation			
Ileostomy:			
Maintenance			
GENITOURINARY			
Catheterization:			
Insertion—Male			
Insertion—Female			
Irrigation			

continues

Exhibit B–2 continued

SKILL	*Initial* Competency Demonstrated (Enter Date)	Evaluation Method DO–Direct Observation SIM–Simulation CA–Chart Audit CT–Cognitive Testing (indicate score)	*Ongoing* Competency Assessment Dates/Evaluation Method
Ureterostomy:			
Maintenance			
Nephrostomy:			
Maintenance			
Suprapubic catheter:			
Maintenance			
Biliary tube:			
Maintenance			
Flushing			
INFECTIOUS DISEASE			
Culture collection:			
Throat			
Wound			
INTEGUMENTARY			
Application of Compression Bandage			
Suture/Staple removal			
Wound Irrigation			
Removal of JP drain			
EQUIPMENT			
Pulse oximeter:			
Application			
Set-up			
Troubleshooting			
Nebulizers:			
Application			
Administration			
Tracheal			
Troubleshooting			

continues

Exhibit B–2 continued

SKILL	*Initial* Competency Demonstrated (Enter Date)	Evaluation Method DO–Direct Observation SIM–Simulation CA–Chart Audit CT–Cognitive Testing (indicate score)	*Ongoing* Competency Assessment Dates/Evaluation Method
Suction Machine:			
Set-up			
Operation			
Trouble shooting			
Enteral pumps:			
Set up			
Operation			
Troubleshooting			
Intravenous pumps: (List all used by geographical region)			
Glucometers: (List all used by geographical region)			

Place pre/post test scores, class dates in ongoing column.

Employee Signature _____

Evaluator's Signatures, Titles, and Initials: _____

Source: Adapted from Astarita, T.M., Competency Based Orientation in Home Care: One Agency's Approach, *Home Health Care Management and Practice*, Vol. 8, No. 4, pp. 43–44, © 1996, Aspen Publishers, Inc.

Exhibit B–3 LPN Competency Template

Name _____   Date of Hire _____   Employee ID # _____

I. Pre-Hire Professional Competency Verification:

Copy of Diploma(s) in HR File ❏	Comments:
Copy of License in HR File ❏	
Copy of Current CPR card in HR File ❏	
Competent Performance verified by previous employer ❏	

II. Core Clinical Skills Competency—Initial and Ongoing

SKILL	Initial Competency Demonstrated (Enter Date)	Evaluation Method DO–Direct Observation SIM–Simulation CA–Chart Audit CT–Cognitive Testing (indicate score)	Ongoing Competency Assessment Dates/ Evaluation Methods
1. Demonstrate strategies to minimize safety risks in the community.			
2. Demonstrate correct bag technique.			
3. Demonstrate standard precautions against blood and body fluid pathogens. (Use of PPE)			
4. Demonstrate handwashing.			
5. Demonstrate timely and accurate communication with colleagues.			
6. Demonstrate an effective working plan for time management and organization.			
7. Demonstrate at least minimal documentation proficiency.			
8. Demonstrate, organize, and effectively complete at least one home visit.			
9. Incorporate cultural, age-appropriate, family and environmental data into care, teaching, and assessment.			
10. Successfully complete and/or report data appropriately.			
11. Successfully demonstrate map reading and navigational skills.			
12. Monitor and/or report patient response to therapeutic interventions.			
13. Complete mandatory inservice requirements as outlined by organization.			

continues

Exhibit B–3 continued

Name _____   Date of Hire _____

III. LPN Competency Assessment—Initial and Ongoing

SKILL	*Initial* Competency Demonstrated (Enter Date)	Evaluation Method DO–Direct Observation SIM–Simulation CA–Chart Audit CT–Cognitive Testing (indicate score)	*Ongoing* Competency Assessment Dates/Evaluation Method
RESPIRATORY			
Oxygen Therapy:			
Face Mask			
Tracheal Collar			
Transtracheal			
Metered Dose Inhalers			
Suctioning:			
Nasal			
Tracheal			
Tracheostomy:			
Site Care			
Inner Cannula Change			
GASTROINTESTINAL			
Gastric:			
Insertion			
Maintenance			
Colostomy:			
Maintenance			
Irrigation			
Ileostomy:			
Maintenance			
GENITOURINARY			
Catheterization:			
Insertion—Male			
Insertion—Female			
Irrigation			

continues

Exhibit B–3 continued

SKILL	*Initial* Competency Demonstrated (Enter Date)	Evaluation Method DO–Direct Observation SIM–Simulation CA–Chart Audit CT–Cognitive Testing (indicate score)	*Ongoing* Competency Assessment Dates/Evaluation Method
Ureterostomy:			
Maintenance			
Nephrostomy:			
Maintenance			
Suprapubic catheter:			
Maintenance			
Biliary tube:			
Maintenance			
Flushing			
INFECTUOUS DISEASE			
Culture Collection:			
Throat			
Wound			
INTEGUMENTARY			
Application of Compression Bandage			
Suture/Staple removal			
Wound Irrigation			
Removal of JP drain			
EQUIPMENT			
Pulse oximeter:			
Application			
Set-up			
Troubleshooting			
Nebulizers:			
Application			
Administration			
Tracheal			
Troubleshooting			

continues

Exhibit B–3 continued

SKILL	*Initial* Competency Demonstrated (Enter Date)	Evaluation Method DO–Direct Observation SIM–Simulation CA–Chart Audit CT–Cognitive Testing (indicate score)	*Ongoing* Competency Assessment Dates/Evaluation Method
Suction Machine			
Set-up			
Operation			
Troubleshooting			
Enteral pumps:			
Set-up			
Operation			
Troubleshooting			
Intravenous pumps: (List all used by geographical region)			
Glucometers: (List all used by geographical region)			

Place pre/post test scores, class dates in ongoing column.

Employee Signature _____

Evaluator's Signatures, Titles, and Initials: _____

_____

Source: Adapted from Astarita, T.M., Competency Based Orientation in Home Care: One Agency's Approach, *Home Health Care Management and Practice*, Vol. 8, No. 4, pp. 43–44, © 1996, Aspen Publishers, Inc.

Exhibit B–4 PT Competency Template

Name _____ Date of Hire _____ Employee ID # _____

I. Pre-Hire Professional Competency Verification:

Copy of Diploma(s) in HR File ❑	Comments:
Copy of License in HR File ❑	
Copy of Current CPR card in HR File ❑	
Competent Performance verified by previous employer ❑	

II. Core Clinical Skills Competency—Initial and Ongoing

SKILL	*Initial* Competency Demonstrated (Enter Date)	Evaluation Method DO–Direct Observation SIM–Simulation CA–Chart Audit CT–Cognitive Testing (indicate score)	*Ongoing* Competency Assessment Dates/ Evaluation Methods
1. Demonstrate strategies to minimize safety risks in the community.			
2. Demonstrate correct bag technique.			
3. Demonstrate standard precautions against blood and body fluid pathogens. (Use of PPE)			
4. Demonstrate handwashing.			
5. Demonstrate timely and accurate communication with colleagues.			
6. Demonstrate an effective working plan for time management and organization.			
7. Demonstrate at least minimal documentation proficiency.			
8. Demonstrate, organize, and effectively complete at least one home visit.			
9. Incorporate cultural, age-appropriate, family and environmental data into care, teaching, and assessment.			
10. Successfully complete and/or report data appropriately.			
11. Successfully demonstrate map reading and navigational skills.			
12. Monitor and/or report patient response to therapeutic interventions.			
13. Complete mandatory inservice requirements as outlined by organization.			

continues

Exhibit B–4 continued

Name _____ Date of Hire _____

III. PT Competency Assessment—Initial and Ongoing

SKILL	*Initial* Competency Demonstrated (Enter Date)	Evaluation Method DO–Direct Observation SIM–Simulation CA–Chart Audit CT–Cognitive Testing (indicate score)	*Ongoing* Competency Assessment Dates/Evaluation Method
Home Assessment			
CPM Machine			
Manual Muscle Test/Gross Tests			
Goniometry			
Sensory Tests			
Balance			
Tone			
Joint			
Gait Analysis/Training			
Posture Analysis			
Coordination			
Vital Signs			
Skin and Wound			
Subjective Pain			
Orthosis check			
Biomechanical foot			
Pediatric, Age-Specific Guidelines			

Place pre/post test scores, class dates in ongoing column.

Employee Signature_____

Evaluator's Signatures, Titles, and Initials: _____

_____

Exhibit B–5 OT Competency Template

Name _____   Date of Hire _____   Employee ID # _____

I. Pre-Hire Professional Competency Verification:

Copy of Diploma(s) in HR File ❏	Comments:
Copy of License in HR File ❏	
Copy of Current CPR card in HR File ❏	
Competent Performance verified by previous employer ❏	

II. Core Clinical Skills Competency—Initial and Ongoing

SKILL	*Initial* Competency Demonstrated (Enter Date)	Evaluation Method DO–Direct Observation SIM–Simulation CA–Chart Audit CT–Cognitive Testing (indicate score)	*Ongoing* Competency Assessment Dates/ Evaluation Methods
1. Demonstrate strategies to minimize safety risks in the community.			
2. Demonstrate correct bag technique.			
3. Demonstrate standard precautions against blood and body fluid pathogens. (Use of PPE)			
4. Demonstrate handwashing.			
5. Demonstrate timely and accurate communication with colleagues.			
6. Demonstrate an effective working plan for time management and organization.			
7. Demonstrate at least minimal documentation proficiency.			
8. Demonstrate, organize, and effectively complete at least one home visit.			
9. Incorporate cultural, age-appropriate, family and environmental data into care, teaching, and assessment.			
10. Successfully complete and/or report data appropriately.			
11. Successfully demonstrate map reading and navigational skills.			
12. Monitor and/or report patient response to therapeutic interventions.			

continues

Exhibit B–5 continued

Name _____   Date of Hire _____

III. OT Competency Assessment—Initial and Ongoing

SKILL	*Initial* Competency Demonstrated (Enter Date)	Evaluation Method DO–Direct Observation SIM–Simulation CA–Chart Audit CT–Cognitive Testing (indicate score)	*Ongoing* Competency Assessment Dates/Evaluation Method
Functional Evaluation			
ADL Training			
Motor Re-education			
Perceptual Training			
Fine Motor Coordination Training			
Neurological/Reflex Training			
Sensory Training			
Orthotics/Splinting			
Gait Analysis/Training			
Use of adaptive equipment			
Coordination Testing			
Vital Signs			
Skin and Wound			
Subjective Pain			
Strength Conditioning			
Specific Pediatric Tools: Vestibular board, Developmental toys, etc			
Pediatric Assessment Tools: Gesell, HELP, DeGangi-Berk, etc.			

Place pre/post test scores, class dates in ongoing column.

Employee Signature_____

Evaluator's Signatures, Titles, and Initials: _____

_____

Exhibit B–6 ST Competency Template

Name _____ Date of Hire _____ Employee ID # _____

I. Pre-Hire Professional Competency Verification:

Copy of Diploma(s) in HR File ❏	Comments:
Copy of License in HR File ❏	
Copy of Current CPR card in HR File ❏	
Competent Performance verified by previous employer ❏	

II. Core Clinical Skills Competency—Initial and Ongoing

SKILL	*Initial* Competency Demonstrated (Enter Date)	Evaluation Method DO–Direct Observation SIM–Simulation CA–Chart Audit CT–Cognitive Testing (indicate score)	*Ongoing* Competency Assessment Dates/ Evaluation Methods
1. Demonstrate strategies to minimize safety risks in the community.			
2. Demonstrate correct bag technique.			
3. Demonstrate standard precautions against blood and body fluid pathogens. (Use of PPE)			
4. Demonstrate handwashing.			
5. Demonstrate timely and accurate communication with colleagues.			
6. Demonstrate an effective working plan for time management and organization.			
7. Demonstrate at least minimal documentation proficiency.			
8. Demonstrate, organize, and effectively complete at least one home visit.			
9. Incorporate cultural, age-appropriate, family and environmental data into care, teaching, and assessment.			
10. Successfully complete and/or report data appropriately.			
11. Successfully demonstrate map reading and navigational skills.			
12. Monitor and/or report patient response to therapeutic interventions.			
13. Complete mandatory inservice requirements as outlined by organization.			

continues

Exhibit B–6 continued

Name _____ Date of Hire _____

III. ST Competency Assessment—Initial and Ongoing

SKILL	*Initial* Competency Demonstrated (Enter Date)	Evaluation Method DO–Direct Observation SIM–Simulation CA–Chart Audit CT–Cognitive Testing (indicate score)	*Ongoing* Competency Assessment Dates/Evaluation Method
Evaluation and Assessment			
Voice Disorder Treatment			
Speech Articulation Disorder Treatment			
Use of Electrolarynx			
Use of Communication boards/books			
Use of Specialized pacifiers, nipples, bottles, electric toothbrushes with infants			
Aural rehabilitation			
Dysphagia treatments: swallowing, thermal sour stimulation, gag reflex			
Language disorder treatment: math skills, written/oral comprehension and expression, sequencing			

Place pre/post test scores, class dates in ongoing column.

Employee Signature_____

Evaluator's Signatures, Titles, and Initials: _____

_____

Exhibit B–7 Social Work Competency Template

Name _____ Date of Hire _____ Employee ID # _____

I. Pre-Hire Professional Competency Verification:

Copy of Diploma(s) in HR File ❏	Comments:
Copy of License in HR File ❏	
Copy of Current CPR card in HR File ❏	
Competent Performance verified by previous employer ❏	

II. Core Clinical Skills Competency—Initial and Ongoing

SKILL	*Initial* Competency Demonstrated (Enter Date)	Evaluation Method DO–Direct Observation SIM–Simulation CA–Chart Audit CT–Cognitive Testing (indicate score)	*Ongoing* Competency Assessment Dates/ Evaluation Methods
1. Demonstrate strategies to minimize safety risks in the community.			
2. Demonstrate correct bag technique.			
3. Demonstrate standard precautions against blood and body fluid pathogens. (Use of PPE)			
4. Demonstrate handwashing.			
5. Demonstrate timely and accurate communication with colleagues.			
6. Demonstrate an effective working plan for time management and organization.			
7. Demonstrate at least minimal documentation proficiency.			
8. Demonstrate, organize, and effectively complete at least one home visit.			
9. Incorporate cultural, age-appropriate, family and environmental data into care, teaching, and assessment.			
10. Successfully complete and/or report data appropriately.			
11. Successfully demonstrate map reading and navigational skills.			
12. Monitor and/or report patient response to therapeutic interventions.			
13. Complete mandatory inservice requirements as outlined by organization.			

continues

Exhibit B–7 continued

Name _____ Date of Hire _____

III. SW Competency Assessment—Initial and Ongoing

SKILL	*Initial* Competency Demonstrated (Enter Date)	Evaluation Method DO–Direct Observation SIM–Simulation CA–Chart Audit CT–Cognitive Testing (indicate score)	*Ongoing* Competency Assessment Dates/Evaluation Method
Evaluate client and family's perception/acceptance of needs and emotional responses to current situation			
Provide short-term therapy to address illness-related issues such as anger, depression, anxiety, caregiver burnout, or other			
Assess for and resolve high risk situations as follows: Abuse/neglect, Suicide, Inadequate food/medical supplies			
Successfully complete paperwork for a nursing home referral			
Locate and complete paperwork for appropriate referral to Medical Assistance			
List community resources to assist patients with HIV/AIDS. Drug/Alcohol related problems, teen pregnancy, domestic violence, or other problems			

Place pre/post test scores, class dates in ongoing column.

Employee Signature_____

Evaluator's Signatures, Titles, and Initials: _____

_____

APPENDIX C

Competency-Based Orientation Modules

Exhibit C–1 Aide CBO Module

STANDARD: DATA COLLECTION

Competency Statement: Collects and records data that are comprehensive, accurate, and systematic		
Performance Criteria	Learning Resource	Date Met/Evaluator
1. Collects and records data in standardized, systematic, and concise form		
2. Communicates appropriate data to other persons involved in the individual's or family's care		
3. Meets documentation deadlines per organizational standard		

STANDARD: PLANNING

Competency Statement: Is an efficient member of home care team		
Performance Criteria	Learning Resource	Date Met/Evaluator
1. Establishes time management system and focuses on improving organizational skills in order to increase efficiency		
2. Organizes home visit activities in an efficient and effective manner		
3. Takes into consideration needs of client		
4. Informs patient/caregiver of plan for visit prior to rendering care		

STANDARD: INTERVENTION

Competency Statement: Intervenes to provide comfort, to restore, improve, and promote health		
Performance Criteria	Learning Resource	Date Met/Evaluator
1. Safely provides care		
2. Documents interventions and responses of client/family		

STANDARD: INTERDISCIPLINARY COLLABORATION

Competency Statement: Collaborates with members of home care team		
Performance Criteria	Learning Resource	Date Met/Evaluator
1. Attends interdisciplinary conferences		
2. Communicates changes in patient condition to appropriate personnel		

Source: Portions of this exhibit are data from *Home Care Nursing Standards*, American Nurses Association.

continues

Exhibit C–1 continued

STANDARD: ETHICS

Competency Statement: Portrays ethical code of conduct		
Performance Criteria	Learning Resource	Date Met/Evaluator
1. Treats clients in a dignified, respectful manner		
2. Consults ethics committee with presumed or identified ethical dilemma		
3. Reports incidents in a concise, appropriate, and timely fashion		
4. Maintains client confidentiality		

STANDARD: STRUCTURE AND PROCESS OF HOME CARE ORGANIZATION (organization-specific)

Competency Statement: Demonstrates professional responsibility in the Home Care Aide Role		
Performance Criteria	Learning Resource	Date Met/Evaluator
1. Locates and interprets organizational structure, mission, vision, and goals	*As per organization	
2. List the types of care or services provided by the organization and the referral indicators for each		
3. Locates and interprets the policies and procedures of the organization, specifically: ❏ Advanced Directives ❏ Death and Dying ❏ Patient Confidentiality ❏ Incident Reporting ❏ Inclement Weather ❏ Dress Code ❏ Abuse and Neglect ❏ Personal Safety ❏ Referral Guidelines ❏ Emergency Preparedness ❏ Other:		
4. Identifies geographical service area		
5. Other		
6.		
7.		
8.		
9.		

*e.g., List specific policies, procedures. List pertinent videos, computer-assisted instruction, self-learning modules, primary and secondary references.

Exhibit C–2 PT CBO Module

STANDARD: LEGAL/ETHICAL CONSIDERATIONS

Competency Statement: The home care physical therapist complies with all the legal requirements of jurisdictions regulating the practice of physical therapy, and practices according to the *Code of Ethics* of the American Physical Therapy Association		
Performance Criteria	Learning Resource	Date Met/Evaluator
1. Identifies at least one potential ethical conflicts within home care practice		
2. Verbalizes correct protocol for presumed or identified ethical dilemmas or concerns		
3. Performs initial evaluation including informing patient/caregivers of rights and responsibilities, a clear description of the proposed intervention/treatment, including risks, costs, benefits, and alternatives to the patient/family		

STANDARD: INTERDISCIPLINARY COLLABORATION

Competency Statement: The home care physical therapist collaborates with all appropriate disciplines		
Performance Criteria	Learning Resource	Date Met/Evaluator
1. Attends an interdisciplinary conference involving his patients		
2. Leaves a voice mail with the RN case manager about the plan of care and patient progress		

STANDARD: INITIAL EXAMINATION AND EVALUATION

Competency Statement: The physical therapist performs and documents an initial examination and evaluates the results to identify problems and determine the diagnosis prior to intervention/treatment		
Performance Criteria	Learning Resource	Date Met/Evaluator
1. During orientation, at least one initial evaluation is documented, dated, and signed by the physical therapist		
2. Identifies objective tests and measures used to facilitate outcome measurement		
3. Sufficient data are documented to establish a plan of care		
4. At least one appropriate recommendation is made for additional services to meet the needs of the patient/client		

Source: Portions of this exhibit are data from *American Physical Therapy Association Standards,* © 1996, American Physical Therapy Association.

continues

Exhibit C–2 continued

STANDARD: PLAN OF CARE

Competency Statement: The physical therapist involves the patient/client and appropriate others in the planning, implementation, and assessment of the intervention/treatment program		
Performance Criteria	Learning Resource	Date Met/Evaluator
1. The plan of care includes realistic goals and expected functional outcomes		
2. The plan of care describes intervention/treatment, including frequency and duration		
3. The plan of care includes documentation that is dated and signed by the physical therapist who established the physical therapy plan of care		

STANDARD: INTERVENTION/TREATMENT

Competency Statement: The physical therapist provides, or delegates and supervises, the physical therapy intervention/treatment consistent with the results of the examination, evaluation, and plan of care		
Performance Criteria	Learning Resource	Date Met/Evaluator
1. Delegates appropriately, supervising those who are qualified to provide some aspects of treatment (e.g., PT aide, Home Care Aide)		
2. Revises treatment as indicated by patient progress on either actual patient or simulation		
3. Periodically documents, dates, and signs the patient re-examination and modifications of the plan of care in a simulated or actual case scenario encountered during orientation		

STANDARD: DISCHARGE/DISCONTINUATION OF TREATMENT OR INTERVENTION

Competency Statement: The physical therapist discharges the patient/client from physical therapy intervention/treatment when the goals or projected outcomes for the patient/client have been met, the patient requests discharge, is unable to continue, or the physical therapist determines that intervention/treatment is no longer warranted		
Performance Criteria	Learning Resource	Date Met/Evaluator
1. Discharge documentation includes the status of the patient/client at the time of discharge, the functional outcomes and goals achieved		
2. Discharge documentation is dated, signed, and completed within the time frame specified by the home care organization		
3. Rationale for discharge is included when discharge criteria are not met as per organizational policy. Must demonstrate on at least one discharge during orientation.		

continues

Exhibit C–2 continued

STANDARD: STRUCTURE AND PROCESS OF HOME CARE ORGANIZATION (organization-specific)

Competency Statement: Demonstrates professional responsibility in the Physical Therapist Role		
Performance Criteria	Learning Resource	Date Met/Evaluator
1. Locates and interprets organizational structure, mission, vision, and goals	*As per organization	
2. List the types of care or services provided by the organization and the referral indicators for each		
3. Locates and interprets the policies and procedures of the organization, specifically: ❏ *Advanced Directives* ❏ *Death and Dying* ❏ *Patient Confidentiality* ❏ *Incident Reporting* ❏ *Inclement Weather* ❏ *Dress Code* ❏ *Abuse and Neglect* ❏ *Personal Safety* ❏ *Referral Guidelines* ❏ *Emergency Preparedness* ❏ *Other:*		
4. Identifies geographical service area		
5. Interprets and adheres to payer guidelines		
6. Other		
7.		
8.		
9.		

*e.g., List specific policies, procedures. List pertinent videos, computer-assisted instruction, self-learning modules, primary and secondary references.

Exhibit C–3 OT CBO Module

STANDARD: SCREENING

Performance Criteria	Learning Resource	Date Met/Evaluator
1. Performs initial evaluation on at least one patient during orientation.		
2. Documents evidence of interdisciplinary collaboration, from beginning of service until discharge		
3. At least one appropriate recommendation is made for additional services to meet the needs of the patient/client		

STANDARD: ASSESSMENT

Performance Criteria	Learning Resource	Date Met/Evaluator
1. Completes at least one full assessment of functional capacity, including strengths and weaknesses of patient		
2. Communicates with family and patient the process, purpose, and findings of assessment		
3. Data collection utilizes a combination of observation, interview, record review, and where appropriate, standardized criterion reference tests* as evidenced by documentation within time frame specified by organization.		

STANDARD: PLANNING

Performance Criteria	Learning Resource	Date Met/Evaluator
1. Develops and documents treatment plan based on initial evaluation		
2. Writes goals that are clear, measurable, and behavioral/functional either in clinical or simulated case scenario		
3. Treatment plan includes estimation of potential, strengths and weaknesses, measurable goals, individual differences and needs, input from family/patient, plan for reevaluation, and discharge planning		

STANDARD: INTERVENTION

Performance Criteria	Learning Resource	Date Met/Evaluator
1. Verbalizes resources available to review literature about pertinent topics		
2. Utilizes teaching materials appropriately for patient/family relevant to interventions		
3. Updates interventional strategies appropriately based on patient responses and progress		

Source: Portions of this exhibit are data from *American Occupational Therapy Association Standards*, pp. 129–136, © 1994, American Occupational Therapy Association.

continues

Exhibit C–3 continued

STANDARD: TRANSITION SERVICES

Performance Criteria	Learning Resource	Date Met/Evaluator
1. Discharge planning will be initiated upon admission, providing patient with appropriate information about community resources		
2. Formal discharge plan will be developed based on individual needs as demonstrated on either real or simulated case scenario		
3. Outcomes measurement should evaluate the effectiveness of interventions and provide implications for any services the patient will receive upon discharge from home care. During orientation, at least one sample discharge summary should be completed including these data.		

STANDARD: STRUCTURE AND PROCESS OF HOME CARE ORGANIZATION (organization-specific)

Competency Statement: Demonstrates professional responsibility in the Home Care Physical Therapist Role		
Performance Criteria	Learning Resource	Date Met/Evaluator
1. Locates and interprets organizational structure, mission, vision, and goals		
2. Lists the types of care or services provided by the organization and the referral indicators for each		
3. Locates and interprets the policies and procedures of the organization, specifically: ❏ Advanced Directives ❏ Death and Dying ❏ Patient Confidentiality ❏ Incident Reporting ❏ Inclement Weather ❏ Dress Code ❏ Abuse and Neglect ❏ Personal Safety ❏ Referral Guidelines ❏ Emergency Preparedness ❏ Other:		

continues

Exhibit C–3 continued

STANDARD: STRUCTURE AND PROCESS OF HOME CARE ORGANIZATION (organization-specific) (continued)

Competency Statement: Demonstrates professional responsibility in the Home Care Occupational Therapist Role		
Performance Criteria	Learning Resource	Date Met/Evaluator
4. Identifies geographical service area		
5. Interprets and adheres to payer guidelines		
6. Other		
7.		
8.		
9.		

Data from American Nurses Association Home Care Nursing Standards

*e.g., List specific policies, procedures. List pertinent videos, computer-assisted instruction, self-learning modules, primary and secondary references.

Exhibit C–4 Speech and Audiology CBO Module

STANDARD: ASSESSMENT

Competency Statement: Provides comprehensive discipline-specific assessment techniques.		
Performance Criteria	Learning Resource	Date Met/Evaluator
1. Completes at least one initial evaluation for functional communication ability		
2. Administers at least one standardized criterion-referenced test and interprets results		
3. Administers audiologic tests in the home and documents findings		
4. Evaluates at least one patient utilizing augmented communication or listening assistive devices and their effectiveness.		

STANDARD: TREATMENT

Competency Statement: Provides individualized interventions.		
Performance Criteria	Learning Resource	Date Met/Evaluator
1. In course of initial evaluation, obtains patient/family input when planning treatment, informing of rehabilitation potential		
2. Performs period reassessments within time frame as specified by organization. Simulation or actual case scenario may be utilized to demonstrate		
3. Evaluates fit and efficacy of assistive devices		

STANDARD: INTERDISCIPLINARY COLLABORATION

Competency Statement: The home care speech therapist/audiologist collaborates with all appropriate disciplines		
Performance Criteria	Learning Resource	Date Met/Evaluator
1. Attends an interdisciplinary conference involving his patients		
2. Leaves a voice mail with the RN case manager about the plan of care and patient progress		

Source: Portions of this exhibit are data from *Guidelines for Delivery of Speech Pathology and Audiology Services in Home Care*, pp. IV56–IV57.

continues

Exhibit C–4 continued

STANDARD: LEGAL/ETHICAL CONSIDERATIONS

Competency Statement: The home care speech therapist/audiologist performs in accordance with organizational codes of ethics		
Performance Criteria	Learning Resource	Date Met/Evaluator
1. Identifies at least one potential ethical conflict within home care practice		
2. Verbalizes correct protocol for presumed or identified ethical dilemmas or concerns		
3. Performs initial evaluation including informing patient/caregivers of rights and responsibilities, a clear description of the proposed intervention/treatment, including risks, costs, benefits, and alternatives to the patient/family		

STANDARD: DISCHARGE/DISCONTINUATION OF TREATMENT OR INTERVENTION

Competency Statement:The speech therapist/audiologist discharges the patient/client from therapy intervention/treatment when the goals or projected outcomes for the patient/client have been met, the patient requests discharge, is unable to continue, or the therapist determines that intervention/treatment is no longer warranted		
Performance Criteria	Learning Resource	Date Met/Evaluator
1. Discharge documentation includes the status of the patient/client at the time of discharge, the functional outcomes and goals achieved		
2. Discharge documentation is dated, signed, and completed within the time frame specified by the home care organization		
3. Rationale for discharge is included when discharge criteria are not met as per organizational policy. Must demonstrate on at least one discharge during orientation.		

STANDARD: STRUCTURE AND PROCESS OF HOME CARE ORGANIZATION (organization-specific)

Competency Statement: Demonstrates professional responsibility in the Home Care Speech Therapist/Audiologist role		
Performance Criteria	Learning Resource	Date Met/Evaluator
1. Locates and interprets organizational structure, mission, vision, and goals	*As per organization	

continues

Exhibit C–4 continued

STANDARD: STRUCTURE AND PROCESS OF HOME CARE ORGANIZATION (organization-specific)
(continued)

Competency Statement: Demonstrates professional responsibility in the Home Care Speech Therapist/Audiologist role		
Performance Criteria	Learning Resource	Date Met/Evaluator
2. Lists the types of care or services provided by the organization and the referral indicators for each		
3. Locates and interprets the policies and procedures of the organization, specifically: ❐ *Advanced Directives* ❐ *Death and Dying* ❐ *Patient Confidentiality* ❐ *Incident Reporting* ❐ *Inclement Weather* ❐ *Dress Code* ❐ *Abuse and Neglect* ❐ *Personal Safety* ❐ *Referral Guidelines* ❐ *Emergency Preparedness* ❐ *Other:*		
4. Identifies geographical service area		
5. Interprets and adheres to payer guidelines		
6. Other		
7.		
8.		
9.		

*e.g., List specific policies, procedures. List pertinent videos, computer-assisted instruction, self-learning modules, primary and secondary references.

Exhibit C–5 Social Work CBO Module

Competency Statement: Social workers in home health settings shall have knowledge of chronic, acute, and terminal illnesses, physical disabilities, and the resultant age-specific impact on individual and family systems		
Performance Criteria	Learning Resource	Date Met/Evaluator
1. Assesses for potential sequelae from long-term illnesses, functional losses, social isolation, and economic instability when developing plan for social work, documenting appropriately		
2. Evaluates other factors that affect care (e.g., environment, family, home, work, finances); evaluates their impact and intervenes appropriately		
3. Identifies current coping mechanisms used by the patient, family, and staff, and intervenes appropriately		

Competency Statement: The home health social worker shall integrate social work intervention with that of other members of the interdisciplinary team		
Performance Criteria	Learning Resource	Date Met/Evaluator
1. Educates colleagues from other disciplines regarding the psychosocial needs of the client and family		
2. Documents evidence of interdisciplinary collaboration		

Competency Statement: The home health social worker shall work to achieve an appropriate continuum of care, assuring the clients of ongoing services to meet their needs		
Performance Criteria	Learning Resource	Date Met/Evaluator
1. Lists several referral sources		
2. Establishes factors for discharge		
3. Uses negotiation, persuasion, conflict management, and confrontation skills in a simulated or actual case setting		

Source: Portions of this exhibit are data from National Association of Social Work.

continues

Exhibit C–5 continued

Competency Statement: The functions of the social worker in home health settings shall include specific services to the client population, the staff of the agency, and the community		
Performance Criteria	Learning Resource	Date Met/Evaluator
1. Uses clear, effective, and timely communication with colleagues, clients, and families	*As per organization	
2. Acknowledges and uses the expertise of others through formal and informal consultation		
3. Contributes to overall effectiveness of homecare services as evidenced by adhering to established protocols, policy and procedures		

STANDARD: STRUCTURE AND PROCESS OF HOME CARE ORGANIZATION (organization-specific)

Competency Statement: Demonstrates professional responsibility in the Home Care Social Worker Role		
Performance Criteria	Learning Resource	Date Met/Evaluator
1. Locates and interprets organizational structure, mission, vision, and goals	*As per organization	
2. List sthe types of care or services provided by the organization and the referral indicators for each		
3. Locates and interprets the policies and procedures of the organization, specifically: ❏ Advanced Directives ❏ Death and Dying ❏ Patient Confidentiality ❏ Incident Reporting ❏ Inclement Weather ❏ Dress Code ❏ Abuse and Neglect ❏ Personal Safety ❏ Referral Guidelines ❏ Emergency Preparedness ❏ Other:		
4. Identifies geographical service area		
5. Interprets and adheres to payer guidelines		
6. Other		
7.		
8.		
9.		

*e.g., List specific policies, procedures. List pertinent videos, computer-assisted instruction, self-learning modules, primary and secondary references.

Exhibit C–6 RN CBO Module

STANDARD: THEORY

Competency Statement: Applies theoretical concepts as a basis for decisions in practice		
Performance Criteria	Learning Resource	Date Met/Evaluator
1. Locates resources for referencing conceptual bases for practice		
2. Summarizes organizational policy for continuing education		
3. Examines personal and professional assumptions about home health practice as specialized area of community health nursing		
4. Nursing actions are congruent with recognized nursing theories and established knowledge		
5. Recognized nursing theories and knowledge are evaluated and tested within the practice setting		

STANDARD: DATA COLLECTION

Competency Statement: Collects and records data that are comprehensive, accurate, and systematic		
Performance Criteria	Learning Resource	Date Met/Evaluator
1. Collects and records data in standardized, systematic, and concise form		
2. In conjunction with the family and individual, collects appropriate data		
3. Participates in an ongoing interdisciplinary process of revising and reviewing the data base on the individual and family		
4. Communicates appropriate data to other persons involved in the individual's or family's care		
5. Utilizes nursing information system as instructed		
6. Ensures that appropriate documentation related to patient teaching methods and response to teaching is completed		
7. Portrays knowledge of and follows care maps		
8. Documents strategies and interventions according to organizational standards		
9. Meets documentation deadlines		

Source: Portions of this exhibit are data from *Standards of Home Health Nursing Practice*, © 1997, American Nurses Association.

continues

Exhibit C–6 continued

STANDARD: DIAGNOSIS

Competency Statement: Utilizes health assessment data to determine nursing diagnosis		
Performance Criteria	Learning Resource	Date Met/Evaluator
1. Demonstrates competent assessment skills		
2. Formulates and revises nursing diagnoses through comprehensive and continuing assessment		
3. Collaborates with other health personnel to assure that diagnoses are congruent with the individual's or family's clinical status		
4. Communicates the nursing diagnoses obtained during health assessment to appropriate members of the health care team		
5. Identifies factors that affect care (e.g., environment, safety)		

STANDARD: PLANNING

Competency Statement: Develops care plans that establish goals: Is based upon nursing diagnoses, and incorporates therapeutic, preventative, and rehabilitative nursing actions		
Performance Criteria	Learning Resource	Date Met/Evaluator
1. Initiates development of client care plan in partnership with the client, family, physician, and other appropriate health care professionals		
2. Revises plan as goals and objectives are achieved or changed		
3. Documents plan in a standardized, systematic and concise form		
4. Client care plan reflects relevant theoretical concepts, includes measurable goals including date of accomplishment, identifies sequence of action for achieving goals, and proposes alternatives for continuity of care		

continues

Exhibit C–6 continued

STANDARD: PLANNING (continued)

Competency Statement: Develops care plans that establish goals: Is based upon nursing diagnoses, and incorporates therapeutic, preventative, and rehabilitative nursing actions		
Performance Criteria	Learning Resource	Date Met/Evaluator
5. Selects and demonstrates teaching strategies appropriate to content and level of knowledge		
6. Selects teaching content appropriate to patient level of knowledge		
7. Consults other disciplines before developing a teaching plan		
8. Anticipates potential problems and rapidly identifies emerging problems		
9. Anticipates and projects patient care supplies, equipment, and medication needed to control patient care situation		
10. Goal development focuses on prevention of complications and health promotion		
11. Establishes time management system and focuses on improving organization skills in order to increase efficiency		
12. Establishes priorities for patient care effectively		
13. Projects patient visits		
14. Identifies potential barriers to optimum goal attainment		
15. Develops a time frame for teaching, training, and return demonstrations in order to achieve desired outcomes		
16. Identifies clinical care environmental hazards and intervenes satisfactorily		
17. Demonstrates how and when to terminate skilled nursing services		
18. Develops interventions based upon applicable scientific theories		

continues

Exhibit C–6 continued

STANDARD: INTERVENTION

Competency Statement: Intervenes to provide comfort, to restore, improve, and promote health; to prevent complications and sequelae of illness and to effect rehabilitation		
Performance Criteria	Learning Resource	Date Met/Evaluator
1. Intervenes with the concurrence and or participation of the client and family		
2. Safely administers medically prescribed medication and treatment		
3. Treats physical and psychological responses to changes in health status, level of independence, and treatment		
4. Supervises and evaluates ancillary personnel who provide care to clients and families		
5. Informs the client and family about the client's health status, health care resources, and treatment		
6. Documents interventions and responses of the client/family		
7. Identifies geographical community resources; consults and refers patients when appropriate		
8. Utilizes principles of adult learning when providing patient/caregiver education		
9. Provides patient/caregiver with education materials		

STANDARD: EVALUATION

Competency Statement: Evaluates clients' and families' responses to interventions in order to determine progress toward goal attainment and to revise the database, nursing diagnoses, and plan of care		
Performance Criteria	Learning Resource	Date Met/Evaluator
1. Clearly documents the evaluation results and revision of the plan of care, as well as the results of care		
2. In conjunction with the client and family, revises priorities, goals, and interventions as indicated in the evaluation process		
3. Recognizes variances to patient care delivery and identifies reason for variance		

continues

Exhibit C–6 continued

STANDARD: EVALUATION (continued)

Competency Statement: Evaluates clients' and families' responses to interventions in order to determine progress toward goal attainment and to revise the database, nursing diagnoses and plan of care		
Performance Criteria	Learning Resource	Date Met/Evaluator
4. Evaluates nursing care to determine whether individualized patient care needs are being met and if quality of care is being maintained		
5. Evaluates the effectiveness of teaching on an ongoing basis and updates plan as needed		

STANDARD: CONTINUITY OF CARE

Competency Statement: Provides appropriate and uninterrupted care along the health care continuum, utilizing discharge planning, case management, and coordination of resources		
Performance Criteria	Learning Resource	Date Met/Evaluator
1. Establishes factors for discharge on admission		
2. Assesses the total health care needs of the client and family, including physiological, psychological, intellectual, social, emotional, spiritual, environmental, and education needs		
3. Assesses and coordinates all appropriate services and resources of the client		

STANDARD: INTERDISCIPLINARY COLLABORATION

Competency Statement: Initiates and maintains a liaison relationship with all appropriate health care providers to assure that all efforts effectively complement one another		
Performance Criteria	Learning Resource	Date Met/Evaluator
1. Demonstrates evidence of two-way communication between disciplines		
2. Consults and plans with colleagues, recognizing the team as an integral part of one's own effectiveness		

continues

Exhibit C–6 continued

STANDARD: INTERDISCIPLINARY COLLABORATION (continued)

Competency Statement: Initiates and maintains a liaison relationship with all appropriate health care providers to assure that all efforts effectively complement one another		
Performance Criteria	Learning Resource	Date Met/Evaluator
3. Acknowledges and uses expertise of others through formal and informal consultations for evaluation and planning patient care		
4. Develops mechanism for regular contact with multidisciplinary team members to coordinate care		
5. Solicits prompt responses from physicians		
6. Attends interdisciplinary conferences		
7. Documents interdisciplinary collaboration		

STANDARD: ETHICS

Competency Statement: Utilizes code for nurses established by the ANA as a guide for ethical decision making in practice		
Performance Criteria	Learning Resource	Date Met/Evaluator
1. Provides an example of an ethical dilemma encountered in home care practice		
2. Consults ethics committee with presumed or identified ethical dilemmas or concerns		
3. Reports incidents in concise, appropriate, and timely fashion		
4. Informs patient/caregivers of rights and responsibilities and interacts with patients in manners which uphold the same		
5. Maintains client confidentiality		
6. Obtains informed consent		
7. Intervenes to promote patient safety and security in manners consistent with the ethical and legal parameters of the scope within the nurse practice act		

continues

Exhibit C–6 continued

STANDARD: STRUCTURE AND PROCESS OF HOME CARE ORGANIZATION (organization-specific)

Competency Statement: Demonstrates professional responsibility in the RN Home Care Role		
Performance Criteria	Learning Resource	Date Met/Evaluator
Organization-specific competencies	*As per organization	
1. Locates and interprets organizational structure, mission, vision, and goals		
2. Lists the types of care or services provided by the organization and the referral indicators for each		
3. Locates and interprets the policies and procedures of the organization, specifically: ❏ *Advanced Directives* ❏ *Death and Dying* ❏ *Patient Confidentiality* ❏ *Incident Reporting* ❏ *Inclement Weather* ❏ *Dress Code* ❏ *Abuse and Neglect* ❏ *Personal Safety* ❏ *Referral Guidelines* ❏ *Emergency Preparedness* ❏ *Other:*		
4. Identifies geographical service area		
5. Interprets and adheres to payer guidelines		
6. Other		
7.		
8.		
9.		

*e.g., List specific policies, procedures. List pertinent videos, computer-assisted instruction, self-learning modules, primary and secondary references.

Exhibit C–7 LPN CBO Module

STANDARD: DATA COLLECTION

Competency Statement: Collects and records data that are comprehensive, accurate, and systematic		
Performance Criteria	Learning Resource	Date Met/Evaluator
1. Collects and records data in standardized. systematic, and concise form		
2. In conjunction with the family and individual, collects appropriate data		
3. Communicates appropriate data to other persons involved in the individual's or family's care		
4. Utilizes nursing information system as instructed		
5. Ensures that appropriate documentation related to patient teaching methods and response to teaching is completed		
6. Utilizes nursing information system as instructed		
7. Portrays knowledge of and follows care maps		
8. Documents strategies and interventions according to organizational standards		
9. Meets documentation deadlines		

STANDARD: PLANNING

Competency Statement: Develops care plans that establish goals: Is based upon nursing diagnoses, and incorporates therapeutic, preventative, and rehabilitative nursing actions		
Performance Criteria	Learning Resource	Date Met/Evaluator
1. Documents plan in a standardized, systematic, and concise form		
2. Selects and demonstrates teaching strategies appropriate to content and level of knowledge		
3. Selects teaching content appropriate to patient level of knowledge		
4. Anticipates potential problems and rapidly identifies emerging problems		
5. Anticipates and projects patient care supplies, equipment, and medication needed to control patient care situation		
6. Establishes time management system and focuses on improving organization skills in order to increase efficiency		

Source: Portions of this exhibit are data from *Standards of Home Health Nursing Practice,* © 1997, American Nurses Association.

continues

Exhibit C–7 continued

STANDARD: PLANNING (continued)

Competency Statement: Develops care plans that establish goals: Is based upon nursing diagnoses, and incorporates therapeutic, preventative, and rehabilitative nursing actions		
Performance Criteria	Learning Resource	Date Met/Evaluator
7. Establishes priorities for patient care effectively		
8. Identifies potential barriers to optimum goal attainment		
9. Identifies clinical care environmental hazards and intervenes satisfactorily		

STANDARD: DIAGNOSIS

Competency Statement: Utilizes health assessment data to determine nursing diagnosis		
Performance Criteria	Learning Resource	Date Met/Evaluator
1. Demonstrates competent assessment skills		
2. Identifies factors that affect care (e.g., environment, safety)		

STANDARD: INTERVENTION

Competency Statement: Intervenes to provide comfort, to restore, improve, and promote health; to prevent complications and sequelae of illness and to affect rehabilitation		
Performance Criteria	Learning Resource	Date Met/Evaluator
1. Intervenes with the concurrence and or participation of the client and family		
2. Safely administers medically prescribed medication and treatment		
3. Treats physical and psychological responses to changes in health status, level of independence, and treatment		
4. Informs the client and family about the client's health status, health care resources, and treatment		
5. Documents interventions and responses of the client/family		

continues

Exhibit C–7 continued

STANDARD: INTERVENTION (continued)

Competency Statement: Intervenes to provide comfort, to restore, improve, and promote health; to prevent complications and sequelae of illness and to effect rehabilitation		
Performance Criteria	Learning Resource	Date Met/Evaluator
6. Identifies geographical community resources; consults and refers patients when appropriate		
7. Utilizes principles of adult learning when providing patient/caregiver education		
8. Provides patient/caregiver with educational materials		

STANDARD: EVALUATION

Competency Statement: Evaluates clients' and families' responses to interventions in order to determine progress toward goal attainment and to revise the database, nursing diagnoses, and plan of care		
Performance Criteria	Learning Resource	Date Met/Evaluator
1. Provides data to assist RN in the evaluation of the plan of care		
2. Recognizes variances to patient care delivery and identifies reason for variance		
3. Evaluates the effectiveness of teaching on an ongoing basis		

STANDARD: INTERDISCIPLINARY COLLABORATION

Competency Statement: Initiates and maintains a liaison relationship with all appropriate health care providers to assure that all efforts effectively complement one another		
Performance Criteria	Learning Resource	Date Met/Evaluator
1. Demonstrates evidence of two-way communication between disciplines		
2. Consults and plans with colleagues, recognizing the team as an integral part of one's own effectiveness		

continues

Exhibit C–7 continued

STANDARD: INTERDISCIPLINARY COLLABORATION (continued)

Competency Statement: Initiates and maintains a liaison relationship with all appropriate health care providers to assure that all efforts effectively complement one another		
Performance Criteria	Learning Resource	Date Met/Evaluator
3. Solicits prompt responses from physicians		
4. Attends interdisciplinary conferences		
5. Documents interdisciplinary collaboration		

STANDARD: ETHICS

Competency Statement: Utilizes code for nurses established by the ANA as a guide for ethical decision making in practice.		
Performance Criteria	Learning Resource	Date Met/Evaluator
1. Provides an example of an ethical dilemma encountered in home care practice		
2. Consults ethics committee with presumed or identified ethical dilemmas or concerns		
3. Reports incidents in concise, appropriate, and timely fashion		
4. Maintains client confidentiality		

STANDARD: STRUCTURE AND PROCESS OF HOME CARE ORGANIZATION (organization-specific)

Competency Statement: Demonstrates professional responsibility in the LPN Home Care Role		
Performance Criteria	Learning Resource	Date Met/Evaluator
Organization-specific competencies	*As per organization	
1. Locates and interprets organizational structure, mission, vision, and goals		
2. List the types of care or services provided by the organization and the referral indicators for each		

continues

Exhibit C–7 continued

STANDARD: STRUCTURE AND PROCESS OF HOME CARE ORGANIZATION (organization-specific)

Competency Statement: Demonstrates professional responsibility in the RN Home Care Role		
Performance Criteria	Learning Resource	Date Met/Evaluator
3. Locates and interprets the policies and procedures of the organization, specifically: ❏ *Advanced Directives* ❏ *Death and Dying* ❏ *Patient Confidentiality* ❏ *Incident Reporting* ❏ *Inclement Weather* ❏ *Dress Code* ❏ *Abuse and Neglect* ❏ *Personal Safety* ❏ *Referral Guidelines* ❏ *Emergency Preparedness* ❏ *Other:*		
4. Identifies geographical service area		
5. Interprets and adheres to payer guidelines		
6. Other		
7.		
8.		
9.		

*e.g., List specific policies, procedures. List pertinent videos, computer-assisted instruction, self-learning modules, primary and secondary references.

NOTE: CBO should reflect individual state vocational/practical nurse law.

Resources

RESOURCES FOR STAFF DEVELOPMENT—MATERIALS

Periodicals

Adult Learning
American Association for Adult and Continuing Education
1200 19th Street NW, Suite 300
Washington, DC 20036

American Nurses Publishing
Marketing Services
P.O. Box 2224
Waldorf, MD 20604-2244

Journal of Nursing Staff Development
Lippincott-Raven Publishers
12107 Insurance Way, Suite 114
Hagerstown, MD 21740

Nursing Management
Springhouse Corporation
Circulation Department
434 West Downer
Aurora, IL 60506

The Journal of Continuing Education in Nursing
6900 Grove Road
Thorofare, NJ 08086

Audiovisuals and Books

Jossey-Bass Publishers Catalog
350 Sansome Street
San Francisco, CA 94104

NLN Books and Videos Catalog
National League for Nursing
350 Hudson Street
New York NY 10014

OSHA Publications
US Department of Labor
200 Constitution Avenue NW
Room N3101
Washington, DC 20210
http://www.osha.gov/

The Info-Line Collection
Practical Guidelines for Training and Development Professionals
American Society for Training and Development
1640 King Street, Box 1443
Alexandria, VA 22313-2043

Williams & Wilkins
Electronic Media for Healthcare Education
428 East Preston Street
Baltimore, MD 21202

Training Ideas

Resource Guide and Product Catalog
Talico
2320 S Third Street, Suite 5
Jacksonville Beach, FL 32250

Lakewood Publications, Inc.
50 South 9th Street
Minneapolis, MN 55402
1 (800) 707-7769

American Society for Training and
Development
1640 Duke Street, Box 1443
Alexandria, VA 22313-2043

HOME CARE EDUCATOR RESOURCE LIST

American Association for Continuity of Care
11250 Roger Bacon Drive
Suite 8
Reston, VA 22090-5202
(703) 437-4377

American Federation of Home Health Agencies
1320 Fenwick Lane
Suite 100
Silver Spring, MD 20910
(301) 588-1454

American Nurses Association Council
for Professional Nursing
Education and Development
American Nurses Association
600 Maryland Avenue SW
Washington, DC 20024
(202) 554-4444

American Nurses Credentialing Center
600 Maryland Avenue SW
Suite 100 West
Washington, DC 20024
1 (800) 284-2378
http://www.nursingworld.org/ancc/html

American Society for Training and Development
1640 Duke Street, Box 1443
Alexandria, VA 22313-2043
(703) 683-8100

Associated Home Health Nurses of America, Inc.
555 East Ocean Boulevard
Suite 203
Long Beach, CA 90802
(562) 437-5773
http://www.ahhna.com

Computers in Nursing
University of Southern Maine
96 Falmouth Street, Box 9300
Portland, ME 04103

HCARENURSE@LISTSERV.MEDEC.com

Home H. Care Extranet @
www.telemedical.com/telemedicine/home.
html
(Communication, collaboration, teaching,
and management for all home health care
participants)

Joint Commission on Accreditation of
Healthcare Organizations
One Renaissance Boulevard
Oakbrook Terrace, IL 60181
(630) 792-5000
http://www.jcaho.org

Martindale's Health Science Guide
http://www.sci.lib.uc.edu/HSG/
Nursing.html
(Nursing and medical health information,
news updates, research updates, tutorials,
interactive classes and multiple health
resources and weblinks

National League for Nursing
350 Hudson Street, 4th floor
New York, NY 10019
(212) 989-9393

Nursing Staff Development & Continuing Education
http://www.mich.edu.esn
University of Michigan web site with information, articles, communication, and continuing education tutorials

REHABNET
http://www.rehab.net/whatis.html
(Information, communication, and links to web sources for physical therapy, occupational therapy, speech therapy)

Speech Therapy Online
http://www.speechtherapist.com
(Communication, information, and links for speech therapists)

Sigma Theta Tau Nursing Honor Society
550 North St.
Indianapolis, IN 46202
(317) 634-8171
http://stti-web.upui.edu

Visiting Nurse Associations of America
3801 East Florida Avenue, Suite 900
Denver, CO 80210
(303) 753-0218

LIST OF PROFESSIONAL ASSOCIATIONS

American Dietetic Association
216 West Jackson Boulevard
Chicago, IL 60606-6995
1 (800) 877-1600

American Medical Association
515 North State Street
Chicago, IL 60610
(312) 464-4755

American Nurses Association
600 Maryland Avenue, SW
Washington, DC 20024
(800) 274-4262

American Occupational Therapy Association
4720 Montgomery Lane
P.O. Box 31220
Bethesda, MD 20824-1220
(301) 652-2682

American Physical Therapy Association
1111 North Fairfax
Alexandria, VA 22314
(800) 999-2782

American Speech, Language, and Hearing Association
10801 Rockville Pike
Rockville, MD 20852
(301) 897-5700

Home Healthcare Nurses Association
437 Twin Bay Drive
Pensacola, FL 32534-1350
1 (800) 558-4462

Intravenous Nurses Society
Two Brighton Street
Belmont, MA 02178
(617) 489-5205

National Association of Social Workers
750 First Street, NE
Suite 700
Washington, DC 20002-4241
(202) 408-8600
(800) 638-8799

National Association for Home Care
228 Seventh Street, SE
Washington, DC 20003-4306
(202) 547-7424

National Nursing Staff Development Organization
437 Twin Bay Drive
Pensacola, FL 32534-1350
1 (800) 489-1995

Index